Simulation and Game-Based Learning for the Health Professions

Rachel Umoren
University of Washington, USA

A volume in the Advances in Medical Education, Research, and Ethics (AMERE) Book Series

IGI Global
PUBLISHER of TIMELY KNOWLEDGE

Published in the United States of America by
IGI Global
Medical Information Science Reference (an imprint of IGI Global)
701 E. Chocolate Avenue
Hershey PA, USA 17033
Tel: 717-533-8845
Fax: 717-533-8661
E-mail: cust@igi-global.com
Web site: http://www.igi-global.com

Library of Congress Cataloging-in-Publication Data

Names: Umoren, Rachel A., 1979- author.
Title: Simulation and game-based learning for the health professions / by Rachel A. Umoren.
Description: Hershey, PA : Medical Information Science Reference, [2022] | Includes bibliographical references and index. | Summary: "This authored publication focuses on simulation-based education for the health professions and the role of school-business-community collaboration to promote the translation of simulation skills to clinical and public health practice by introducing the principles of simulation education and adult learning theories that apply to simulation and gaming for health professionals"-- Provided by publisher.
Identifiers: LCCN 2021049784 (print) | LCCN 2021049785 (ebook) | ISBN 9781799843788 (hardcover) | ISBN 9781799843795 (ebook)
Subjects: LCSH: Medical personnel. | Educational games. | Computer-assisted instruction.
Classification: LCC R690 .U46 2022 (print) | LCC R690 (ebook) | DDC 610.73/7--dc23/eng/20211102
LC record available at https://lccn.loc.gov/2021049784
LC ebook record available at https://lccn.loc.gov/2021049785

This book is published in the IGI Global book series Advances in Medical Education, Research, and Ethics (AMERE) (ISSN: 2475-6601; eISSN: 2475-661X)

British Cataloguing in Publication Data
A Cataloguing in Publication record for this book is available from the British Library.

For electronic access to this publication, please contact: eresources@igi-global.com.

Advances in Medical Education, Research, and Ethics (AMERE) Book Series

ISSN:2475-6601
EISSN:2475-661X

MISSION

Humans are living longer now than ever as a result of advances in the medical field. Having the tools available to train knowledgeable and ethical future generations of doctors and medical researchers is essential to continuing to advance our understanding of the human body and develop new ways of treating and curing sickness and disease.

The **Advances in Medical Education, Research, and Ethics (AMERE)** book series highlights publications pertaining to advancements in pedagogical practice for developing future healthcare professionals, research methods, and advancements in the medical field, as well as moral behavior and practice of healthcare professionals, students, and researchers. Featuring research-based book publications that are highly relevant to the healthcare community, this series is ideally designed for library inclusion at medical universities and research institutions as well as personal use by medical professionals, researchers, and upper-level students entering the field.

COVERAGE

- Clinical Research
- Conflicts of Interest
- Ethics in Medicine
- Healthcare Pedagogy
- Medical Curricula
- Medical Simulation
- Patient Data
- Professional Development
- Research Methods
- Scientific Misconduct

IGI Global is currently accepting manuscripts for publication within this series. To submit a proposal for a volume in this series, please contact our Acquisition Editors at Acquisitions@igi-global.com or visit: http://www.igi-global.com/publish/.

The Advances in Medical Education, Research, and Ethics (AMERE) Book Series (ISSN 2475-6601) is published by IGI Global, 701 E. Chocolate Avenue, Hershey, PA 17033-1240, USA, www.igi-global.com. This series is composed of titles available for purchase individually; each title is edited to be contextually exclusive from any other title within the series. For pricing and ordering information please visit http://www.igi-global.com/book-series/advances-medical-education-research-ethics/132365. Postmaster: Send all address changes to above address.

Titles in this Series

For a list of additional titles in this series, please visit:
http://www.igi-global.com/book-series/advances-medical-education-research-ethics/132365

Handbook of Research on Developing Competencies for Pre-Health Professional Students, Advisors, and Programs
Rohini Ganjoo (The George Washington University, USA) and Lisa S. Schwartz (The George Washington Universty, USA)
Medical Information Science Reference • © 2022 • 435pp • H/C (ISBN: 9781668459690) • US $425.00

Handbook of Research on Improving Allied Health Professions Education Advancing Clinical Training and Interdisciplinary Translationa Research
Rui Pedro Pereira Almeida (University of Algarve, Portugal)
Medical Information Science Reference • © 2022 • 409pp • H/C (ISBN: 9781799895787) • US $395.00

Handbook of Research on Advising and Developing the Pre-Health Professional Student
Lisa S. Schwartz (The George Washington University, USA) and Rohini Ganjoo (The George Washington University, USA)
Information Science Reference • © 2022 • 390pp • H/C (ISBN: 9781799896173) • US $425.00

Instructional Design Exemplars in eHealth and mHealth Education Interventions
Suha R. Tamim (University of South Carolina, USA)
Medical Information Science Reference • © 2022 • 323pp • H/C (ISBN: 9781799894902) • US $295.00

Contemporary Issues in Global Medicine and Moving Toward International Healthcare Equity
Nick Comninellis (University of Missouri-Kansas City, USA) and Steven D. Waldman (University of Missouri-Kansas City School of Medicine, USA)
Medical Information Science Reference • © 2022 • 305pp • H/C (ISBN: 9781799884903) • US $295.00

For an entire list of titles in this series, please visit:
http://www.igi-global.com/book-series/advances-medical-education-research-ethics/132365

IGI Global
PUBLISHER of TIMELY KNOWLEDGE

701 East Chocolate Avenue, Hershey, PA 17033, USA
Tel: 717-533-8845 x100 • Fax: 717-533-8661
E-Mail: cust@igi-global.com • www.igi-global.com

Table of Contents

Section 3
Sustainability and Global Dissemination of Simulation Education

Preface

Simulation education is used all over the world. Since the seminal Institute of Medicine study "To Err is Human," healthcare organizations in high resource settings have increased their use of simulation with the goal of enhancing healthcare delivery and patient outcomes. While much is known about the short- and long-term effects of simulation education in high-resource situations, there remain gaps in knowledge and uptake in low-resource environments. Healthcare agencies, organizations, and other stakeholders' policies influence the usage of simulation in educational settings. While there is little doubt that simulation is useful, the cost of offering it, particularly in these contexts, may be prohibitive. While recognizing these constraints, the target audience of this book on *Simulation and Game-Based Learning for the Health Professions* is healthcare educators with an interest in simulation education in both high and low resource settings.

This book contains a total of ten chapters and is broken up into three sections. The chapters that make up Section 1 serve as an introduction to simulation education and scenario development. The process of simulation education and assessment is the primary topic of discussion in Section 2. This section, which is comprised of Chapters 5 through 7, gives an overview of the methods and approach to simulation instruction. This includes the process of preparing, facilitating, and debriefing simulation scenarios. In order to run productive simulation sessions, facilitators need to plan not only the content of the simulation but also the logistics, including things like the equipment needed and the location of the simulation event. In the third section, we investigate the ideas of long-term viability and the global application of simulation education. This section examines the critical steps that must be taken in order to translate and integrate simulation education on a global scale including academic-industry partnerships and costs. It is comprised of Chapters 8 through 10.

The first section of Chapter 1 provides a concise summary of the history of health professional simulation, which can be traced back to ancient times. Definitions are provided for both manikin-based and virtual simulation, also known as simulation games. In addition, fundamental issues such as in-situ simulation, simulation quality, and simulation technology, as well as an approach to simulation education, are discussed in the first chapter of this book. Both the connection between simulation and patient safety as well as the impact that the military and aviation industries have had on the modern-day simulation practice are topics that are investigated. Last but not least, a global review of the use of simulation in learning and evaluation in health professional education serves as the chapter's conclusion.

The theories of adult learning and the ideas behind game-based learning along with their applications to simulation are discussed in Chapter 2. Specifically, the chapter focuses on how these concepts can be applied to the development of simulation education curricula. The idea that players can learn from playing games provides the conceptual foundation for a wide variety of different kinds of virtual simulation games. Adult learners are distinct from child learners in a number of important ways. Teachers have a responsibility to be aware of these distinctions and modify their instructional strategies appropriately. Simulation and game-based learning are two types of educational solutions that are based on the theory of adult learning. This chapter discusses adult learning theories in the context of simulation education, as well as how knowledge of these concepts can be applied to the development, implementation, and assessment of simulation curricula. Simulation-based learning lends itself well to the implementation of a wide variety of learning theories. While the chapter covers a range of adult learning theories, including andragogy, Kolb's experiential learning theory, Bandura's idea of self-efficacy, and Mezirow's theory of transformative learning, there are a large number of additional potentially applicable theories, and educators who design and develop simulation curricula frequently employ a wide variety of concepts. Although it is possible that some simulation instructors are not familiar with these principles, they are essential for designing activities that are not only fun but also instructive for students who have varying levels of experience and exposure to game-based learning. It is possible to increase the effectiveness of simulation-based learning for both pre-service and in-service educators by increasing the amount of exposure to the concepts discussed in this article and by intentionally applying these concepts in real-world settings.

The third and fourth chapters discuss various methods for the creation of scenarios, as well as the various types of manikin-based and virtual simulation, as well as numerous applications in healthcare. The type of manikin to use is determined by the learning objectives and learner characteristics, as well as the facilitator's experience and comfort level. The first thing that instructors need to do is determine the learning goals, then select appropriate simulation equipment and environments. Simulation educators may also devise new simulation scenarios or modify existing ones to accomplish these aims. The methodology for the development of scenarios for manikin-based simulation is discussed in Chapter 3. Manikin-based simulation refers to the practice of performing procedures on dolls or humanoid figurines called manikins (mannequins) that would normally be performed on a human patient. This chapter discusses the many different types of manikin-based simulation, including high-fidelity and low-fidelity manikins and how these tools can be used in various simulation settings. The learning goals, the characteristics of the learners, the experience level of the facilitator, and the comfort level of the facilitator all play a role in determining the type of manikin that should be used. The learning objectives can be satisfied by either adapting existing scenarios or creating new ones. New scenarios need to be based on evidence, have clearly defined learning goals, and go through extensive testing to ensure that they are easy to implement and effective for the population of learners for whom they are designed. In conclusion, the chapter provides a description of the approach to developing basic simulation scenarios for manikin-based simulation.

In Chapter 4, an overview of the approach to developing virtual simulation scenarios and best practices for debriefing and providing feedback on virtual simulations are presented. Simulation training that utilizes computer-generated 3D models and environments is what is referred to as virtual simulation. This chapter covers two distinct categories of virtual simulations: virtual reality (VR) and augmented reality (AR). Virtual Reality (VR) and Augmented Reality (AR) Smartphones, head-mounted displays, and other types of headsets are just some of the devices that can be used to experience virtual reality and augmented reality simulations. The type of device that should be used depends on the learning objectives, the characteristics of the learners, the availability of devices for the learners, as well as the level of experience and comfort level of the facilitator. It is possible to construct or adapt virtual scenarios in order to meet learning objectives. To ensure that the learning objectives are met, new scenarios need to be developed with the assistance of subject matter experts. Additionally, early end-user testing of the newly constructed scenarios needs to be carried out to ensure that the newly developed scenarios are user-friendly and productive for the target audience of learners. Teamwork training, standardized virtual patients, and procedure-based training are some of the other applications of virtual simulation in healthcare.

Chapter 5 provides an overview of simulation instruction methodologies and processes, including simulation scenario design, facilitation, and debriefing during simulation sessions. Instructors must give scenario information, while simulation debriefers take learners through a reflective session based on the learning objectives. This chapter examines the practical procedures for organizing simulations and the foundations for various simulation debriefing methodologies. The success of a simulation session is directly proportional to the amount of planning that goes into the session. In order to be effective, facilitators need to be well-organized and knowledgeable. It is recommended to carry out professional simulation scenarios that are equipped with clear educational goals and provide guarantees of a risk-free learning environment. Debriefing sessions should be learner-centered and concentrate on objective facts in order to reinforce appropriate actions and discover strategies for improving future performance.

The tools that can be used to evaluate the performance of manikin-based and virtual simulations through direct and indirect observation, surveys, and other metrics of data capture are discussed in Chapter 6. Formative and summative evaluations of student performance can both be accomplished through the use of simulations. This chapter presents tools and methodologies for evaluating the performance of manikin-based and virtual simulations through direct and indirect observation, video review, and other data acquisition measures. Instructors are guided through a process for evaluating the performance of teams using methods that have been verified. The effect of stress on performance, the elimination of bias, and the evaluation of large groups of learners are all mentioned as special issues that arise when assessing the individual and team performance of individuals and teams. meticulous data gathering by skilled observers using approved technologies. Evaluation of learner performance during simulation is supported by the use of video recordings for retrospective review, as well as by keeping the ratio of facilitators to students as low as possible. Through the use of virtual simulations, the performance of large groups of learners can be objectively evaluated.

Chapter 7 provides an overview of telesimulation, remote facilitation and debriefing. Telesimulation is the practice of conducting simulation-based education over the internet utilizing either generic or custom video platforms. The learners and the facilitator or debriefer are in different parts of the country. Training via telesimulation may cover a wide range of topics, from realistic clinical scenarios to in-depth technical instruction on how to operate various telemedicine platforms and the most effective procedures. This chapter covers the fundamental elements and classifications of video conferencing platforms, as well as their applications in telesimulation facilitation and debriefing, remote learner assessment, and telementoring, respectively. Considerations pertaining to technology, such as hardware, applications, connectivity to the internet, and technical support, are brought up. Telesimulation is a developing subfield of simulation-based education that may provide students who have not previously had access to simulation education with the opportunity to acquire additional support through remote facilitation and/or teledebriefing. This is because telesimulation can be carried out remotely. Learners have demonstrated a willingness to experiment with telesimulation, despite the fact that it requires fundamental technical expertise, advance preparation, and on-site support considerations. To fully understand the impact that telesimulation training has on clinical practice, additional research is required. The use of telemedicine and other technological advances, on the other hand, will be beneficial to the expansion of the rapidly developing field of simulation education.

Chapter 8 begins with a discussion of the intersection of school-business-community collaboration and its impact on translation of skills from simulation to clinical practice. The process of learning, perfecting, analyzing, and researching one's skills can all be accomplished through the use of simulation education. Any educational strategy should promote learning, and in the case of healthcare simulation, it should also facilitate the transfer of learned skills to clinical practice. Research that demonstrates how simulation assists students in transferring their abilities from the classroom to the clinical setting is receiving a growing amount of attention in the pursuit of the goal of improving patient outcomes. It's possible that the way and setting in which the simulation education is carried out could help with the transfer of skills. Cooperation between academic institutions, private businesses, and local communities creates an environment that is conducive to the building and furnishing of simulation facilities, as well as the execution of in-situ simulation in clinical environments. This chapter looks at the importance of collaboration between schools, businesses, and communities in the process of translating skills learned in simulation into clinical practice, with a particular emphasis on improving the care of patients.

The advancement of simulation education and clinical practice is dependent on the results of simulation research, which is why Chapter 9 of this book is dedicated to describing research and data collection strategies for simulation educators. This chapter provides instruction on fundamental research principles and methodologies for simulation faculty members who are engaged in research or other forms of scholarly work. One of the things that are included is an overview of how to begin a scholarly project, how to ask research questions that are clearly defined, and how to explicitly identify study objectives. This chapter also discusses how to collect quantitative and qualitative data during simulation sessions, as well as how to interpret and report simulation results. Additionally, the chapter covers how to conduct simulation research. Obtaining approval from an institutional review board to conduct research on human subjects and becoming a member of a collaboration network for simulation research are two additional things to consider. In conclusion, the process of designing a research project for educational purposes, carrying out data collection, and disseminating the findings is analogous to that of a clinical research project. It is necessary to take into consideration not only the ethical standards of research, which include the protection of human subjects, but also the organization and evaluation of the data that is gathered. Finally, as the field of simulation develops, the options for disseminating research findings to other educators and educational audiences will expand. One of the most significant areas of progress is the establishment of networks of simulation instructors and researchers. Research that is carried out in collaboration using simulations will be of great assistance to the profession in its ongoing search for the most effective methods of educating and assessing students.

The strategies for ensuring the long-term viability of simulation education and expanding its reach across the globe are discussed in Chapter 10. In order for simulation to be an effective and long-term sustainable educational method, establishments need to have appropriate and continuous availability of training resources, educated instructors, and curricula. This chapter discusses the various considerations that should be given to stakeholders prior to the adoption and implementation of a simulation program. Later on in the chapter, the costs of both manikin-based and virtual simulations, as well as the amount of revenue generated and the return on investment. The widespread implementation of simulation education at both the pre-service and in-service levels of training is being driven by institutions of higher education for health professionals, hospitals, certifying bodies, and organizations representing health professionals. In this chapter, the roles that faculty development and simulation research play in the widespread adoption of simulation education around the world are explored. Economic evaluations of simulation education in high and low resource settings are encouraged and will add value to the current practice of simulation education. This is the case even in high resource settings with adequate support for the fixed and variable costs of simulation. In addition, economic evaluations of simulation education in low resource settings are likely to highlight the benefits of simulation education and increase uptake.

In conclusion, academic-industry-community collaborations are essential to the efficiency of simulation education as well as its continued viability in the long run. These connections can be utilized to safeguard simulation space within hospitals, provide access to simulation and medical equipment for more lifelike simulation experiences, and provide assistance for simulation events. Training on a simulator should hopefully lead to better outcomes for patients. This can be accomplished in a variety of ways, including improving technical skills through procedural competency, fostering team communication and non-technical skills, and improving system performance by identifying and addressing root causes of failure, reducing active failures, and minimizing latent safety threats. These are just a few of the many ways that this can be done. It is necessary to cultivate partnerships between educational institutions, healthcare organizations, and community partners in order to advance equality and sustainability. This can be accomplished through open communication, exploration, and regular reevaluation of the goals and objectives of each partner.

Simulation education has been acknowledged and utilized by healthcare and training institutions as a highly desirable and effective method of training health professionals for many decades. This recognition and use of this method dates back to the 1980s. Even though simulation has been around since ancient times, both the theory behind it and the actual practice of it have developed in tandem with adult educational thought. In recent years, there has been a lot of support for using health professional simulation to improve patient safety and reduce medical errors. This support comes from both patients and medical professionals. As a direct consequence of this, simulation education is now incorporated into both the pre-service and the ongoing training of health professionals at all levels. A significant amount of money has been invested in simulation education as a result of collaboration between academic institutions, healthcare organizations, and industry partners. As a result, learners in the health professional field now have access to this resource thanks to the establishment of simulation centers in academic settings.

Learners in both low-resource and high-resource environments have the opportunity to participate in a wide range of simulation experiences, such as virtual simulation and simulation based on manikins. However, awareness is a barrier to the widespread application and utilization of simulation. Because simulation is now used in high- and low-resource settings, there is now a significant opportunity for academic evaluation of simulation education as a method for acquiring and keeping healthcare worker skills up to date. This opportunity was created as a result of the extension of simulation to multiple disciplines. This book was written utilizing a frame of reference that takes into consideration the characteristics of simulation education and how they apply to both high-resource and low-resource settings. Additionally, this book takes into consideration the facilitators and hurdles that exist in these settings with regard to the adoption of simulation. This book's contribution to the body of research on faculty development for simulation education will improve simulation facilitation and debriefing skills, leading to simulation sessions of higher quality that are centered on the learner and leading to improved educational outcomes. In healthcare simulations, where the objective is to ensure the safety of patients as a result of the knowledge gained from simulated experiences, translation to practice is an extremely important component. When there are no experienced facilitators available on-site, learners in settings that are geographically remote can potentially benefit from new insights into individual and team performance through the use of telesimulation.

The use of more complicated methods for data collection during the simulation, such as monitoring the subject's physiological state and tracking their motion and gaze, is gaining popularity. Because more and more virtual simulations and virtual simulated patients are becoming available, teachers now have access to a wide range of tools that enable them to conduct and evaluate simulations with varying sizes of groups of students, including both small and large ones. When it comes to communication and teamwork training, facilitators have access to a wide variety of tried-and-true methods that can be customized to fit the needs of their specific setting and the participants in their classes. As innovative methods of evaluating and providing objective, performance-based feedback to learners continue to develop, it is possible that artificial intelligence or crowd-sourced evaluation of audio and video data will be used to alleviate some of the stress that is placed on educators tasked with completing these evaluations.

In conclusion, while simulation-based education is a very effective technique for health professional education, organizational acceptance of simulation education is heavily influenced by cost considerations. When calculating the return on investment of simulation instruction, healthcare companies that value patient safety must include both immediate and long-term outcomes. Faculty development opportunities, accreditation requirements, the expansion of evidence-based curricula, corporate support, and an increase in the evidence base supporting the use of simulation methodologies are all driving the global expansion of simulation.

Rachel Umoren
University of Washington, USA

Acknowledgment

I would like to acknowledge the inspiration provided by simulation colleagues and learners around the world and the enduring support of my family which led to successful completion of this work.

Section 1

Introduction to Simulation Education and Scenario Development

Chapter 1
Introduction to Simulation in the Healthcare Professions

ABSTRACT

This chapter begins with a brief history of health professional simulation which had its origins in antiquity. The types of simulation and various approaches to simulation-based education including manikin-based and virtual simulation (also known as simulation games) are described. The chapter also introduces an approach to simulation education and basic concepts such as in situ simulation, simulation fidelity, and simulation technology. The relationships between simulation and patient safety and the influence of the military and aviation industry on modern day practice of simulation are explored. Finally, the chapter concludes with an overview of the global application of simulation to learning and evaluation in health professional education.

INTRODUCTION

Simulation has been utilized in various forms for centuries. However, the current approaches to simulation education date back to the 19th century with the use of obstetric simulators to train midwives and obstetricians in how to recognize and treat childbirth complications. The growth of simulation education has been fostered by an increased focus on patient safety events. While the traditional approaches to learning in the health professions have relied on observation and practice in the clinical setting, simulation allows learners to practice their skills and make mistakes without harming a patient.

DOI: 10.4018/978-1-7998-4378-8.ch001

Manikin-based simulation involves the use of humanoid simulators by trained simulation faculty who facilitate simulation scenarios in simulation centers i.e., dedicated locations for simulation, or in clinical settings. Other simulation modalities such as telesimulation and virtual simulation are accessible by remote facilitators and learners. The "fidelity" of the simulation experience represents the degree to which it matches a clinical experience. While historically, manikins were crude representations of the human form, today's manikins come in all sizes and portray realistic physiologic responses. The concepts of high-fidelity and low-fidelity as well as high-technology and low-technology simulation are explored in Chapter 3 titled "Scenario Development for Manikin-based Simulation" and Chapter 4 titled "Scenario Development for Virtual Simulation".

Origins of Health Professional Simulation

Early Simulators

For centuries, clay and stone models of humans have been described in many cultures (Owen, 2012). One of the earliest surviving clay models to show anatomy was the Early Classic Maya head which represents in two parts, the head in life and a skull (Owen, 2012). In China, the imperial physician Wang Wei-Yi (987-1067) used two life-sized bronze statutes for teaching surface anatomy and acupuncture points. The models were covered in wax and filled with a liquid so a drip when the acupuncture needle was removed indicated the correct location of the acupuncture point (Maciocia, 1982). Antique diagnostic dolls have been described that were used in China to enable patients wishing to preserve their modesty to describe their symptoms by pointing to the corresponding sites on the dolls which represented naked women reclining sideways on a wooden bed (Bause, 2010).

18th Century Simulators

The current system of health professional education derived its roots in the fifteenth century when Henry VIII decreed that to address the practice of medicine by "ignorant persons [with] …no manner of insight… nor any other kind of learning", those wishing to practice medicine, should undergo examinations (Magee, 2004). In 1522, the College of Physicians was founded by Thomas Linacre. This was followed in 1540, by the establishment of examination processes for Surgeons. Other groups that gained recognition during this period were apothecaries who dispensed medicines and midwives who looked after the delivery of infants (Magee, 2004). Around this time, the study of anatomy was facilitated by anatomic models. The first wax anatomic model was created in 1598 by Ludovico Cardi (also known as Cigoli) as a small carved human figure made out of red wax with careful rendering of the external musculature (Ballestriero, 2010). The wax anatomic workshop in Florence called La Specola made "remarkably attractive [models]; bodies seemed to be alive, pulsating" and "animated eyes: colored irises and candid whites give the impression of the eyes of a living person, or at least those belonging to a still warm body" (Owen, 2012). Intricate simulators were developed in the 18th century for obstetric training (Owen, 2012).

19th Century Simulators

For many medical schools clinical obstetric experience was scarce in the 19th century as many women delivered at home. Obstetric simulators were made of skeletal material including pelvic bones covered with fabric and leather and which could leak amniotic fluid and blood were used to train midwives and obstetricians to recognize and manage obstetric complications (Owen, 2012; Owen & Pelosi, 2013). The Budin-Pinard simulator was described in 1877 and was used to demonstrate the application of forceps to the fetal head (Owen & Pelosi, 2013). There were two versions, with and without a moveable sacrum. It was marketed "for learning touch, palpation, the operations in general, versions by both external and internal manipulations, ...etc., with uterus, artificial bag of waters..." (Owen & Pelosi, 2013).

20th Century Simulators

However, in the early 20th century, the use of stillborn cadavers was still promoted over fetus simulators (Reed, 1931). Moreover, as more women began to deliver in hospitals, learners had the opportunity to learn from a large population of obstetrics patients and relied less on simulators (Owen, 2012; Owen & Pelosi, 2013). The first simulator used to teach nurses was a life-sized manikin called Mrs. Chase. In 1911, she was used to train nurses how to dress, turn and transfer patients (Aebersold, 2016). Nurses were taught to give injections using Arabella in 1914. In the 1940s, a male manikin was used by the U.S. Army to teach the techniques of hospital care (Aebersold,

2016). In 1960, the first manikin to train on mouth-to-mouth ventilation and chest compressions was developed called Rescue Annie [Laerdal Medical] (Aebersold, 2016). One of the first high-fidelity simulators was developed for use in anesthesia, Sim One [Sierra Engineering Company] was also developed in the 1960s. In 1968, during the American Heart Association Scientific Sessions, Doctor Michael Gordon from the University of Miami Medical School presented "Harvey, the Cardiology Patient Simulator" (Cooper & Taqueti, 2008). Harvey was followed by several high-fidelity simulators in the 1990s (Aebersold, 2016). In 2000, Laerdal Medical developed SimMan (Aebersold, 2016). Medical simulation has a long history, but the rapid technological advances of the last decade have brought a remarkable realism to the science of simulation.

Table 1. History of simulator development

Time period	Material	Educational focus	References
Pre-18th Century	Clay, stone, wood, ivory	Surface anatomy	Owen, 2012 Maciocia, 1982 Bause, 2010
18th Century	Wax, wood, human skeleton	Anatomy	Magee, 2004 Ballestriero, 2010 Owen, 2012
19th Century	Human skeleton, fabric, leather	Obstetrics	Owen, 2012 Owen & Pelosi, 2013
20th Century	Wood, metal, plastic	Resuscitation, Nursing, Internal Medicine	Cooper & Taqueti, 2008 Owen, 2012 Owen & Pelosi, 2013 Aebersold, 2016
21st Century	Plastic, metal, computer electronics, fiberglass	Multiple specialties including Surgery, Internal Medicine, Obstetrics and Pediatrics	Jones et al., 2015 Cooper & Taqueti, 2008 Padilha et al., 2019 Mills, Williams, et al., 2013 Mills, Wu, et al., 2013 Nelissen et al., 2017

21st Century Simulators

Today, three major companies: Gaumard, CAE and Laerdal Medical lead the field of simulator development to meet the needs of healthcare students and professionals. Although they were quite advanced at the time, the human patient simulators of the early 2000s were relatively simple when compared to current models. Current human patient simulators possess life-like features including pulse, blood pressure, temperature, respiration rate, heart and lung sounds, blood and urine return, glucose tolerance, the ability to sweat, drool, cry, in addition to the ability to speak, respond and describe symptoms (Cooper & Taqueti, 2008; Jones et al., 2015). The manikin's lungs can have a different sound in each lobe, or the heart can have an isolated sound in a specific chamber (Cooper & Taqueti, 2008; Padilha et al., 2019).

Clinical simulation centers became popular in the early to mid-2000s. Institutions created models of hospital rooms, patient examination, and emergency rooms for simulated patient treatment. These collaborative training environments allow healthcare students and practicing health professionals to apply their knowledge to the care of simulated patients (patient actors or human-manikin simulators) without taking the risk of jeopardizing patient safety (Jones et al., 2015). Simulation provides the hands-on training in advanced emergency response techniques that prepares the learners to carry out potentially dangerous procedures and to improve patient safety (Mills, Williams, et al., 2013; Mills, Wu, et al., 2013). The benefits of simulation-based training have been demonstrated in both high and low resource settings. Curricula on adult and pediatric resuscitation have been used globally and obstetric simulation-based training was associated with a 38% reduction in incidence of post-partum hemorrhage and improved clinical performance of basic delivery skills and management of post-partum hemorrhage in the clinical setting (Nelissen et al., 2017).

Virtual Simulation

Virtual simulations with a focus on medical history taking and physical examination use virtual patients in dynamic and immersive clinical environments ranging from prehospital environments to environments in the community (Eyikara & Baykara, 2018; Nicolaou et al., 2019; Umoren et al., 2014). In some cases, these virtual patients are controlled by simulation facilitators operating simulated systems, but in other cases they are computer controlled "non-player characters" (NPCs) (Marei et al., 2019; Sweigart & Hodson-Carlton, 2013). While these virtual patients may be depicted on a computer touchscreen, it is also feasible to simulate patients using virtual reality and augmented reality (Kononowicz et al., 2019; Motz et al., 2018). There is great flexibility afforded by the ability to access virtual patients that depict patients of different ages and ethnic backgrounds through a variety of multimedia, with dynamic patient scenarios, supported by physiological algorithms (Huwendiek, 2019). For example, the clinical virtual simulator (Body Interact) presents virtual patients with an underlying physiological algorithm that recreates a dynamic health condition that responds to user interventions (Padilha et al., 2019). Virtual laparoscopic simulators have broad utility in surgical specialties and serious games have been used as training tools to improve surgical dexterity (Guedes et al., 2019; Overtoom et al., 2017; Paquette et al., 2017; Shim et al., 2018).

There is evidence that simulation games enable significant improvement in students' knowledge retention and clinical reasoning (Kyaw et al., 2019). Simulation games are particularly effective when combined with other strategies such as briefing and debriefing, with learners showing improvement in both initial knowledge retention and knowledge retention over time (Padilha et al., 2019). The use of virtual simulations can also improve student satisfaction with learning without influencing the perception of general efficiency. These benefits can be achieved at comparatively low cost to in-person simulation (Farra et al., 2019; Haerling, 2018; Vishwanath et al., 2017).

Simulation and Patient Safety

Influence by Aviation and the Military

Simulation education is built on several decades of evidence showing a clear link between simulation-based training and safety. Simulation is the industry standard in healthcare education and training. While the use of simulation in medical education has evolved over the decades in the context of meeting training objectives, the application of patient safety objectives to simulation arose from its use in the field of aviation to prevent safety events and near misses leading to plane crashes. The early linkages between simulation and safety were first demonstrated in aviation in the late 1970s and early 1980s (Aebersold, 2016). The use of virtual reality simulators in the setting of aviation also led to the adoption of these technologies in the field of medical simulation. The flight simulator provided a standardized experience that reproduced scenarios of various levels of complexity which allowed learners of different levels of skill to practice responses to infrequently occurring, but high-stakes events.

Similarly, medical simulation has adopted practices first described in military simulation settings including briefs and after action debriefs (Kolbe et al., 2015). At the start of each simulation, the organizers, and staff meet to introduce staff, state expectations and goals, assign roles and responsibilities, and to identify and troubleshoot problems before the simulation begins. Staff introductions are made, and their roles in the simulation described. Participants are also given an agenda of events for the session along with any other information they need to know. Facilitators create a welcoming and positive environment for learners and provide an orientation to the location, type of scenario and equipment to be used (Jones et al., 2015).

Debriefing sessions take place after each simulation is complete. The use of the word "debrief" originated in military settings and first used in 1945 during World War II (Johnson, 2016). Debriefs are events during which simulation facilitators and participants discuss what went right, what went wrong, and whether the goals and expectations were met (Jones et al., 2015; Sawyer et al., 2016; Sawyer et al., 2016). These discussions which are intended to be highly reflective in nature (as opposed to directive feedback sessions) allow participants to reflect on their experience, ask questions of each other and the facilitator and improve their performance during subsequent events. While many approaches to debriefing have been described, most debriefing sessions focus on learner reactions, followed by analysis and ending with a discussion of lessons learned (Bowe et al., 2017; Sawyer et al., 2016). In some cases, debriefing sessions result in the identification of potential safety risks and hazards that apply to clinical practice and a written report is submitted to address these in the clinical setting.

Simulation has been shown to improve clinical training and promote patient safety and is seen as a method of risk-free learning (Kirsch et al., 2019). Although hands-on learning with real patients cannot be completely replaced, simulation scenarios provide a safe environment for learners to make mistakes and practice new skills. Investment in this approach to training has many advantages which help improve healthcare practitioners' skills and competencies, and in return, improve patient safety and reduce health care costs.

Interprofessional Simulation Education

In recent times, Simulation Centers, or Clinical Skills Centers as they are often referred to in undergraduate health professional education, were established to support the health professional and interprofessional training and to promote advances in simulation though the development of innovative research, education, and quality improvement initiatives. Jointly managed simulation centers create an interdisciplinary, multi-specialty environment. Centralizing training in simulation centers enables the centralization of all medical and surgical skills training and simulation activities, facilitating interprofessional education. Simulation Centers support learners from other disciplines including nursing, public health, dentistry, pharmacy, and podiatry, providing simulation-based clinical education and comprehensive professional development for all health professions. In addition to training medical students, medical interns, medical residents, registered nurses, nursing students, and other licensed healthcare workers from all fields of medicine and nursing, clinical skills simulation centers train community healthcare providers including first responders, transport teams, non-licensed caregivers, and home health aides. Interprofessional simulation activities allow for the assessment of critical thinking and clinical reasoning skills, while also encouraging collaboration and shared decision-making (West et al., 2016).

Simulation research has contributed lessons for continuing medical education, undergraduate and graduate medical education and supported the effectiveness of simulation in undergraduate and continuing medical education. The use of simulation to address the gap that exists between theory and skills lab experiences and clinical practice whether in bedside nursing, medicine or other specialties allows both students and new graduates to overcome the difficulties in adjusting to real life practice (Labrague et al., 2019). In view of persistent healthcare workforce shortages, it is important for nurses entering the workforce to be capable of functioning at a high level. Simulation helps to boost learners' confidence when working with a real patient for the first time and virtual simulations can prepare learners for encounters in the simulation center as well as in clinical settings (Bayram & Caliskan, 2019; Eyikara & Baykara, 2018). Working in a simulated environment allows students to make mistakes and understand the potential consequences of their actions without jeopardizing patient safety to prevent such errors from happening in the future (Labrague et al., 2019). Nursing students who take part in education programs involving simulations perform fewer medical mistakes in clinical settings, and are able to better develop their critical thinking and clinical decision-making skills. These findings led to the publication of guidelines supporting the use and integration of simulation in education from the American College of Nursing and American College of Chest Physicians evidence-based educational guidelines (Norman, 2009). However, of the 22 U.S. states that have reported and defined simulation usage, 7 do not allow the full 50% suggested by the NCSBN and many undergraduate nursing programs have not yet formalized the percentage of clinical hours that can be completed through simulation (Bradley et al., 2019; Doolen et al., 2016). Ultimately, the optimal integration of simulation-based medical education into medical student, resident and fellow education is meant to complement direct bedside clinical instruction.

Organizing Simulation Education

It is the responsibility of the Simulation Program Director to ensure and document that simulation faculty are trained in scenario development and qualified to conduct simulation and debriefings. Trained simulation faculty create and facilitate comprehensive medical simulation scenarios with different levels of learners. See Chapter 3 on "Scenario Development for Manikin-based Simulation" and Chapter 5 on "Organizing Simulations for Interprofessional Learners". Through simulation educator courses, faculty learn to effectively utilize various kinds of simulation including high-fidelity medical simulation, simulation with standardized patients, procedural simulation, telesimulation, and virtual simulation (Erich, 2016).

Working alongside simulation faculty are the Operations specialists, also known as, Simulation Technician or Technologists (Gavilanes, 2015). These individuals work behind the scenes to make simulations happen by setting up the simulation environment with the appropriate manikin and clinical supplies needed for the selected scenario. They also make adjustments to reflect the manikin physiologic responses and are indispensable members of the simulation team, supporting educational programs with a diverse and varied set of skills (Gantt, 2016). Simulation faculty and specialists have expertise in the creation of 3D printed models and the use of medical moulage, i.e., makeup to increase the realism of the scenario (Stokes-Parish et al., 2018). Thoughtfully designed and facilitated simulations mimic the clinical setting with a high degree of fidelity to help the learner develop problem-solving and decision-making skills.

Clinical Simulation Environments

Simulation facilities can be used to simulate a hospital, home, and primary care settings. The facility is often designed to cater to specific specialties and/or partitioned by activity type and learner skill level (Mendiratta-Lala et al., 2015). For example, certain rooms may be designated as nursing skills practice labs or obstetrics or perioperative simulation suites. There can be large training classrooms as well as smaller rooms designed for small group debriefing. Hybrid simulation rooms incorporate virtual and manikin-based simulation while mid-fidelity and high-fidelity labs feature manikins with low and high technology features. Simulation facilities designed to represent primary care office settings are distinguished in furniture set-up and available supplies. Other settings that represent home environments are used for training on home assessments and nutrition will require typical home furnishing. Clinical simulation facilities designed to simulate hospital rooms are fully equipped with hospital beds, gurneys or exam tables, monitors, IV poles, defibrillators, blood pressure cuffs, simulated oxygen ports, otoscopes and ophthalmoscopes and all equipment and supplies required to respond to medical and nursing interventions, including emergencies. Nursing skills practice areas are fully equipped for students to practice clinical nursing skills at all levels of nursing practice that may occur with diverse clients across the lifespan.

The requirements and design of simulation facilities have evolved due to the introduction of advanced human manikin simulators. The environmental considerations include optimal temperature, protection from humidity and dust and constant electricity to support high-fidelity manikin performance. Further, the involvement of remote learners through telesimulation, and the increasing use of virtual and augmented reality (Thomas et al., 2021; Yu et al., 2017) have also led to changes in the type of equipment needed and networking requirements to support a diverse range of simulation activities and technologies for in person and remote learners and instructors. In addition to clinical equipment, simulation rooms are equipped with video- and audio-recording capabilities to allow recording of skills and scenarios. The debriefing rooms are set up as small conference rooms equipped with audio-visual capabilities, projectors or large screen monitors where facilitators and healthcare students review the video recording of the scenario and engage in a reflective discussion of on the events that occurred during the simulation (Dufrene & Young, 2014; Levett-Jones & Lapkin, 2014; Lyons et al., 2015; Maestre & Rudolph, 2015).

Figure 1. Simulation session conducted in a simulation center

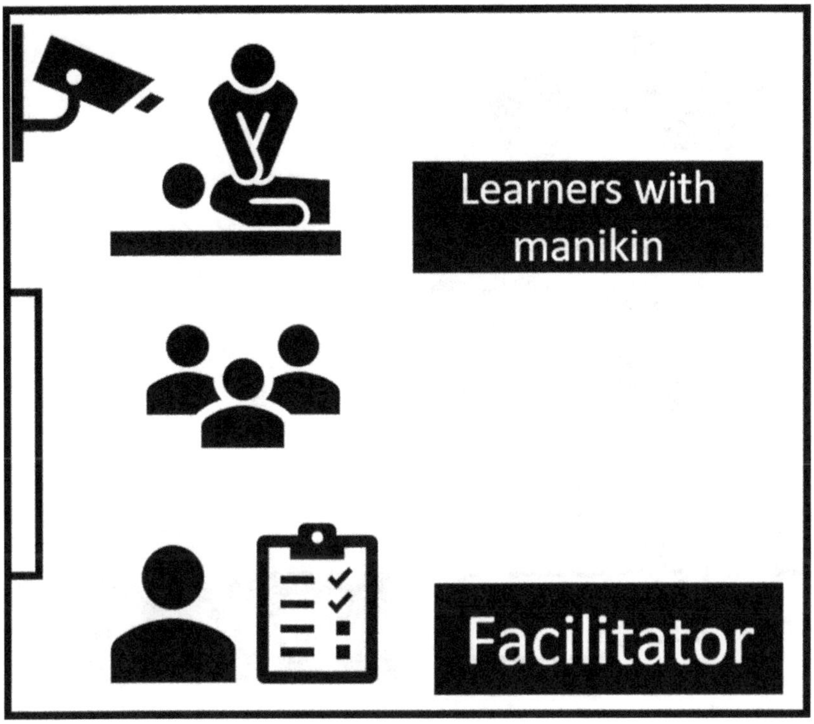

While simulation and clinical skills centers offer benefits in creating a dedicated space for simulation, simulation programs can operate effectively "in-situ" or within the hospital/workplace setting. These in situ simulations may have added benefits of identifying safety hazards that would not be easily noted in an educational space (Kerner et al., 2016; Wetzel et al., 2013). However, the timing and location of simulations conducted in the actual clinical environment may be limited by patient care needs and privacy concerns (Holtschneider, 2013).

Figure 2. Simulation session conducted in situ within the clinical environment

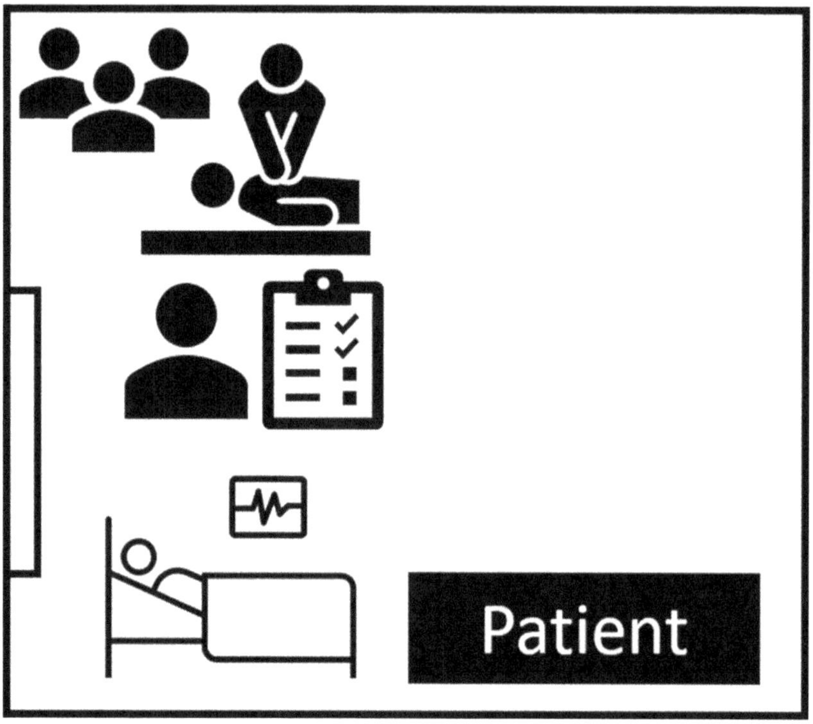

Global Application of Simulation to Learning and Evaluation

Simulation-based learning gives educators the ability to prepare health care students with advanced professional skills before they enter the workforce and to support continuing education for practicing health professionals (Park et al., 2020). While older, more traditional learning mechanisms, like lectures, apprenticeships and practice-based learning, continue to provide students with the foundational knowledge required for future success, the rise of simulation-based training has revolutionized medical education. Participants will learn faster, become familiar with advanced technology, improve their clinical skills, enhance critical thinking, and become more self - assured in their skills while under the supervision of trained instructors (Nichols et al., 2019). Moreover, the use of virtual simulation training modules can help them to perfect their skills at hours and pace convenient to them and at times even in the absence of an instructor (Zgoura et al., 2019).

The Clinical Skills Center is a place of instruction for health professional students where they learn patient interviewing and how to perform physical examinations and practice procedural skills and teamwork in the years prior to graduation. In many instances, the same facilities are used for both training and evaluation of medical students in these areas. In U.S. medical education, simulation plays a significant role in assessments that occur at the end of the third year of medical school in which the objectives are to: 1. Evaluate the students' ability to interview and communicate with patients; 2. Assess the students' physical examination skills; 3. Gauge the students' ability to synthesize data and present it in written format; 4. Provide feedback to students on their clinical skills; 5. Measure the skills of the class as a whole, so that individual and curricular deficiencies can be addressed; 6. Create the opportunity to experience a timed clinical skills examination like the standardized assessments previously required by the USMLE Step 2 Clinical Skills examination (Alvin, 2016; Gilliland et al., 2008; Langendyk, 2006).

Evaluation may occur by direct observation or with the assistance of standardized patients (SPs) who are trained actors that facilitate the assessment of history taking, physical examination skills, communications skills, and approach of the learner (Ju et al., 2015). SPs may engage with learners in person or virtually. In some instances, computer-programmed virtual simulated patients are used (Kononowicz et al., 2015). Simulated patient interactions, when added to traditional coursework, improved student counseling aptitude and knowledge retention scores (Bowers et al., 2017). Virtual simulated patients have also been demonstrated to have a positive impact on knowledge gain and student motivation (Kleinert et al., 2015). Standardized patients (SPs) are trained in interview, communication, physical examination, and feedback techniques. Simulated patient encounters are an important feature of clinical simulation. Clinical simulation centers can also serve as locations where standardized patients who are trained in a standardized manner to portray a patient in scenarios in which history-taking, physical examination, counseling and/or relationship building are important learning objectives. The role of standardized patients differs from human-patient simulators in that simulators are typically used in high-risk scenarios such as those involving severe hemorrhaging or cardiac arrest. In these instances, students learn to assess changes in a patient's status and react to those changes with appropriate interventions such as cardiac compressions, endotracheal intubation, positive pressure ventilation and the administration of vasoactive medications if performed in a simulated setting would be harmful to a patient actor. A study of student nurses' performance and stress in deteriorating patient simulations with SPs did not vary from similar scenarios using high-fidelity patient simulators (Ignacio et al., 2015).

Video debriefing allows learners to watch their simulation performance and work to understand with their colleagues and simulation facilitator what they were thinking and feeling at that moment when the events occurred (Zhang et al., 2019). This is a powerful learning tool. There are specialized video capture systems available that allow for annotation and note taking during the session which facilitate the discussion and debrief by allowing debriefers to fast-forward the video to the specific area of interest. However, simple video cameras can also be used. In addition to facilitating video debriefing, the presence of video cameras in the simulation rooms can also be used record and transmit the simulations to observation rooms that can be co-located within the simulation center or located elsewhere off-site in which students and faculty can view or facilitate the simulation in real time (Ohta et al., 2017). In a pilot study by Ohta et al., a pediatric acute care simulation by remote facilitation significantly improved students' performance and was as effective as a traditional, locally facilitated simulation (Ohta et al., 2017).

The growth of simulation education is limited by the availability of trained simulation facilitators. Participating in simulation electives as a medical student, resident or other health professional learner expands exposure to simulation and demonstrates investment and interest in the educational modality. Electives are not required activities, but they increase learners' preparation for a simulation fellowship for advanced training on simulation facilitation, debriefing and research (Kotal et al., 2015). Simulation fellowships are designed to provide advanced training in the emerging field of simulation-based medical education (Ahmed et al., 2017). Learners in a simulation rotation or fellowship participate in simulation sessions, and the development and implementation of simulation curricula and simulation-based research (Ahmed et al., 2017). Medical Simulation Fellows have also pursued Masters' degrees in Medical Education, Healthcare Simulation Science, or Public Health.

SOLUTIONS AND RECOMMENDATIONS

The role of simulation technology is seen as the enhancement of medical education through the development, application, and assessment of learner-centered educational methods. Institutions that incorporate simulation technologies across the entire medical education continuum highlight the high priority of clinical performance education. A growing emphasis on the need of patient safety has been a driving force behind the expansion of simulation education. When it comes to learning in the medical field, the traditional methods have depended on observation and practice in a clinical setting. However, simulation gives students the opportunity to practice their abilities and make mistakes without endangering a real patient.

The usage of humanoid simulators in manikin-based simulation is performed by trained simulation faculty in simulation centers, also known as dedicated places for simulation, or in clinical settings. These simulation faculty members facilitate simulation scenarios using the simulators. Learners and facilitators who are located remotely have access to a variety of other simulation modalities, including telesimulation and virtual simulation. The "fidelity" of the simulation experience refers to the degree to which it is similar to the experience of being in a clinical setting. In the past, manikins were merely crude approximations of the human body. However, manikins available now come in a variety of sizes and exhibit physiological reactions that are more accurate. Prominent global manufacturers utilize direct and indirect marketing to ensure that their products visible to simulation experts.

Global trends in the use of simulation have led to medical simulation market analyses reports with respect to aspects such as the volume of sales, valuation forecast, market size, and the market competition trends as well as the market concentration rate on basis of the key contributing countries. The acknowledgment and funding of simulation education by the leadership of an organization is essential to the development of simulation as a method. However, acknowledging the savings made possible by simulation as well as the return on investment (ROI) made possible by simulation is a significant contributor to the long-term viability of the method. After all, the ratio of instructors to students in simulations is quite high, and the demands placed on the logistics of the situation in terms of equipment, space, and time are considerable. The value proposition of simulation in comparison to various other educational approaches needs to be presented to decision-makers. Along with the direct and indirect costs, the potential savings from events or complications that did not occur as a result of the simulation, such as central line infections or pericardial effusions, must be considered.

The expansion of simulation is constrained by a lack of qualified instructors. As a health care professional learner, participating in simulation electives broadens one's exposure to simulation and shows commitment to and interest in the educational method. Fellowships in simulation-based medical education provide advanced training in this rapidly developing field.

Increasing opportunities for learners to engage in a simulation rotation or fellowship, participate in simulation sessions, create simulation curricula and engage in simulation-based research will increase the number of qualified faculty available to support simulation programs.

FUTURE RESEARCH DIRECTIONS

Despite its long history, medical simulation has recently gained a new level of realism thanks to rapid technological advances over the last decade. Clay and stone models of humans were used for centuries. Wax anatomical models were created in the 18th century. In the 19th century, obstetric simulators that leaked amniotic fluid and blood were used to train midwives and obstetricians on how to recognize and treat obstetrical complications. While the human patient simulators of the early 2000s were quite advanced at the time, today's simulators have many lifelike features including the ability to speak, respond, and describe symptoms.

While the evidence around the use of simulation in health professional education is strong, there are many gaps in our knowledge of how various types of simulation can be best applied to pre-service and in-service education. The use of virtual simulation is continually evolving as the technologies that support it become more accessible and the imagery more realistic. Simulation games are particularly effective when combined with other strategies such as briefing, simulation, and debriefing, with learners showing improvement in both initial knowledge retention and knowledge retention over time (Padilha et al., 2019). The use of virtual simulations can also improve student satisfaction with their educational experiences (Farra et al., 2019; Haerling, 2018; Vishwanath et al., 2017). Learners are placed in dynamic and immersive environments ranging from prehospital settings to community settings (Eyikara & Baykara, 2018; Nicolas et al., 2019); some are controlled by simulation facilitators using simulated systems, while others are controlled by computers (Umoren et al., 2014; Guedes et al., 2019; Shim et al., 2018).

The use of simulation for team training and to reinforce communication and behavioral skills continues to evolve. The use of simulation to address the gap that exists between theory and skills lab experiences and clinical practice, whether in bedside nursing, medicine, or other specialties, allows both students and new graduates to overcome the difficulties in adjusting to their new environments. Simulation research has contributed lessons for continuing medical education, undergraduate and graduate medical education, and supported the effectiveness of simulation in undergraduate and continuing medical education. However, the measurement tools for interprofessional team performance skills have been relatively static.

It wasn't long ago that manikins were nothing more than crude representations of the human anatomy. Manikins are now available in a wide range of sizes and can mimic a wider range of physiological reactions. In addition, there are now opportunities to incorporate robotics, artificial intelligence and other novel technologies for analyzing facial expression, and empathic communication and other communication-oriented behaviors during simulation training. Additionally, clinical simulation centers can be used as locations where standardized patients who are trained to portray a patient in scenarios where history-taking, physical examination, counseling, and/or relationship-building are important learning objectives can be practiced in a standardized manner. Finally, the use of technology and telemedicine devices that allow for telesimulation and remote facilitation of simulations will expand in the coming decade and the experience and educational outcomes of learners trained in this manner will need to be compared with those of in-person simulation.

CONCLUSION

Simulation education is a highly desirable and effective approach to training health professionals that has been recognized and utilized by healthcare and training institutions for many decades. While the origins of simulation date back to antiquity and the principles and practice of simulation have evolved in line with adult educational theory. The use of simulation in medical education has evolved over the years in the context of meeting training objectives. However, the global application and use of simulation is limited by awareness and access to programs for simulation instructor training.

Simulation is currently the industry standard in healthcare education and training. Simulation education is built on several decades of evidence showing a clear link between simulation-based training and safety. However, the application of patient safety objectives to simulation arose from its use in the field of aviation to prevent safety events and near misses. In recent times, use of health professional simulation has received significant support from an impetus to increase patient safety and decrease medical errors. This has led to the integration of simulation education at all levels of pre-service and in-service health professional training.

While there is no substitute for real-world experience, simulations offer a safe way for students to try out new skills and learn from their mistakes. There are numerous benefits to using this method of training to improve the abilities of healthcare providers and, as a result, improve patient safety and lower healthcare costs. The range of simulation experiences including manikin-based simulation and virtual simulation are available to learners in high-resource settings, but not always in lower resource settings. Virtual and manikin-based simulations can be found in hybrid simulation rooms, while mid- and high-fidelity clinical simulation labs use manikins with varying levels of technology.

Investment in this method of training has many advantages that help improve healthcare practitioners' skills and competencies, and in return, this improves patient safety. When compared to other types of education, the return on investment for simulation education is higher because it has a longer-term impact on the safety of patients and the outcomes of their care. However, investors in simulation training may need to adjust their expectations for returns because a commitment to the sustainable development of human resources may have more modest earnings results in the near term.

REFERENCES

Aebersold, M. (2016). The history of simulation and its impact on the future. *AACN Advanced Critical Care*, *27*(1), 56–61. doi:10.4037/aacnacc2016436 PMID:26909454

Ahmed, R. A., Frey, J. A., Hughes, P. G., & Tekian, A. (2017). Simulation fellowship programs in graduate medical education. *Academic Medicine*, *92*(8), 1214. doi:10.1097/ACM.0000000000001780 PMID:28590944

Alvin, M. D. (2016). The USMLE step 2 CS: Time for a change. *Medical Teacher*, *38*(8), 854–856. doi:10.3109/0142159X.2016.1147539 PMID:27007882

Ballestriero, R. (2010). Anatomical models and wax Venuses: Art masterpieces or scientific craft works? *Journal of Anatomy*, *216*(2), 223–234. doi:10.1111/j.1469-7580.2009.01169.x PMID:20002228

Bause, G. S. (2010). Antique Chinese diagnostic dolls. *Anesthesiology*, *112*(3), 513–513. doi:10.1097/01.anes.0000368880.41177.27 PMID:20179494

Bayram, S. B., & Caliskan, N. (2019). Effect of a game-based virtual reality phone application on tracheostomy care education for nursing students: A randomized controlled trial. *Nurse Education Today*, *79*, 25–31. doi:10.1016/j.nedt.2019.05.010 PMID:31102793

Bowe, S. N., Johnson, K., & Puscas, L. (2017). Facilitation and Debriefing in Simulation Education. *Otolaryngologic Clinics of North America*, *50*(5), 989–1001. doi:10.1016/j.otc.2017.05.009 PMID:28822579

Bowers, R., Tunney, R., Kelly, K., Mills, B., Trotta, K., Wheeless, C. N., & Drew, R. (2017). Impact of Standardized Simulated Patients on First-Year Pharmacy Students' Knowledge Retention of Insulin Injection Technique and Counseling Skills. *American Journal of Pharmaceutical Education*, *81*(6), 113–113. doi:10.5688/ajpe816113 PMID:28970614

Bradley, C. S., Johnson, B. K., Dreifuerst, K. T., White, P., Conde, S. K., Meakim, C. H., Curry-Lourenco, K., & Childress, R. M. (2019). Regulation of simulation use in United States prelicensure nursing programs. *Clinical Simulation in Nursing*, *33*, 17–25. doi:10.1016/j.ecns.2019.04.004

Cooper, J., & Taqueti, V. (2008). A brief history of the development of mannequin simulators for clinical education and training. *Postgraduate Medical Journal*, *84*(997), 563–570. doi:10.1136/qshc.2004.009886 PMID:19103813

Doolen, J., Mariani, B., Atz, T., Horsley, T. L., O'Rourke, J., McAfee, K., & Cross, C. L. (2016). High-fidelity simulation in undergraduate nursing education: A review of simulation reviews. *Clinical Simulation in Nursing*, *12*(7), 290–302. doi:10.1016/j.ecns.2016.01.009

Dufrene, C., & Young, A. (2014). Successful debriefing - best methods to achieve positive learning outcomes: A literature review. *Nurse Education Today*, *34*(3), 372–376. doi:10.1016/j.nedt.2013.06.026 PMID:23890542

Erich, J. (2016). The Secrets of a Successful Simulation Program. Technology and tools can improve the experience, but optimizing the benefit for training EMS providers requires a bit more. *EMS World*, *45*(5), 16–22. https://pubmed.ncbi.nlm.nih.gov/27337829 PMID:27337829

Eyikara, E., & Baykara, Z. G. (2018). Effect of simulation on the ability of first year nursing students to learn vital signs. *Nurse Education Today*, *60*, 101–106. doi:10.1016/j.nedt.2017.09.023 PMID:29078202

Farra, S. L., Gneuhs, M., Hodgson, E., Kawosa, B., Miller, E. T., Simon, A., Timm, N., & Hausfeld, J. (2019). Comparative Cost of Virtual Reality Training and Live Exercises for Training Hospital Workers for Evacuation. *Computers, Informatics, Nursing, 37*(9), 446–454. doi:10.1097/CIN.0000000000000540 PMID:31166203

Gantt, L. (2016). Simulation operations specialists job descriptions composition, negotiation, and processes. In *Healthcare Simulation: A Guide for Operations Specialists* (pp. 131–136). Wiley. doi:10.1002/9781118949443

Gavilanes, J. S. (2015). Evolution of the Simulation Operations Specialist (SOS). *Healthcare Simulation: A Guide for Operations Specialists*, 15.

Gilliland, W. R., Rochelle, J. L., Hawkins, R., Dillon, G. F., Mechaber, A. J., Dyrbye, L., Papp, K. K., & Durning, S. J. (2008). Changes in clinical skills education resulting from the introduction of the USMLE™ step 2 clinical skills (CS) examination. *Medical Teacher, 30*(3), 325–327. doi:10.1080/01421590801953026 PMID:18484462

Guedes, H. G., Câmara Costa Ferreira, Z. M., Ribeiro de Sousa Leão, L., Souza Montero, E. F., Otoch, J. P., & Artifon, E. L. A. (2019). Virtual reality simulator versus box-trainer to teach minimally invasive procedures: A meta-analysis. *International journal of surgery (London, England), 61*, 60–68. doi:10.1016/j.ijsu.2018.12.001 PMID:30529216

Haerling, K. A. (2018). Cost-Utility Analysis of Virtual and Mannequin-Based Simulation. *Simulation in Healthcare: Journal of the Society for Simulation in Healthcare, 13*(1), 33-40. doi:10.1097/SIH.0000000000000280

Holtschneider, M. E. (2013). Simulation programs versus simulation centers in the hospital/workplace setting: It's not about the space. *Journal for Nurses in Professional Development, 29*(4), 213–213. doi:10.1097/NND.0b013e31829c521e PMID:23877294

Huwendiek, S. (2019). Design and implementation of virtual patients for learning of clinical reasoning. *GMS Journal for Medical Education, 36*(4), Doc33–Doc33. doi:10.3205/zma001241 PMID:31544133

Ignacio, J., Dolmans, D., Scherpbier, A., Rethans, J.-J., Chan, S., & Liaw, S. Y. (2015). Comparison of standardized patients with high-fidelity simulators for managing stress and improving performance in clinical deterioration: A mixed methods study. *Nurse Education Today, 35*(12), 1161–1168. doi:10.1016/j.nedt.2015.05.009 PMID:26047602

Johnson, W. B. (2016). *Military settings.* Academic Press.

Jones, F., Passos-Neto, C. E., & Braghiroli, O. F. M. (2015). Simulation in Medical Education: Brief history and methodology. *Principles and Practice of Clinical Research, 1*(2).

Ju, M., Berman, A. T., & Vapiwala, N. (2015). Standardized Patient Training Programs: an Efficient Solution to the Call for Quality Improvement in Oncologist Communication Skills. *Journal of cancer education: the official journal of the American Association for Cancer Education, 30*(3), 466-470. doi:10.1007/s13187-014-0715-x

Kerner, R. L., Jr., Gallo, K., Cassara, M., D'Angelo, J., Egan, A., & Simmons, J. G. (2016). Simulation for Operational Readiness in a New Freestanding Emergency Department: Strategy and Tactics. *Simulation in Healthcare: Journal of the Society for Simulation in Healthcare, 11*(5), 345-356. doi:10.1097/SIH.0000000000000180

Kirsch, V., Johannsen, W., Thrien, C., Herzig, S., & Matthes, J. (2019). "Hopefully, I will never forget that again" - sensitizing medical students for drug safety by working on cases and simulating doctor-patient communication. *GMS Journal for Medical Education, 36*(2), Doc17–Doc17. doi:10.3205/zma001225 PMID:30993175

Kleinert, R., Heiermann, N., Plum, P. S., Wahba, R., Chang, D.-H., Maus, M., Chon, S.-H., Hoelscher, A. H., & Stippel, D. L. (2015). Web-Based Immersive Virtual Patient Simulators: Positive Effect on Clinical Reasoning in Medical Education. *Journal of Medical Internet Research, 17*(11), e263–e263. doi:10.2196/jmir.5035 PMID:26577020

Kolbe, M., Grande, B., & Spahn, D. R. (2015). Briefing and debriefing during simulation-based training and beyond: Content, structure, attitude and setting. *Best Practice & Research. Clinical Anaesthesiology, 29*(1), 87–96. doi:10.1016/j.bpa.2015.01.002 PMID:25902470

Kononowicz, A. A., Woodham, L. A., Edelbring, S., Stathakarou, N., Davies, D., Saxena, N., Tudor Car, L., Carlstedt-Duke, J., Car, J., & Zary, N. (2019). Virtual Patient Simulations in Health Professions Education: Systematic Review and Meta-Analysis by the Digital Health Education Collaboration. *Journal of Medical Internet Research, 21*(7), e14676. doi:10.2196/14676 PMID:31267981

Kononowicz, A. A., Zary, N., Edelbring, S., Corral, J., & Hege, I. (2015). Virtual patients—What are we talking about? A framework to classify the meanings of the term in healthcare education. *BMC Medical Education, 15*(1), 11–11. doi:10.118612909-015-0296-3 PMID:25638167

Kotal, E. R., Sivertson, R. M., Wolfe, S. P., Lammers, R. L., & Overton, D. T. (2015). A survey of simulation fellowship programs. *The Journal of Emergency Medicine, 48*(3), 351–355. doi:10.1016/j.jemermed.2014.10.004 PMID:25456774

Kyaw, B. M., Saxena, N., Posadzki, P., Vseteckova, J., Nikolaou, C. K., George, P. P., Divakar, U., Masiello, I., Kononowicz, A. A., Zary, N., & Tudor Car, L. (2019). Virtual Reality for Health Professions Education: Systematic Review and Meta-Analysis by the Digital Health Education Collaboration. *Journal of Medical Internet Research, 21*(1), e12959. doi:10.2196/12959 PMID:30668519

Labrague, L. J., McEnroe-Petitte, D. M., Bowling, A. M., Nwafor, C. E., & Tsaras, K. (2019). High-fidelity simulation and nursing students' anxiety and self-confidence: A systematic review. *Nursing Forum, 54*(3), 358–368. doi:10.1111/nuf.12337 PMID:30852844

Langendyk, V. (2006). Not knowing that they do not know: Self-assessment accuracy of third-year medical students. *Medical Education, 40*(2), 173–179. doi:10.1111/j.1365-2929.2005.02372.x PMID:16451246

Levett-Jones, T., & Lapkin, S. (2014). A systematic review of the effectiveness of simulation debriefing in health professional education. *Nurse Education Today, 34*(6), e58–e63. doi:10.1016/j.nedt.2013.09.020 PMID:24169444

Lyons, R., Lazzara, E. H., Benishek, L. E., Zajac, S., Gregory, M., Sonesh, S. C., & Salas, E. (2015). Enhancing the effectiveness of team debriefings in medical simulation: More best practices. *Joint Commission Journal on Quality and Patient Safety, 41*(3), 115–125. doi:10.1016/S1553-7250(15)41016-5 PMID:25977127

Maciocia, G. (1982). History of acupuncture. *Journal of Chinese Medicine, 9*, 9–15.

Maestre, J. M., & Rudolph, J. W. (2015). Theories and styles of debriefing: The good judgment method as a tool for formative assessment in healthcare. *Revista Española de Cardiología (English Ed.), 68*(4), 282–285. doi:10.1016/j.rec.2014.05.018 PMID:25239179

Magee, R. (2004). Medical practice and medical education 1500– 2001: An overview. *ANZ Journal of Surgery*, *74*(4), 272–276. doi:10.1111/j.1445-2197.2004.02960.x PMID:15043741

Marei, H. F., Donkers, J., Al-Eraky, M. M., & Van Merrienboer, J. J. G. (2019). Collaborative use of virtual patients after a lecture enhances learning with minimal investment of cognitive load. *Medical Teacher*, *41*(3), 332–339. doi:10.1080/0142159X.2018.1472372 PMID:29798713

Mendiratta-Lala, M., Williams, T. R., Mendiratta, V., Ahmed, H., & Bonnett, J. W. (2015). Simulation center training as a means to improve resident performance in percutaneous noncontinuous CT-guided fluoroscopic procedures with dose reduction. *AJR. American Journal of Roentgenology*, *204*(4), W376–W383. doi:10.2214/AJR.14.13420 PMID:25794086

Mills, D. M., Williams, D. C., & Dobson, J. V. (2013). Simulation training as a mechanism for procedural and resuscitation education for pediatric residents: A systematic review. *Hospital Pediatrics*, *3*(2), 167–176. doi:10.1542/hpeds.2012-0041 PMID:24340419

Mills, D. M., Wu, C. L., Williams, D. C., King, L., & Dobson, J. V. (2013). High-fidelity simulation enhances pediatric residents' retention, knowledge, procedural proficiency, group resuscitation performance, and experience in pediatric resuscitation. *Hospital Pediatrics*, *3*(3), 266–275. doi:10.1542/hpeds.2012-0073 PMID:24313097

Motz, P., Gray, M., Sawyer, T., Kett, J., Danforth, D., Maicher, K., & Umoren, R. (2018). Virtual Antenatal Encounter and Standardized Simulation Assessment (VANESSA): Pilot Study. *JMIR Serious Games*, *6*(2), e8. doi:10.2196/games.9611 PMID:29752249

Nelissen, E., Ersdal, H., Mduma, E., Evjen-Olsen, B., Twisk, J., Broerse, J., van Roosmalen, J., & Stekelenburg, J. (2017). Clinical performance and patient outcome after simulation-based training in prevention and management of postpartum haemorrhage: An educational intervention study in a low-resource setting. *BMC Pregnancy and Childbirth*, *17*(1), 301–301. doi:10.118612884-017-1481-7 PMID:28893211

Nichols, A., Wiley, S., Morrell, B. L., Jochum, J. E., Moore, E. S., Carmack, J. N., Hetzler, K. E., Toon, J., Hess, J. L., Meer, M., & Moore, S. M. (2019). Interprofessional Healthcare Students' Perceptions of a Simulation-Based Learning Experience. *Journal of Allied Health*, *48*(3), 159–166. https://pubmed.ncbi.nlm.nih.gov/31487353 PMID:31487353

Nicolaou, P., McCrorie, P., & Nicolaou, S. A. (2019). Using virtual patients to integrate physiology, pathophysiology, and pharmacology in preclinical teaching. *Advances in Physiology Education*, *43*(3), 277–281. doi:10.1152/advan.00010.2019 PMID:31166125

Norman, G. (2009). The American College of Chest Physicians evidence-based educational guidelines for continuing medical education interventions: A critical review of evidence-based educational guidelines. *Chest*, *135*(3), 834–837. doi:10.1378/chest.09-0036 PMID:19265092

Ohta, K., Kurosawa, H., Shiima, Y., Ikeyama, T., Scott, J., Hayes, S., Gould, M., Buchanan, N., Nadkarni, V., & Nishisaki, A. (2017). The Effectiveness of Remote Facilitation in Simulation-Based Pediatric Resuscitation Training for Medical Students. *Pediatric Emergency Care*, *33*(8), 564–569. doi:10.1097/PEC.0000000000000752 PMID:27261952

Overtoom, E. M., Jansen, F.-W., van Santbrink, E. J. P., Schraffordt Koops, S. E., Veersema, S., & Schreuder, H. W. R. (2017). Training in Basic Laparoscopic Surgical Skills: Residents Opinion of the New Nintendo Wii-U Laparoscopic Simulator. *Journal of Surgical Education*, *74*(2), 352–359. doi:10.1016/j.jsurg.2016.10.004 PMID:27789193

Owen, H. (2012). Early use of simulation in medical education. *Simulation in Healthcare*, *7*(2), 102–116. doi:10.1097/SIH.0b013e3182415a91 PMID:22374231

Owen, H., & Pelosi, M. A. II. (2013). A historical examination of the Budin-Pinard phantom: What can contemporary obstetrics education learn from simulators of the past? *Academic Medicine*, *88*(5), 652–656. doi:10.1097/ACM.0b013e31828b0464 PMID:23524924

Padilha, J. M., Machado, P. P., Ribeiro, A., Ramos, J., & Costa, P. (2019). Clinical virtual simulation in nursing education: Randomized controlled trial. *Journal of Medical Internet Research*, *21*(3), e11529. doi:10.2196/11529 PMID:30882355

Paquette, J., Lemyre, M., Vachon-Marceau, C., Bujold, E., & Maheux-Lacroix, S. (2017). Virtual Laparoscopy Simulation: a Promising Pedagogic Tool in Gynecology. *JSLS: Journal of the Society of Laparoendoscopic Surgeons, 21*(3), e2017.00048. doi:10.4293/JSLS.2017.00048

Park, C., Grant, J., Dumas, R. P., Dultz, L., Shoultz, T. H., Scott, D. J., Luk, S., Abdelfattah, K. R., & Cripps, M. W. (2020). Does simulation work? Monthly trauma simulation and procedural training are associated with decreased time to intervention. *The Journal of Trauma and Acute Care Surgery*, *88*(2), 242–248. doi:10.1097/TA.0000000000002561 PMID:31804411

Reed, C. B. (1931). *Operative obstetrics on the manikin for students and practitioners*. P. Blakiston's Son & Company, Incorporated.

Sawyer, T., Eppich, W., Brett-Fleegler, M., Grant, V., & Cheng, A. (2016). More Than One Way to Debrief: A Critical Review of Healthcare Simulation Debriefing Methods. *Simulation in Healthcare: Journal of the Society for Simulation in Healthcare, 11*(3), 209-217. doi:10.1097/SIH.0000000000000148

Sawyer, T., Loren, D., & Halamek, L. P. (2016). Post-event debriefings during neonatal care: why are we not doing them, and how can we start? *Journal of Perinatology: Official Journal of the California Perinatal Association, 36*(6), 415-419. doi:10.1038/jp.2016.42

Shim, J. S., Noh, T. I., Kim, J. Y., Pyun, J. H., Cho, S., Oh, M. M., Kang, S. H., Cheon, J., Lee, J. G., Kim, J. J., & Kang, S. G. (2018). Predictive Validation of a Robotic Virtual Reality Simulator: The Tube 3 module for Practicing Vesicourethral Anastomosis in Robot-Assisted Radical Prostatectomy. *Urology*, *122*, 32–36. doi:10.1016/j.urology.2018.08.013 PMID:30144481

Stokes-Parish, J. B., Duvivier, R., & Jolly, B. (2018). Investigating the impact of moulage on simulation engagement—A systematic review. *Nurse Education Today*, *64*, 49–55. doi:10.1016/j.nedt.2018.01.003 PMID:29459192

Sweigart, L., & Hodson-Carlton, K. (2013). Improving student interview skills: The virtual avatar as client. *Nurse Educator*, *38*(1), 11–15. doi:10.1097/NNE.0b013e318276df2d PMID:23222623

Thomas, A., Burns, R., Sanseau, E., & Auerbach, M. (2021). Tips for Conducting Telesimulation-Based Medical Education. *Cureus*, *13*(1). PMID:33552792

Umoren, R., Stadler, D. J., Gasior, S. L., Al-Sheikhly, D., Truman, B., & Lowe, C. (2014). Global collaboration and team-building through 3D virtual environments. *Innovations in Global Medical and Health Education*, 1.

Vishwanath, A., Kam, M., & Kumar, N. (2017). Examining low-cost virtual reality for learning in low-resource environments. *Proceedings of the 2017 Conference on Designing Interactive Systems.*

West, C., Graham, L., Palmer, R. T., Miller, M. F., Thayer, E. K., Stuber, M. L., Awdishu, L., Umoren, R. A., Wamsley, M. A., Nelson, E. A., Joo, P. A., Tysinger, J. W., George, P., & Carney, P. A. (2016). Implementation of interprofessional education (IPE) in 16 U.S. medical schools: Common practices, barriers and facilitators. *Journal of Interprofessional Education & Practice*, *4*, 41–49. doi:10.1016/j.xjep.2016.05.002

Wetzel, E. A., Lang, T. R., Pendergrass, T. L., Taylor, R. G., & Geis, G. L. (2013). Identification of latent safety threats using high-fidelity simulation-based training with multidisciplinary neonatology teams. *Joint Commission Journal on Quality and Patient Safety*, *39*(6), 268–273. doi:10.1016/S1553-7250(13)39037-0 PMID:23789165

Yu, H., Zhang, C. Y., Zhang, S. H., Cheng, H., & Chen, J. (2017). Virtual Simulation Teaching Centre in Dental Education: a Report from Fujian Medical University, China. *The Chinese Journal of Dental Research: The Official Journal of the Scientific Section of the Chinese Stomatological Association (CSA)*, *20*(3), 173-177. doi:10.3290/j.cjdr.a38773

Zgoura, P., Hettich, D., Natzel, J., Özcan, F., & Kantzow, B. (2019). Virtual Reality Simulation in Peritoneal Dialysis Training: The Beginning of a New Era. *Blood Purification*, *47*(1-3), 265–269. doi:10.1159/000494595 PMID:30522112

Zhang, H., Mörelius, E., Goh, S. H. L., & Wang, W. (2019). Effectiveness of Video-Assisted Debriefing in Simulation-Based Health Professions Education: A Systematic Review of Quantitative Evidence. *Nurse Educator*, *44*(3), E1–E6. doi:10.1097/NNE.0000000000000562 PMID:30015683

KEY TERMS AND DEFINITIONS

Augmented Reality: Computer generated holographic images can be viewed by the learner in the physical environment using a mobile device or specially designed headset.

High-Fidelity Manikin: This term refers to a technology-enabled manikin with features such as mechanical respiration and heart rate.

Low-Fidelity Manikin: This is typically a low cost, low technology manikin with minimal features.

Objective Structured Clinical Examination (OSCE): An approach to assessment that involves defined objectives and anticipated actions, often with an accompanying checklist for assessment.

Simulation Debriefer: A simulation instructor who leads the learners through a reflective analysis of simulation events.

Simulation Facilitator: A simulation instructor who guides the learners through the scenario with the goal of meeting learning objectives.

Simulation Technician/Specialist: An individual who supports the practice of simulation through setting up and managing simulation manikins and supplies.

Teledebriefing: Teledebriefing describes a process in which learners who are participating in a simulation scenario undergo debriefing with a facilitator located at an off-site location.

Telefacilitation: The conduct of a telesimulation by a remote facilitator.

Telesimulation: Telesimulation is a process by which telecommunication and simulation resources are utilized to provide education, training, and/or assessment to learners at an off-site location.

Video-Assisted Debriefing: The practice of using video captured during simulation sessions for reflective discussions on learner and team performance.

Virtual Environment: 3D computer generated objects that can be viewed on a screen or in a head-mounted display.

Virtual Reality: Computer generated 3D images viewed by a learner in a virtual environment using a low-cost or high-end head mounted display.

Chapter 2
Theory of Simulation and Gaming for Health Professional Education

ABSTRACT

Simulation and game-based learning are educational strategies that are grounded in adult learning theory. Adult learners differ from young learners in many ways. Instructors must recognize these differences and tailor their instructional strategies accordingly. While there are many theories of adult learning, no single theory fully explains how and why adults learn through simulation-based methods. This chapter introduces adult learning theories that have been described in the context of simulation education and how the awareness of these concepts can be applied to simulation curriculum development, implementation, and assessment in health professional learners.

INTRODUCTION

Training for health professionals, both those about to enter the field (pre-service) and those already working in the field (in-service), is increasingly including simulation-based instruction (Coburn et al., 2020; Glenn & Claman, 2020; Mossenson et al., 2020; Park et al., 2020). One of the driving reasons for the growth of simulation education has been the recognition that medical errors lead to as many as 400,000 deaths in the U.S. each year (Deering et al., 2011; Harvey et al., 2013; Motycka et al., 2018; Riley et al., 2011). Clinical

DOI: 10.4018/978-1-7998-4378-8.ch002

simulations can reduce medical errors by increasing staff comfort with both common and rare high-risk situations requiring specific skills (Bierer et al., 2018; McArdle et al., 2018; Motycka et al., 2018; Stout-Aguilar et al., 2018). Healthcare simulations can also focus on teamwork and improving the communication between team members (Fewster-Thuente & Batteson, 2016; Sweigart et al., 2016; Umoren et al., 2017).

Simulation is a place where learners and instructors can engage in conversation and interaction within the context of a simulation. The simulation scenario provides an opportunity for learners to try out brand new ideas and experiment with new concepts and approaches (Davis et al., 2017). Simulation experiences are used to emphasize the facts and theory from didactic sessions and independent study (Barry Issenberg et al., 2005). Debriefing is a process that takes place after each simulation scenario is completed, and it is led by qualified simulation facilitators. Participants in the simulation talk about their experiences with the debriefing process. A debriefing is an opportunity for reflection and a discussion of strategies to improve results and reduce the likelihood of future errors (Salik & Paige, 2020; Zhang et al., 2019). In the same way that simulation in the military improved battlefield preparedness and flight simulators in aviation have been used to reduce the number of plane crashes, simulation in healthcare has provided opportunities for health professional learners to improve their procedural skills and practice their teamwork and clinical decision-making abilities (Aebersold, 2016; Everett et al., 2017).

Adult education can be defined as the purposeful and systematic process of teaching and learning that enables a person to acquire new values, attitudes, knowledge, skills, and disciplines in order to fulfill the responsibilities of their adult roles (Merriam, 2001; Prakash et al., 2019). Adult learners have a need to know why they must learn something. It is essential for adult students to understand the relevance of the material they are studying. The education they receive must have a value or benefit for them and lead to an improvement in their lives (Knowles et al., 2005). Further, it is important for instructors to emphasize the advantages that adult learners will have once they have learned the material (Knowles et al., 2005).

Capable instructors in any field of education should have a number of characteristics, the most important of which are a strong knowledge base, experience, and the ability to teach students with patience while also giving them agency (Rashid, 2017). Each learner group is made up of individuals with distinct personalities and backgrounds, as well as a variety of individual learning styles and varied degrees of preparation for learning (Kolb & Kolb, 2005). Each participant in an educational event learns at a different speed, utilizes a different mode of learning, and comes into the event with gaps in their understanding of fundamental abilities. This indicates that teachers have a responsibility to detect and correct these knowledge gaps as they construct new information and urge students to reflect on how this knowledge applies to their clinical context and practice.

During pre-service education, the instructor is responsible for setting goals and objectives, learning is organized around predetermined teaching plans, and there is very little of an emphasis placed on reflection (Grossman & Conelius, 2015; Merriam, 2001). However, while this method might be successful for students who are younger or less experienced, the environment in which people learn is very different. This is because adults almost always choose to study, which is a very different motivator than being required to learn in school (Rashid, 2017). Adult students are responsible for their own education and are more concerned with the practical application of what they study (Merriam, 2001; Prakash et al., 2019). They favor independence and may give the impression of being resistant to acquiring new skills (Merriam, 2001). The pace is particularly important for practicing healthcare professionals, since they frequently have to strike a balance between school, job, and personal difficulties (Rashid, 2017).

BACKGROUND

Simulations tell "stories" that provide meaning to the learning experience. In healthcare, these stories allow learners to experience a high acuity event, team dynamic or situation in a controlled fashion with lessons that they can apply to their work or learning environment (Haubruck et al., 2018; Haugland & Reime, 2018; Hege et al., 2018). While manikin-based simulation is the prevailing form of simulation-based education, virtual simulations or simulation games are a complementary pedagogical strategy to manikin-based simulation (M.-S. Bracq et al., 2019; Foronda et al., 2020; Guedes et al., 2019). These virtual simulations provide the opportunity to improve clinical reasoning skills in students through exposure to a large number of clinical scenarios, other tools and strategies, such as case studies and problem-based learning (Chen & Hu, 2018; Haubruck et al., 2018; Kowalewski et al., 2017). Virtual simulations may be more appropriate than manikin-based simulations for some purposes, particularly disaster simulations. They have also been described for simulations that focus on teamwork and communication skills as well as procedural skills training (Banaszek et al., 2017; Berman et al., 2017; Bernardo, 2017; Gray et al., 2020; Motz et al., 2018; Umoren et al., 2017).

In health professional education, learners begin with a theoretical knowledge base, then progress to using virtual and manikin-based simulated experiences in a simulation center or in situ within the clinical environment, then start to observe real-world activity before beginning the immersive experience of becoming part of that world and growing professionally within that environment (Rashid, 2017). While the approach to exposing learners to these modalities may be sequential or repetitive, the use of simulation and/ or observation generally precedes clinical practice for health professional learners (Jeffers & Poling, 2019; Matterson et al., 2018; Offiah et al., 2019; Park et al., 2020; Rowse & Dearani, 2019). A sentinel study on simulation-based learning using a manikin simulator, Harvey, showed students trained

Figure 1. Simulation and observation precede clinical practice for health professional learners

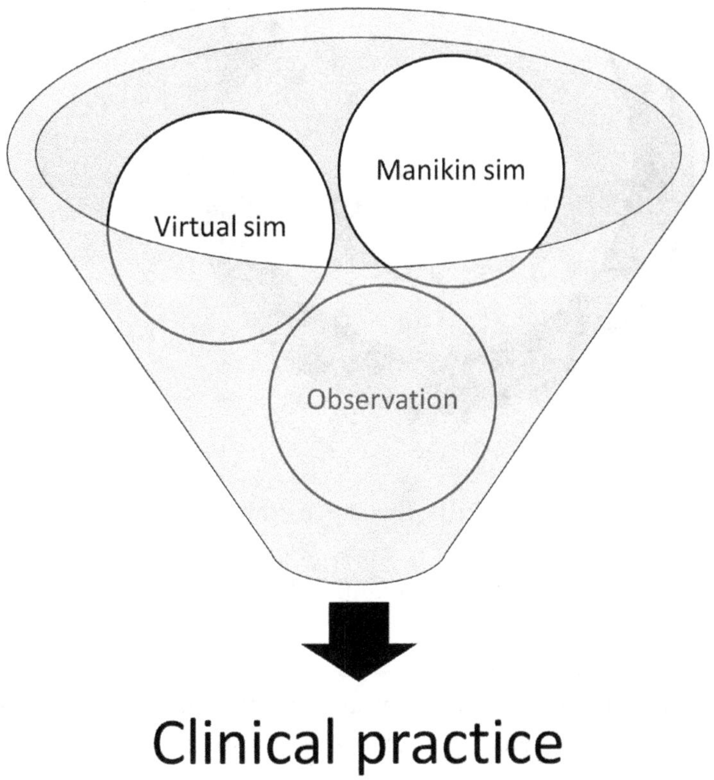

with manikins and real patients performed better than those who interacted with real patients only (Issenberg & Scalese, 2008). See Figure 1.

On the other hand, for healthcare practitioners undergoing continuing

Figure 2. Simulation experiences complement clinical practice for experienced healthcare practitioners

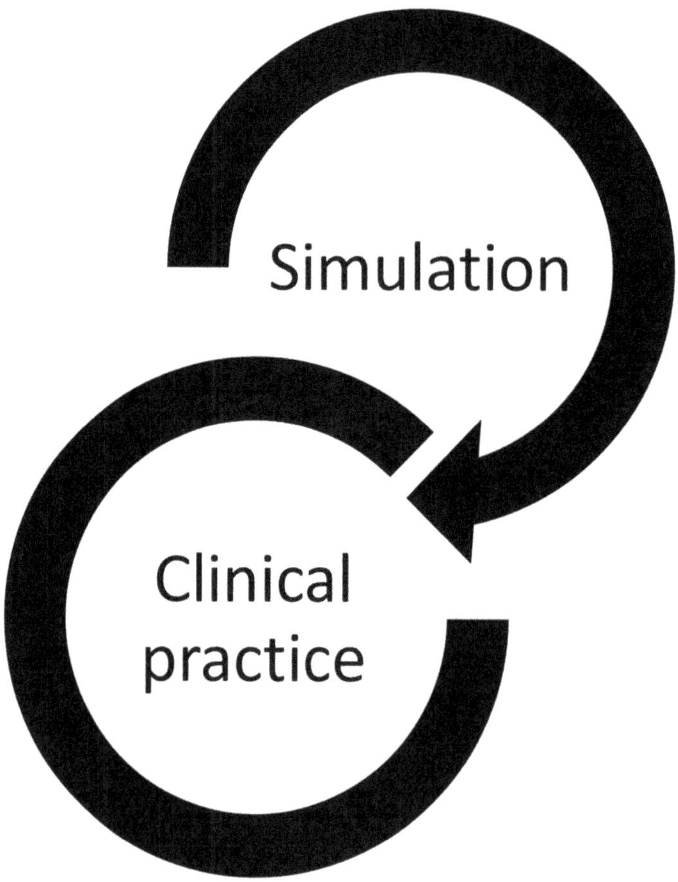

education to maintain their skills, the use of simulation complements clinical practice. See Figure 2.

The use of virtual simulations or games that involve simulation is not new, but the technologies that are employed in virtual simulation have progressed considerably throughout the course of recent history. This technological evolution has led to an increase in the availability and accessibility of virtual reality and augmented reality simulation software and hardware, which has made the technology more accessible to students at all levels of training, including primary, secondary, and tertiary institutions, as well as healthcare facilities in low- and high-income settings (Umoren RA, 2020). The traditional methods of learning, such as lectures and videos, which take a more passive approach, have recently received increased attention due to concerns that these methods result in poor retention and transfer to practice. Simulation games, on the other hand, have received increased attention recently (Cook et al., 2011). In addition, the amount of information that must be reliably communicated to learners is growing, while the learners' time and attention spans are becoming increasingly constrained. This is especially true for adult learners, whose participants often come from a wide range of life stages and have a large number of additional obligations. E-learning modules need to be very interactive if they are to appeal to the present generation of students, who have grown up playing video games from a very young age. These interactive and goal-oriented training solutions may satisfy the demands of learners and fill the void, particularly in situations when options for in-person simulation are limited. As gamified cooperative and learning strategies make their way into educational curriculum, there has been an increase in the number of instances in which avatars, role playing games, point systems, badges, and leaderboards are used (Kapp, 2012; Malone, 1981). Nevertheless, gamification is not limited to the addition of these badges, points, and incentives to educational activities, and it is not an ideal solution for all types of educational settings (Kapp, 2012). Simulation games, on the other hand, are attempts to find solutions to problems while simultaneously engaging learners and boosting retention through the utilization of game-based thinking and approaches (Malone, 1981). The creation of virtual simulation games, often known as serious games, occurs when traditional educational content is gamified. In addition to adult learning theory, the tenets of game-based theory are applicable to the process of acquiring knowledge through participation in virtual simulations (Kapp, 2012; Malone, 1981).

ADULT LEARNING THEORY AND SIMULATION EDUCATION

The adult learning theory begins with the concept that adults require an explanation of why they are being taught a particular topic. Adult education activities need to be well-organized and interactive, and they should consider the diversity of their students. Andragogy, experiential learning, self-directed learning, social cognitive theory, and transformational learning are just few of the many educational philosophies that have been developed to explain adult education (Knowles et al., 2005; Merriam, 2001; Rashid, 2017). In the early 1970s, Knowles coined the term "andragogy" to describe the distinct differences between the educational experiences of children and those of adult learners (Knowles et al., 2005). Adults, in terms of their orientation toward learning, are said to be task-centered and problem-centered, according to Knowles (Knowles et al., 2005). Adults, in comparison to younger learners, bring a different motivation and experiences to the learning process. Additionally, adults have a better ability for reflection in comparison to younger learners (Knowles et al., 2005; Merriam, 2001). Training and education that disregards the principles of adult learning has the potential to stifle their motivation (Knowles et al., 2005). Adults are prepared to acquire the knowledge and skills necessary to effectively deal with the challenges and opportunities presented by real-life scenarios (Knowles et al., 2005). Although adult learning theory has been shown to play an important part in both education and practice, the majority of simulation research do not specify an explicit learning theory (Lavoie et al., 2018). Only 16 out of a total of 120 simulation studies were found to offer a learning theory that explained why simulation was utilized. This was discovered through a systematic review of simulation research (Kaakinen & Arwood, 2009; Lavoie et al., 2018). Experiential learning, social cognitive theory, and transformative learning theory are important learning theories that have been investigated in relation to simulation-based learning.

Experiential Learning

The experiential learning theory developed by David Kolb is frequently cited as being among the most prominent learning theories connected with simulation (Kolb & Kolb, 2005; Manolis et al., 2013). Kolb's learning theory depicts learning as occurring in 4 stages representing how learners interact with the experience or environment. In this cycle, a concrete experience leads to reflective observation which then lead to abstract conceptualization (or concept formation) that is then used in problem solving and decision making also known as the active experimentation stage (Kolb & Kolb, 2005). Simulation studies often report knowledge acquisition and retention and associate the simulation session with a concrete experience or active experimentation that prompts reflective observation and abstract conceptualization (as part of debriefing), which then leads to future actions. The use of deliberate

Table 1. Relationship between the stages of Kolb's experiential learning theory and simulation education

Kolb's experiential learning theory		Application to simulation education
Stage 1	Concrete experience	Learner participates in a challenging simulation scenario
Stage 2	Reflective observation	Encounter leads to self-evaluation. Facilitated or self-debrief promotes reflection on performance.
Stage 3	Abstract conceptualization	Active participation in debriefing process with facilitator and other learners leads to discussion and change in perspective. Reflection and discussion lead to identification of new ideas, concepts, or lessons learned.
Stage 4	Active experimentation	Learner considers ways to apply lessons learned in future scenarios or practice.

practice has been demonstrated to improve learning outcomes and aligns with Ericsson's deliberate practice theory (Ericsson, 2004; Stocker et al., 2014).

The Kolb Learning Style Inventory describes four learning styles (accommodating, assimilating, converging and diverging) which are designed to help individuals identify the way they learn from experiences (Manolis et al., 2013). These learning styles are assessed based on a learners' emphasis on abstractness over concreteness and action over reflection (Shinnick & Woo, 2015). Each learning style is described as having unique educational styles and needs. While there is mixed evidence on whether learning styles are associated with learning outcomes, some studies indicate higher effect sizes of simulation for assimilating and diverging learners than for accommodating and converging learners (Shinnick & Woo, 2015). Other instruments that have been used to determine learning style preference are the Honey and Mumford Learning Style Questionnaire (Honey, 2001) and the Dunn and Dunn Learning Style Questionnaire (Dunn et al., 1995).

Social Cognitive Theory

Bandura's social cognitive theory suggests that learners observe and extract information from others' behavior and this learning then guides later action (Lavoie et al., 2018). Observational learning occurs through attention, retention through symbolic coding operations or skill practice, reproduction, and motivation. Simulation provides opportunity for learners to self-regulate their behavior and learn. In these studies, simulation is considered a strategy that can promote health professional learners' self-efficacy through mastery of specific skills and learning through the experiences of others including social persuasion. Bandura's concept of self-efficacy is defined as the "belief in one's capabilities to organize and execute the courses of action required to manage prospective situations" (Lavoie et al., 2018). The concept of self-efficacy is closely related to goal setting and achievement (Chan et al., 2019). Some of the scales used to measure self-efficacy include the General Self-efficacy Scale (Chen et al., 2001) and the Trans-cultural Self-efficacy Tool (Jeffreys, 2000). According to Bandura, observing what can happen and drawing conclusions from experiences of others can also provide knowledge to the learner and influence self-efficacy (Lavoie et al., 2018; Stocker et al., 2014). Learners utilize these experiences to appraise their own abilities to deal with a variety of scenarios and develop self-efficacy, which subsequently becomes fundamental to their actions while participating in further simulation experiences or in clinical practice settings (Stocker et al., 2014).

Transformative Learning Theory

According to Mezirow's theory of transformative learning, learning is the process of using a prior interpretation to construe a new or revised interpretation of the meaning of one's experience in order to guide future action. This new or revised interpretation of the meaning of one's experience is used to guide future action (Briese et al., 2020; Kerins et al., 2020). The first phase described by Mezirow is that of a 'disorienting dilemma' in which the individual is faced with an experience that challenges his or her prior assumptions. This corresponds with a learners' experience of a simulation scenario where they are asked to perform an assessment or resuscitation. The next phases relate to self-examination (phase 2) and critical reflection (phase 3), open discussion and development of a new perspective (phase 4)

Table 2. Relationship between the phases of Mezirow's transformative learning theory and simulation education

Mezirow's transformative learning theory		Application to simulation education
Phase 1	Disorienting dilemma	Learner participates in a challenging simulation scenario
Phase 2	Self-examination	Encounter leads to self-evaluation
Phase 3	Critical reflection	Facilitated or self-debrief promotes reflection on performance
Phase 4	Open discussion and development of a new perspective	Active participation in debriefing process with facilitator and other learners leads to discussion and change in perspective
Phase 5	Exploration of new roles	Reflection and discussion lead to identification of new ideas, concepts, or lessons learned.
Phase 6	Planning a course of action	Learner considers ways to apply lessons learned in future scenarios or practice.

which prompts the exploration of new roles (phase 5) and planning a course of action (phase 6) (Briese et al., 2020; Kerins et al., 2020).

APPLICATION OF ADULT LEARNING THEORY TO SIMULATION EDUCATION

As adult learners are the focus of healthcare simulation education, it is important to consider how healthcare educators can apply the principles and strategies of adult learning theory when designing and implementing simulation education. In many nursing studies, another frequently cited theory is the instructional design framework called the Jeffries Simulation Framework. The five individual components of the Jeffries Simulation Framework are: facilitator, participant, educational practices, outcomes, and simulation design characteristics (Adamson, 2015). Unlike young learners, adult learners are not a homogeneous group of students at a particular academic level. While this heterogeneity can create some challenges, using adult learning principles, simulation instructors provide learning tasks that require learners to 'construct' their own understanding by relating new knowledge to what they already know (Murad et al., 2010; Rashid, 2017). This experience allows the learner to enter into a situation where they actually have to process the information directly in their own minds through reflection (Poore et al., 2019). This reflection promotes learning from the simulation experience and will let the learner recall it more easily. When the learner encounters a situation like the simulated one, they can apply what they learned through further experimentation. Through simulation, learners see the impact of their decisions and actions and are better able to adjust their current practices. While simulation can be conducted individually, scenarios are often designed for a group or team.

Application to Procedural Simulation

Learning to do something technically or procedurally requires structure in order to guarantee the acquisition of skills that are necessary for safe practice (Ramesh M. Nataraja et al., 2018; R. M. Nataraja et al., 2018; Rashid, 2017). For instance, when health professionals are being trained on a novel piece of equipment or process, it is important to let the learners attempt to use the equipment or the process in a simulated setting before using it in a clinical setting on an actual patient. This is because using the equipment or the process on an actual patient could result in serious injury or even death.

The beginning of educational theories that assist the acquisition of technical skills may be traced back to the 1950s, when Bloom et al. recognized the three educational domains of cognitive, emotional, and psychomotor learning (Irvine, 2017). A 7-step process of procedural learning as applied to trauma and surgical training was developed based on this work (Dave, 1970; Davis et al., 2017; Simpson, 1966). This process involved the steps of: 1) Conceptualization; 2) Visualization; 3) Verbalization; 4) Guided practice; 5) Feedback; 6) Skill mastery; and 7) Autonomy (Davis et al., 2017). These concepts can be applied to various procedural skills such as endotracheal intubation, chest tube placement and resuscitation training. Studies have shown increased self-efficacy through a combination of mastery performance and observational learning (Stocker et al., 2014). Manikin-based simulations are discussed in more detail in Chapter 3 on “Scenario Development for Manikin-based Simulation”.

Application to Team Training

Simulations for the purpose of team training can be run either in specialized centers or out in the field or in-situ. Team composition may mimic an interprofessional clinical team or learners may be placed in atypical roles. Simulation within interprofessional teams may foster organizational learning and culture change (Stocker et al., 2014). Socio-cultural learning theories suggest that in-situ team training simulation sessions improve effectiveness and efficacy of learning in preference to training in a simulation center (Stocker et al., 2014). The impact of using real teams versus improvised teams on the learning process in simulated training (Stocker et al., 2014). Interprofessional simulations with participants in the role of simulated providers enhance the fidelity of scenarios, because various provider roles do not routinely practice without interaction with other health care providers for patient care. Incorporating other professions in the simulations mirrors what learners would expect to find in the clinical environment (Greenwood & Ewell, 2018). Interprofessional simulation supports learners to provide more "patient-centered care," give "people choices," and be "a better listener to patients" (Greenwood & Ewell, 2018). Each simulated event must challenge team members by challenging their skills and even triggering failures in order to optimize efficiency of adult learning (Stocker et al., 2014). For sustained improvement of team performance or individual skills, simulation training should include regular, repeated practice sessions (Matterson et al., 2018).

Application to Virtual Simulation

Virtual simulation, one of the most prominent forms of eLearning in the field of health professional education, requires learners to draw on what they've been taught in the classroom setting and begin applying their problem-solving skills (M.-S. Bracq et al., 2019; Cerezo Espinosa et al., 2019; de Boer et al., 2019). Virtual simulation provides a safe, effective, and simple online environment to practice critical-thinking and decision-making skills (Braun et al., 2019; Harrington et al., 2018; Woodham et al., 2019). Virtual simulation allows instructors to overcome the difficulties of managing physical space and scheduling, enabling training institutions to expand the number of clinical scenarios available for student training (Umoren et al., 2014).

These software simulations present goals, which in turn generate purpose and focus, and when coupled to measurable outcomes, establish skills that are prerequisites (Bayram & Caliskan, 2019; M. S. Bracq et al., 2019). Once the target has been accomplished, the game is ended, and the learner progresses to the following stage of the instruction (Foronda et al., 2018). The goal of constructing environments in simulation games is to encourage learners to engage in conflict, competition, or collaboration. These environments can be used to engage either individual learners or groups of learners. Learners are said to be engaged in competitive behavior when they are required to focus their attention on improving their performance in order to beat their fellow students at the game by being quicker or more talented than they are. On the other hand, cooperation necessitates working together in order to accomplish what is intended or reach the objectives that have been set. The learner has to put in a lot of effort in order to keep from losing to the game system or to another player in a simulation game that uses conflict principles. A high score, accumulating points, or winning awards all provide support for the respective conflict, cooperation, and collaboration systems (Kapp, 2012). The development of scenarios for virtual simulations is the topic of discussion in Chapter 4: Scenario Development for Virtual Simulations.

APPLICATION OF ADULT LEARNING THEORY TO SIMULATION CURRICULUM DEVELOPMENT

When developing any kind of simulation course, it is critical to have a solid understanding of adult learning theory to serve as the foundation for the course's design. This tactic can be of assistance to simulation teachers in the process of planning courses in a manner that will make learning easier at each stage of the planning process: conception, development, and implementation. In order to facilitate this process, the simulation instructor needs to establish a risk-free learning environment in which students are encouraged to experiment with different strategies and gain knowledge from their experiences, and the class needs to be incorporated into a well-organized educational program (Barry Issenberg et al., 2005).

Applications of adult learning theory to designing simulation courses rely heavily on autonomy, collaboration, and self-direction (Rashid, 2017). The principle of Autonomy relies on whether the learner feels like they were viewed as capable and allowed to do what they could (Rashid, 2017). Adult learners prefer self-directed learning and simulation instructors must create training that allows them to independently problem-solve and set personal goals (Merriam, 2001; Murad et al., 2010). The ability to generate different scenarios in a simulation is also aligned with the theory of self-direction (Murad et al., 2010). Studies in adult learners indicate that there is a preference for self-directed and self-designed learning projects over group-learning experiences (Murad et al., 2010). Adult learners also prefer more than one medium for learning, and they desire to control the timing and pace of learning experiences (Knowles et al., 2005). Simulation instructors should allow learners to discover things for themselves, providing guidance and help when mistakes are made (Bowe et al., 2017; Cheng et al., 2017; Keskitalo et al., 2014). Instructors may find surveying learners to assess technical knowledge and skills prior to beginning the training course will allow them to adjust instruction accordingly and address learners with different levels of experience (Brown et al., 2012).

In practical terms, andragogy means that instruction for adults needs to focus more on the process and less on the instructional content (Merriam, 2001). While the design of in-person and eLearning simulation courses is important, the delivery is equally so. There is broad agreement regarding the applicability of the Kolb's learning cycle on the structure of a simulated training session (Kolb & Kolb, 2005). Debriefing after each simulation is needed to encourage reflection during and post-event (Rashid, 2017; Salik & Paige, 2020; Sawyer et al., 2016). As described by Kolb, the need to address specific actions performed during the simulation event that may impact patient safety drives reflective observation, conceptualization and experimental activity which leads learners to test new approaches (Kolb & Kolb, 2005). While reflection on our actions is not atypical following an event, in simulation, learners are provided with the option to share, process and learn from this reflection (Sawyer et al., 2016). The act of critical reflection which is important to both experiential and transformative learning involves questioning one's conceptual framework, then engaging in experimentation by testing, refining and retesting various solutions (Briese et al., 2020; Kolb & Kolb, 2005).

The goal of simulation learning is to teach concepts by placing learners in situations or simulations that are similar to those in which they will use the concepts they are learning in their clinical practice. Learners are engaged, motivated to take action, learning is promoted, and problems are solved through the use of game-based mechanics and aesthetics in virtual simulations (Ghoman, Patel, et al., 2020; Nasiri et al., 2019). The use of slides in traditional classroom instruction is very similar to the interactive e-learning technology. For instance, interactive learning software may include 'drag and drop' activities rather than 'multiple choice' questions, or it may incorporate videos, which research suggests may have a "somewhat positive impact" on the learning process (Cooper & Higgins, 2015). The technology generates an immersive experience, which can be constructed on a framework that evaluates the performance of the learner and offers individualized feedback.

In order to cater to the needs of the learner, the difficulty of the simulations can also be altered (Hart et al., 2018; Hayden et al., 2018). The simulation should not be very challenging nor overly simplistic. The majority of virtual simulations activities include a demonstration or practice mode, which is designed to assist new students in understanding the goals and game mechanics of the activity. When learners participate in the activity in person, it may take them some time to grow accustomed to the components of the simulation environment, such as the high-fidelity manikin. The use of hints and instructions provides novice learners with the ability to practice new abilities while receiving advice and feedback from the instructor. This could pave the way for a mode in which students are not provided with any direction. Learners with varying amounts of previous training and expertise might benefit from the utilization of a variety of various difficulty levels. Learning through virtual simulations has the significant advantage over learning in person since it may be engaged in at the learners' whim, unlike in-person learning. The learner is granted license to fail with low repercussions, which encourages autonomy and discovery-based learning. Do-overs and replays provide this opportunity. It is possible that completing the virtual simulation without experiencing any setbacks or having the opportunity to try again might be considered unsatisfying to the learner. Obtaining success after a number of failed efforts gives one a sense of having accomplished something. However, there is a balance to this approach because, if a learner is unable to recover from setbacks, they will eventually give up, and will not come back. Because of this, instructional designers for virtual simulations frequently employ the scaffolding method, which begins with more direction and gradually provides less guidance as the learner becomes more independent in finding solutions to issues (Kapp, 2012; Zigmont et al., 2011).

SIMULATION ASSESSMENT EVALUATION AND FEEDBACK

Assessment of learners, facilitators and the educational experience should be conducted as part of any simulation program. Assessment processes have evolved over time and now include a variety of technical and non-technical competency assessments including communication, critical thinking, teamwork and collaboration, clinical judgment, caring, safety, and patient centered care (Rashid, 2017). Other outcomes include learner perception and satisfaction, knowledge, procedural skills and attitudes, self-confidence and self-efficacy, simulation performance, learning transfer into clinical settings, learner stress and anxiety and other measures such as grades and written examination performance (Alfred et al., 2019; Ghoman, Cutumisu, et al., 2020; Meerkov et al., 2019; Wooding et al., 2020). Learner assessment is expected for a teaching program and regular, longitudinal assessments are generally recommended to demonstrate impact on learning and knowledge transfer to clinical settings to have an impact on patient safety. Validated tools for evaluation of simulation performance are covered in more detail in Chapter 6.

Theories that support competency-based education in simulation are oriented to the attainment of learning outcomes. A multi-pronged approach is utilized to determine whether learning outcomes have been achieved and to provide feedback on competency (Lavoie et al., 2018). In simulation, competencies are typically characterized as task-specific behaviors demonstrated during the simulation scenario, often in the context of milestones indicating a progression of expertise from novice to expert performance. There is broad agreement regarding the necessity of debriefing and guided reflection after the simulated experience (Salik & Paige, 2020). To facilitate this process, one of the key requirements for manikin-based simulation is for the simulation facilitator to be present and available, to give advice, if required, and ensure that the learning objectives are accomplished (Rashid, 2017). It is important for the simulation facilitator to provide positive feedback as well as to facilitate reflection on aspects of the simulation that did not go as well as planned (Rashid, 2017).

To achieve this goal, facilitators of simulations place a strong emphasis on the use of open-ended questions, which are designed to spark conversation and encourage participants to share information and experience that is pertinent to the topic at hand (Barry Issenberg et al., 2005). The learner will be more inclined to accept and implement the learning when they are given the opportunity to investigate their own feelings and come to the realization on their own that their acts, the ramifications of those actions, and the need to modify this behavior in the course of future occurrences. It's possible that there won't be a real-life teacher present if you're using a virtual simulation. On the other hand, the simulation is frequently developed with the intention of delivering either instant informational feedback or delayed input, as well as consequences dependent on the learner's performance (Kapp, 2012). Although being at the top of the score leaderboard is one form of feedback, feedback also occurs throughout the simulation game as a result of the detection and representation of activity. This activity includes the location of the player, the amount of time that is still available, how well other players are doing, and so on (Kapp, 2012). Both the informative feedback and the consequences are connected to the educational goals, and they are intended to elicit the appropriate behavior or actions (Koivisto et al., 2018). Both in-person and online simulations highlight relationships and "cause and effect" to cut down on the amount of time needed to understand new ideas, even when dealing with complicated systems. In either scenario, time compression and other techniques that simulate the faster passage of time can be utilized to demonstrate the results of activities in a more expedient manner (Kapp, 2012).

The involvement of the learner in each stage of the learning process is ensured by the incorporation of learning objectives and self-evaluation plans into the instructional materials. The confirmation that the learning goals have been accomplished is the responsibility of the teacher, and the learner relies on the instructor for performance-based feedback. On the other hand, the teacher is reliant on the learner for feedback regarding the course material as well as the instructor's facilitation of the simulation scenario and debriefing of the exercise (Barry Issenberg et al., 2005). It is essential to put in place consistent feedback mechanisms that allow students to communicate with their instructors about the aspects of their education that work best for them, as well as what they want and need to learn. The input ought to be incorporated into the design of, as well as the ongoing updating of, the simulation courses.

SOLUTIONS AND RECOMMENDATIONS

Simulation-based education is premised on adult learning theory. Simulation in health professions education has been used in both pre-service and in-service education of healthcare professionals. The application of adult learning theory has been described in procedural training, team training and virtual simulation. It is important for simulation facilitators to be familiar with the theoretical basis of simulation as this knowledge will inform their development and implementation of simulation curricula. Simulation curricula should be focused on learning objectives and enable learners to gain new skills from experiences that they can relate to, and that are useful for their practice.

Learners should be given the opportunity for structured self-reflection during debriefing as this is a key element of both experiential and transformative learning. Many strategies to encourage self-reflection have been described and include debriefing techniques that feature open-ended questions in a safe environment. Simulation assessment should utilize a multi-faceted approach with validated tools for evaluation and feedback. The continuum of scenario development, assessment and session feedback should involve learners who can provide valuable input and inform the iterative development of simulation curricula.

One of the most important requirements for a simulation session is that the simulation facilitator must be always present and available in order to ensure that the learning objectives are met. However, in cases where the simulation facilitator is unavailable, automated manikin-based or computer-based feedback and guided reflection may be a way to increase accessibility of simulation education. Finding new ways to provide learners with objective, yet constructive criticism and encourage in-depth consideration of any areas of the exercise that did not go according to plan are opportunities for future applications of adult learning theory to simulation education.

FUTURE RESEARCH DIRECTIONS

The relationship between the adult learning theory and simulation design and implementation is an area of ongoing research. In particular, understanding the relationship of game-based learning theory to healthcare virtual simulations will enable the development of compelling, interactive learning experiences that will enable instructors and students to meet their learning goals. While, the objective assessment of surgical technical and non-technical skills continues to challenge instructors, the development of validated tools in this area continues to expand and is an area for future research. Validated tools enable instructors to teach key skills progressively and provide feedback to learners when they have achieved pre-specified milestones or competencies.

Since the advent of virtual simulations and games based on simulation, the technology used to create these simulations have evolved significantly. As a result of this technological advancement, virtual and augmented reality simulation software and hardware have become more widely available and accessible to students at all educational levels. Concerns about the poor recall and application of traditional learning techniques like lectures and films have recently raised focus to more active methods. The applications of these methods which include various kinds of virtual simulations including virtual reality, mixed reality, augmented reality, screen-based simulations, and haptic-enabled simulations such as laparoscopic simulations continue to be an active area of research. As learners who have been engaged in primary and secondary education using gamified collaborative and learning strategies advance into the higher education curriculum, avatars, role play games, point systems, badges, and leaderboards and other forms of gamification may play an increasing role. These gamification techniques may have varying utility and educational efficacy depending on the learning objectives. As such, simulation educators must ensure that their approaches to curriculum development remain grounded in adult learning theory.

CONCLUSION

The realization that preventable medical mistakes are responsible for a significant number of deaths annually in the United States has been one of the primary forces propelling the expansion of simulation education. Clinical simulations have the potential to cut down on medical errors by making personnel more familiar with both typical and unique high-risk circumstances that call for specialized expertise and communication between members of the team. Adult learners' preferences for self-directed and self-designed learning projects over group learning experiences have been documented in several studies. Adults prefer to learn in a variety of ways, and they want to be in charge of the schedule and speed of their education. Students should be allowed to discover things on their own, but instructors should be on hand to help them if mistakes are made. There are many learning theories that apply to simulation-based education. This chapter highlighted prominent adult learning theories such as andragogy, Kolb's experiential learning theory, Bandura's concept of self-efficacy, and Mezirow's theory of transformative learning. However, there are many other potentially applicable theories and instructors designing and developing simulation curricula often utilize several principles in their design. Game-based learning provides the theoretical basis for many virtual simulation games. While instructors many be less familiar with these principles, they are essential to creating activities that are not just entertaining but educational for learners at various levels of experience and exposure to game-based learning. In conclusion, increased exposure to these concepts and their application to practice will help to make simulation-based learning more effective for pre-service and in-service health professionals.

REFERENCES

Adamson, K. (2015). A systematic review of the literature related to the NLN/Jeffries simulation framework. *Nursing Education Perspectives*, *36*(5), 281–291. doi:10.5480/15-1655 PMID:26521495

Aebersold, M. (2016). The history of simulation and its impact on the future. *AACN Advanced Critical Care*, *27*(1), 56–61. doi:10.4037/aacnacc2016436 PMID:26909454

Alfred, M. C., Neyens, D. M., & Gramopadhye, A. K. (2019). Learning in simulated environments: An assessment of 4-week retention outcomes. *Applied Ergonomics*, *74*, 107–117. doi:10.1016/j.apergo.2018.08.002 PMID:30487089

Banaszek, D., You, D., Chang, J., Pickell, M., Hesse, D., Hopman, W. M., Borschneck, D., & Bardana, D. (2017). Virtual Reality Compared with Bench-Top Simulation in the Acquisition of Arthroscopic Skill: A Randomized Controlled Trial. *The Journal of Bone and Joint Surgery. American Volume*, *99*(7), e34–e34. doi:10.2106/JBJS.16.00324 PMID:28375898

Barry Issenberg, S., Mcgaghie, W. C., Petrusa, E. R., Lee Gordon, D., & Scalese, R. J. (2005). Features and uses of high-fidelity medical simulations that lead to effective learning: A BEME systematic review. *Medical Teacher*, *27*(1), 10–28. doi:10.1080/01421590500046924 PMID:16147767

Bayram, S. B., & Caliskan, N. (2019). Effect of a game-based virtual reality phone application on tracheostomy care education for nursing students: A randomized controlled trial. *Nurse Education Today*, *79*, 25–31. doi:10.1016/j.nedt.2019.05.010 PMID:31102793

Berman, A. H., Biguet, G., Stathakarou, N., Westin-Hägglöf, B., Jeding, K., McGrath, C., Zary, N., & Kononowicz, A. A. (2017). Virtual Patients in a Behavioral Medicine Massive Open Online Course (MOOC): A Qualitative and Quantitative Analysis of Participants' Perceptions. *Academic Psychiatry: The Journal of the American Association of Directors of Psychiatric Residency Training and the Association for Academic Psychiatry, 41*(5), 631-641. doi:10.1007/s40596-017-0706-4

Bernardo, A. (2017). Virtual Reality and Simulation in Neurosurgical Training. *World Neurosurgery*, *106*, 1015–1029. doi:10.1016/j.wneu.2017.06.140 PMID:28985656

Bierer, J., Memu, E., Leeper, W. R., Fortin, D., Fréchette, E., Inculet, R., & Malthaner, R. (2018). Development of an In Situ Thoracic Surgery Crisis Simulation Focused on Nontechnical Skill Training. *The Annals of Thoracic Surgery*, *106*(1), 287–292. doi:10.1016/j.athoracsur.2018.01.058 PMID:29499178

Bowe, S. N., Johnson, K., & Puscas, L. (2017). Facilitation and Debriefing in Simulation Education. *Otolaryngologic Clinics of North America, 50*(5), 989–1001. doi:10.1016/j.otc.2017.05.009 PMID:28822579

Bracq, M.-S., Michinov, E., & Jannin, P. (2019). Virtual Reality Simulation in Nontechnical Skills Training for Healthcare Professionals: A Systematic Review. *Simulation in Healthcare: Journal of the Society for Simulation in Healthcare, 14*(3), 188-194. doi:10.1097/SIH.0000000000000347

Bracq, M. S., Michinov, E., & Jannin, P. (2019). Virtual Reality Simulation in Nontechnical Skills Training for Healthcare Professionals: A Systematic Review. *Simulation in Healthcare: Journal of the Society for Simulation in Healthcare, 14*(3), 188-194. doi:10.1097/SIH.0000000000000347

Braun, L. T., Borrmann, K. F., Lottspeich, C., Heinrich, D. A., Kiesewetter, J., Fischer, M. R., & Schmidmaier, R. (2019). Scaffolding clinical reasoning of medical students with virtual patients: Effects on diagnostic accuracy, efficiency, and errors. *Diagnosis (Berlin, Germany), 6*(2), 137–149. doi:10.1515/dx-2018-0090 PMID:30772868

Briese, P., Evanson, T., & Hanson, D. (2020). Application of Mezirow's Transformative Learning Theory to Simulation in Healthcare Education. *Clinical Simulation in Nursing, 48*, 64–67. doi:10.1016/j.ecns.2020.08.006

Brown, R., Rasmussen, R., Baldwin, I., & Wyeth, P. (2012). Design and implementation of a virtual world training simulation of ICU first hour handover processes. *Australian Critical Care: Official Journal of the Confederation of Australian Critical Care Nurses, 25*(3), 178-187. doi:10.1016/j.aucc.2012.02.005

Cerezo Espinosa, C., Segura Melgarejo, F., Melendreras Ruiz, R., García-Collado, Á. J., Nieto Caballero, S., Juguera Rodríguez, L., Pardo Ríos, S., García Torrano, S., Linares Stutz, E., & Pardo Ríos, M. (2019). Virtual reality in cardiopulmonary resuscitation training: a randomized trial [La realidad virtual como método de enseñanza de la reanimación cardiopulmonar: un estudio aleatorizado]. *Emergencias: Revista de la Sociedad Espanola de Medicina de Emergencias, 31*(1), 43-46. https://pubmed.ncbi.nlm.nih.gov/30656873

Chan, R., Booth, R., Strudwick, G., & Sinclair, B. (2019). Nursing Students' Perceived Self-Efficacy and the Generation of Medication Errors with the Use of an Electronic Medication Administration Record (eMAR) in Clinical Simulation. *International Journal of Nursing Education Scholarship, 16*(1). doi:10.1515/ijnes-2019-0014

Chen, G., Gully, S. M., & Eden, D. (2001). Validation of a new general self-efficacy scale. *Organizational Research Methods*, *4*(1), 62–83. doi:10.1177/109442810141004

Chen, X., & Hu, J. (2018). A review of haptic simulator for oral and maxillofacial surgery based on virtual reality. *Expert Review of Medical Devices*, *15*(6), 435–444. doi:10.1080/17434440.2018.1484727 PMID:29865882

Cheng, A., Grant, V., Huffman, J., Burgess, G., Szyld, D., Robinson, T., & Eppich, W. (2017). Coaching the Debriefer: Peer Coaching to Improve Debriefing Quality in Simulation Programs. *Simulation in Healthcare: Journal of the Society for Simulation in Healthcare, 12*(5), 319-325. doi:10.1097/SIH.0000000000000232

Coburn, C. V., Gilland, D., & Stahl, K. (2020). High-Fidelity Simulation in an Undergraduate Ambulatory Care Nursing Course. *Nursing Education Perspectives*, *41*(1), 54–56. doi:10.1097/01.NEP.0000000000000427 PMID:31860491

Cook, D. A., Hatala, R., Brydges, R., Zendejas, B., Szostek, J. H., Wang, A. T., Erwin, P. J., & Hamstra, S. J. (2011). Technology-enhanced simulation for health professions education: A systematic review and meta-analysis. *Journal of the American Medical Association*, *306*(9), 978–988. doi:10.1001/jama.2011.1234 PMID:21900138

Cooper, D., & Higgins, S. (2015). The effectiveness of online instructional videos in the acquisition and demonstration of cognitive, affective and psychomotor rehabilitation skills. *British Journal of Educational Technology*, *46*(4), 768–779. doi:10.1111/bjet.12166

Dave, R. H. (1970). Psychomotor levels. *Developing and Writing Educational Objectives*, 33-34.

Davis, A. J., Fierro, L., Guptill, M., Kiemeney, M., Brown, L., Smith, D. D., & Young, T. P. (2017). Practical Application of Educational Theory for Learning Technical Skills in Emergency Medicine. *Annals of Emergency Medicine*, *70*(3), 402–405. doi:10.1016/j.annemergmed.2017.04.026 PMID:28601275 de Boer, I. R., Lagerweij, M. D., Wesselink, P. R., & Vervoorn, J. M. (2019). The Effect of Variations in Force Feedback in a Virtual Reality Environment on the Performance and Satisfaction of Dental Students. *Simulation in Healthcare: Journal of the Society for Simulation in Healthcare, 14*(3), 169-174. doi:10.1097/SIH.0000000000000370

Deering, S., Rosen, M. A., Ludi, V., Munroe, M., Pocrnich, A., Laky, C., & Napolitano, P. G. (2011). On the front lines of patient safety: Implementation and evaluation of team training in Iraq. *Joint Commission Journal on Quality and Patient Safety*, *37*(8), 350–356. doi:10.1016/S1553-7250(11)37045-6 PMID:21874970

Dunn, R., Griggs, S. A., Olson, J., Beasley, M., & Gorman, B. S. (1995). A meta-analytic validation of the Dunn and Dunn model of learning-style preferences. *The Journal of Educational Research*, *88*(6), 353–362. doi:10.1080/00220671.1995.9941181

Ericsson, K. A. (2004). Deliberate practice and the acquisition and maintenance of expert performance in medicine and related domains. *Academic Medicine*, *79*(10, Suppl), S70–S81. doi:10.1097/00001888-200410001-00022 PMID:15383395

Everett, T. C., MacKinnon, R., de Beer, D., Taylor, M., & Bould, M. D. (2017). Ten years of simulation-based training in pediatric anesthesia: The inception, evolution, and dissemination of the Managing Emergencies in Pediatric Anesthesia (MEPA) course. *Paediatric Anaesthesia*, *27*(10), 984–990. doi:10.1111/pan.13224 PMID:28815823

Fewster-Thuente, L., & Batteson, T. (2016). Teaching Collaboration Competencies to Healthcare Provider Students Through Simulation. *Journal of Allied Health*, *45*(2), 147–151. https://pubmed.ncbi.nlm.nih.gov/27262473 PMID:27262473

Foronda, C., Fernandez-Burgos, M., Nadeau, C., Kelley, C., & Henry, M. (2020). Virtual Simulation in Nursing Education: A Systematic Review Spanning 1996 to 2018. *Simulation in Healthcare: The Journal of the Society for Simulation in Healthcare*, *15*(1), 46–54. doi:10.1097/SIH.0000000000000411 PMID:32028447

Foronda, C. L., Swoboda, S. M., Henry, M. N., Kamau, E., Sullivan, N., & Hudson, K. W. (2018). Student preferences and perceptions of learning from vSIM for Nursing™. *Nurse Education in Practice*, *33*, 27–32. doi:10.1016/j.nepr.2018.08.003 PMID:30223110

Ghoman, S. K., Cutumisu, M., & Schmölzer, G. M. (2020). Simulation-Based Summative Assessment of Neonatal Resuscitation Providers Using the RETAIN Serious Board Game—A Pilot Study. *Frontiers in Pediatrics*, *8*, 14. doi:10.3389/fped.2020.00014 PMID:32083041

Ghoman, S. K., Patel, S. D., Cutumisu, M., von Hauff, P., Jeffery, T., Brown, M. R., & Schmölzer, G. M. (2020). Serious games, a game changer in teaching neonatal resuscitation? A review. *Archives of Disease in Childhood. Fetal and Neonatal Edition*, *105*(1), 98–107. doi:10.1136/archdischild-2019-317011 PMID:31256010

Glenn, A. D., & Claman, F. (2020). Using a Low-Fidelity Simulation to Enhance Cultural Awareness and Emotional Intelligence in Nursing Students. *Nursing Education Perspectives*, *41*(1), 63–64. doi:10.1097/01.NEP.0000000000000425 PMID:31860495

Gray, M. M., Thomas, A. A., Burns, B., & Umoren, R. A. (2020). Evacuation of vulnerable and critical patients: Multimodal simulation for nurse-led patient evacuation. *Simulation in Healthcare*, *15*(6), 382–387. doi:10.1097/SIH.0000000000000451 PMID:32371747

Greenwood, K. C., & Ewell, S. B. (2018). Faculty development through simulation-based education in physical therapist education. *Advances in Simulation (London, England)*, *3*(1), 1–12. doi:10.118641077-017-0060-3 PMID:29450027

Grossman, S., & Conelius, J. (2015). Simulation Pedagogy With Nurse Practitioner Students: Impact of Receiving Immediate Individualized Faculty Feedback. *Creative Nursing*, *21*(2), 100–109. doi:10.1891/1078-4535.21.2.100 PMID:26094373

Guedes, H. G., Câmara Costa Ferreira, Z. M., Ribeiro de Sousa Leão, L., Souza Montero, E. F., Otoch, J. P., & Artifon, E. L. A. (2019). Virtual reality simulator versus box-trainer to teach minimally invasive procedures: A meta-analysis. *International journal of surgery (London, England)*, *61*, 60–68. doi:10.1016/j.ijsu.2018.12.001 PMID:30529216

Harrington, C. M., Kavanagh, D. O., Quinlan, J. F., Ryan, D., Dicker, P., O'Keeffe, D., Traynor, O., & Tierney, S. (2018). Development and evaluation of a trauma decision-making simulator in Oculus virtual reality. *American Journal of Surgery, 215*(1), 42–47. doi:10.1016/j.amjsurg.2017.02.011 PMID:28262203

Hart, D., Bond, W., Siegelman, J. N., Miller, D., Cassara, M., Barker, L., Anders, S., Ahn, J., Huang, H., Strother, C., & Hui, J. (2018). Simulation for Assessment of Milestones in Emergency Medicine Residents. *Academic Emergency Medicine: Official Journal of the Society for Academic Emergency Medicine, 25*(2), 205-220. doi:10.1111/acem.13296

Harvey, E. M., Wright, A., Taylor, D., Bath, J., & Collier, B. (2013). TeamSTEPPS(®) simulation-based training: An evidence-based strategy to improve trauma team performance. *Journal of Continuing Education in Nursing, 44*(11), 484–485. doi:10.3928/00220124-20131025-92 PMID:24199639

Haubruck, P., Nickel, F., Ober, J., Walker, T., Bergdolt, C., Friedrich, M., Müller-Stich, B. P., Forchheim, F., Fischer, C., Schmidmaier, G., & Tanner, M. C. (2018). Evaluation of App-Based Serious Gaming as a Training Method in Teaching Chest Tube Insertion to Medical Students: Randomized Controlled Trial. *Journal of Medical Internet Research, 20*(5), e195–e195. doi:10.2196/jmir.9956 PMID:29784634

Haugland, V. L., & Reime, M. H. (2018). Scenario-based simulation training as a method to increase nursing students' competence in demanding situations in dementia care. A mixed method study. *Nurse Education in Practice, 33*, 164–171. doi:10.1016/j.nepr.2018.08.008 PMID:30224221

Hayden, E. M., Wong, A. H., Ackerman, J., Sande, M. K., Lei, C., Kobayashi, L., Cassara, M., Cooper, D. D., Perry, K., Lewandowski, W. E., & Scerbo, M. W. (2018). Human Factors and Simulation in Emergency Medicine. *Academic Emergency Medicine: Official Journal of the Society for Academic Emergency Medicine, 25*(2), 221-229. doi:10.1111/acem.13315

Hege, I., Kononowicz, A. A., Berman, N. B., Lenzer, B., & Kiesewetter, J. (2018). Advancing clinical reasoning in virtual patients - development and application of a conceptual framework. *GMS Journal for Medical Education, 35*(1), Doc12–Doc12. doi:10.3205/zma001159 PMID:29497697

Honey, P. (2001). *Honey and Mumford learning styles questionnaire*. Peter Honey Learning.

Irvine, J. (2017). A Comparison of Revised Bloom and Marzano's New Taxonomy of Learning. *Research in Higher Education*, 33.

Issenberg, S. B., & Scalese, R. J. (2008). Simulation in health care education. *Perspectives in Biology and Medicine*, *51*(1), 31–46. doi:10.1353/pbm.2008.0004 PMID:18192764

Jeffers, J. M., & Poling, S. (2019). The development and implementation of a 12-month simulation-based learning curriculum for pediatric emergency medicine fellows utilizing debriefing with good judgment and rapid cycle deliberate practice. *BMC Medical Education*, *19*(1), 22–22. doi:10.118612909-018-1417-6 PMID:30646903

Jeffreys, M. R. (2000). Development and psychometric evaluation of the transcultural self-efficacy tool: A synthesis of findings. *Journal of Transcultural Nursing*, *11*(2), 127–136. doi:10.1177/104365960001100207 PMID:11982045

Kaakinen, J., & Arwood, E. (2009). Systematic review of nursing simulation literature for use of learning theory. *International Journal of Nursing Education Scholarship*, *6*(1). Advance online publication. doi:10.2202/1548-923X.1688 PMID:19492985

Kapp, K. M. (2012). *The gamification of learning and instruction: Game-based methods and strategies for training and education*. John Wiley & Sons.

Kerins, J., Smith, S. E., Phillips, E. C., Clarke, B., Hamilton, A. L., & Tallentire, V. R. (2020). Exploring transformative learning when developing medical students' non-technical skills. *Medical Education*, *54*(3), 264–274. doi:10.1111/medu.14062 PMID:31954079

Keskitalo, T., Ruokamo, H., & Gaba, D. (2014). Towards meaningful simulation-based learning with medical students and junior physicians. *Medical Teacher*, *36*(3), 230–239. doi:10.3109/0142159X.2013.853116 PMID:24261916

Knowles, M. S., Holton, E., & Swanson, R. (2005). *The adult learner: the definitive classic in adult education and human resource development (6th ed.)*. Elsevier. doi:10.4324/9780080481913

Koivisto, J. M., Haavisto, E., Niemi, H., Haho, P., Nylund, S., & Multisilta, J. (2018). Design principles for simulation games for learning clinical reasoning: A design-based research approach. *Nurse Education Today*, *60*, 114–120. doi:10.1016/j.nedt.2017.10.002 PMID:29096383

Kolb, A. Y., & Kolb, D. A. (2005). Learning styles and learning spaces: Enhancing experiential learning in higher education. *Academy of Management Learning & Education*, *4*(2), 193–212. doi:10.5465/amle.2005.17268566

Kowalewski, K.-F., Hendrie, J. D., Schmidt, M. W., Proctor, T., Paul, S., Garrow, C. R., Kenngott, H. G., Müller-Stich, B. P., & Nickel, F. (2017). Validation of the mobile serious game application Touch Surgery™ for cognitive training and assessment of laparoscopic cholecystectomy. *Surgical Endoscopy*, *31*(10), 4058–4066. doi:10.100700464-017-5452-x PMID:28281111

Lavoie, P., Michaud, C., Belisle, M., Boyer, L., Gosselin, E., Grondin, M., Larue, C., Lavoie, S., & Pepin, J. (2018). Learning theories and tools for the assessment of core nursing competencies in simulation: A theoretical review. *Journal of Advanced Nursing*, *74*(2), 239–250. doi:10.1111/jan.13416 PMID:28815750

Malone, T. W. (1981). *What makes things fun to learn? A study of intrinsically motivating computer games*. Academic Press.

Manolis, C., Burns, D. J., Assudani, R., & Chinta, R. (2013). Assessing experiential learning styles: A methodological reconstruction and validation of the Kolb Learning Style Inventory. *Learning and Individual Differences*, *23*, 44–52. doi:10.1016/j.lindif.2012.10.009

Matterson, H. H., Szyld, D., Green, B. R., Howell, H. B., Pusic, M. V., Mally, P. V., & Bailey, S. M. (2018). Neonatal resuscitation experience curves: Simulation based mastery learning booster sessions and skill decay patterns among pediatric residents. *Journal of Perinatal Medicine*, *46*(8), 934–941. doi:10.1515/jpm-2017-0330 PMID:29451862

McArdle, J., Sorensen, A., Fowler, C. I., Sommerness, S., Burson, K., & Kahwati, L. (2018). Strategies to Improve Management of Shoulder Dystocia Under the AHRQ Safety Program for Perinatal Care. *Journal of Obstetric, Gynecologic, and Neonatal Nursing*, *47*(2), 191–201. doi:10.1016/j.jogn.2017.11.014 PMID:29304317

Meerkov, M. S., Fischer, J. B., & Saba, T. G. (2019). A simulation procedure curriculum to increase pediatric resident exposure to procedures rarely performed in clinical practice. *Medical Education Online*, *24*(1), 1611305–1611305. doi:10.1080/10872981.2019.1611305 PMID:31056011

Merriam, S. B. (2001). Andragogy and self-directed learning: Pillars of adult learning theory. *New Directions for Adult and Continuing Education*, *2001*(89), 3. doi:10.1002/ace.3

Mossenson, A. I., Tuyishime, E., Rawson, D., Mukwesi, C., Whynot, S., Mackinnon, S. P., & Livingston, P. (2020). Promoting anaesthetisia providers' non-technical skills through the Vital Anaesthesia Simulation Training (VAST) course in a low-resource setting. *British Journal of Anaesthesia*, *124*(2), 206–213. doi:10.1016/j.bja.2019.10.022 PMID:31839255

Motycka, C., Egelund, E. F., Gannon, J., Genuardi, F., Gautam, S., Stittsworth, S., Young, A., & Simon, L. (2018). Using interprofessional medication management simulations to impact student attitudes toward teamwork to prevent medication errors. *Currents in Pharmacy Teaching & Learning*, *10*(7), 982–989. doi:10.1016/j.cptl.2018.04.010 PMID:30236437

Motz, P., Gray, M., Sawyer, T., Kett, J., Danforth, D., Maicher, K., & Umoren, R. (2018). Virtual Antenatal Encounter and Standardized Simulation Assessment (VANESSA): Pilot Study. *JMIR Serious Games*, *6*(2), e8. doi:10.2196/games.9611 PMID:29752249

Murad, M. H., Coto-Yglesias, F., Varkey, P., Prokop, L. J., & Murad, A. L. (2010). The effectiveness of self-directed learning in health professions education: A systematic review. *Medical Education*, *44*(11), 1057–1068. doi:10.1111/j.1365-2923.2010.03750.x PMID:20946476

Nasiri, M., Amirmohseni, L., Mofidi, A., Pires Padilha Paim, C., Bigdeli Shamloo, M. B., & Asadi, M. (2019). Educational games developed for students in perioperative nursing: A systematic review and appraisal of the evidence. *Nurse Education in Practice*, *37*, 88–96. doi:10.1016/j.nepr.2019.05.002 PMID:31129530

Nataraja, R. M., Webb, N., & Lopez, P.-J. (2018). Simulation in paediatric urology and surgery. Part 1: An overview of educational theory. *Journal of Pediatric Urology*, *14*(2), 120–124. doi:10.1016/j.jpurol.2017.12.021 PMID:29567014

Nataraja, R. M., Webb, N., & Lopez, P. J. (2018). Simulation in paediatric urology and surgery, part 2: An overview of simulation modalities and their applications. *Journal of Pediatric Urology*, *14*(2), 125–131. doi:10.1016/j.jpurol.2017.12.009 PMID:29456118

Offiah, G., Ekpotu, L. P., Murphy, S., Kane, D., Gordon, A., O'Sullivan, M., Sharifuddin, S. F., Hill, A. D. K., & Condron, C. M. (2019). Evaluation of medical student retention of clinical skills following simulation training. *BMC Medical Education*, *19*(1), 263–263. doi:10.118612909-019-1663-2 PMID:31311546

Park, C., Grant, J., Dumas, R. P., Dultz, L., Shoultz, T. H., Scott, D. J., Luk, S., Abdelfattah, K. R., & Cripps, M. W. (2020). Does simulation work? Monthly trauma simulation and procedural training are associated with decreased time to intervention. *The Journal of Trauma and Acute Care Surgery*, *88*(2), 242–248. doi:10.1097/TA.0000000000002561 PMID:31804411

Poore, J. A., Dawson, J. C., Dunbar, D.-M., & Parrish, K. (2019). Debriefing Interprofessionally: A Tool for Recognition and Reflection. *Nurse Educator*, *44*(1), 25–28. doi:10.1097/NNE.0000000000000518 PMID:29538051

Prakash, R., Sharma, N., & Advani, U. (2019). Learning process and how adults learn. *International Journal of Academic Medicine*, *5*(1), 75. doi:10.4103/IJAM.IJAM_41_18

Rashid, P. (2017). Surgical education and adult learning: Integrating theory into practice. *F1000 Research*, *6*, 6. doi:10.12688/f1000research.10870.1 PMID:28357046

Riley, W., Davis, S., Miller, K., Hansen, H., Sainfort, F., & Sweet, R. (2011). Didactic and simulation nontechnical skills team training to improve perinatal patient outcomes in a community hospital. *Joint Commission Journal on Quality and Patient Safety*, *37*(8), 357–364. doi:10.1016/S1553-7250(11)37046-8 PMID:21874971

Rowse, P. G., & Dearani, J. A. (2019). Deliberate Practice and the Emerging Roles of Simulation in Thoracic Surgery. *Thoracic Surgery Clinics*, *29*(3), 303–309. doi:10.1016/j.thorsurg.2019.03.007 PMID:31235299

Salik, I., & Paige, J. T. (2020). Debriefing the Interprofessional Team in Medical Simulation. In *StatPearls*. StatPearls Publishing. https://pubmed.ncbi.nlm.nih.gov/32119413 https://www.ncbi.nlm.nih.gov/books/NBK554526/

Sawyer, T., Eppich, W., Brett-Fleegler, M., Grant, V., & Cheng, A. (2016). More Than One Way to Debrief: A Critical Review of Healthcare Simulation Debriefing Methods. *Simulation in Healthcare: Journal of the SOCIETY for Simulation in Healthcare, 11*(3), 209-217. doi:10.1097/SIH.0000000000000148

Shinnick, M. A., & Woo, M. A. (2015). Learning style impact on knowledge gains in human patient simulation. *Nurse Education Today*, *35*(1), 63–67. doi:10.1016/j.nedt.2014.05.013 PMID:24931652

Simpson, E. (1966). *The classification of educational objectives, psychomotor domain*. US Department of Education.

Stocker, M., Burmester, M., & Allen, M. (2014). Optimisation of simulated team training through the application of learning theories: A debate for a conceptual framework. *BMC Medical Education*, *14*(1), 1–9. doi:10.1186/1472-6920-14-69 PMID:24694243

Stout-Aguilar, J., Pittman, A., Bentley, R., Livingston, J., & Watzak, B. (2018). The Effects of Interprofessional Pediatric End-of-Life Simulation on Communication and Role Understanding in Health Professions Students. *Nursing Education Perspectives*, *39*(6), 360–362. doi:10.1097/01.NEP.0000000000000316 PMID:29677043

Sweigart, L. I., Umoren, R. A., Scott, P. J., Carlton, K. H., Jones, J. A., Truman, B., & Gossett, E. J. (2016). Virtual TeamSTEPPS(®) Simulations Produce Teamwork Attitude Changes Among Health Professions Students. *The Journal of Nursing Education*, *55*(1), 31–35. doi:10.3928/01484834-20151214-08 PMID:26812380

Umoren, R., Stadler, D. J., Gasior, S. L., Al-Sheikhly, D., Truman, B., & Lowe, C. (2014). Global collaboration and team-building through 3D virtual environments. *Innovations in Global Medical and Health Education*, 1.

Umoren, R. A. E. F., Ezeaka, C., Ezenwa, B., Fajolu, I., Nafula, M., Makokha, F., Hippe, D., Feltner, J., Patel, S., McGee, A., Asangansi, I., Purkayastha, S., & Bucher, S. (2020, October 2). eHBB: A randomized controlled trial of virtual reality for newborn resuscitation refresher training of healthcare workers in Nigeria and Kenya. *American Academy of Pediatrics National Conference and Exhibition.*

Umoren, R. A., Poore, J. A., Sweigart, L., Rybas, N., Gossett, E., Johnson, M., Allen, M., Scott, P. J., Truman, B., & Das, R. (2017). TeamSTEPPS Virtual Teams: Interactive Virtual Team Training and Practice for Health Professional Learners. *Creative Nursing*, *23*(3), 184–191. doi:10.1891/1078-4535.23.3.184 PMID:28789739

Woodham, L. A., Round, J., Stenfors, T., Bujacz, A., Karlgren, K., Jivram, T., Riklefs, V., Poulton, E., & Poulton, T. (2019). Virtual patients designed for training against medical error: Exploring the impact of decision-making on learner motivation. *PLoS One*, *14*(4), e0215597–e0215597. doi:10.1371/journal.pone.0215597 PMID:31013295

Wooding, E. L., Gale, T., & Maynard, V. (2020). Evaluation of teamwork assessment tools for interprofessional simulation: A systematic literature review. *Journal of Interprofessional Care*, *34*(2), 162–172. doi:10.1080/13561820.2019.1650730 PMID:31552752

Zhang, H., Mörelius, E., Goh, S. H. L., & Wang, W. (2019). Effectiveness of Video-Assisted Debriefing in Simulation-Based Health Professions Education: A Systematic Review of Quantitative Evidence. *Nurse Educator*, *44*(3), E1–E6. doi:10.1097/NNE.0000000000000562 PMID:30015683

Zigmont, J. J., Kappus, L. J., & Sudikoff, S. N. (2011). Theoretical foundations of learning through simulation. *Seminars in Perinatology*, *35*(2), 47–51. doi:10.1053/j.semperi.2011.01.002 PMID:21440810

KEY TERMS AND DEFINITIONS

Augmented Reality: Computer generated holographic images can be viewed by the learner in the physical environment using a mobile device or specially designed headset.

High-Fidelity Manikin: This term refers to a technology-enabled manikin with features such as mechanical respiration and heart rate.

Low-Fidelity Manikin: This is typically a low cost, low technology manikin with minimal features.

Objective Structured Clinical Examination (OSCE): An approach to assessment that involves defined objectives and anticipated actions, often with an accompanying checklist for assessment.

Simulation Debriefer: A simulation instructor who leads the learners through a reflective analysis of simulation events.

Simulation Facilitator: A simulation instructor who guides the learners through the scenario with the goal of meeting learning objectives.

Simulation Technician/Specialist: An individual who supports the practice of simulation through setting up and managing simulation manikins and supplies.

Teledebriefing: Teledebriefing describes a process in which learners who are participating in a simulation scenario undergo debriefing with a facilitator located at an off-site location.

Telefacilitation: The conduct of a telesimulation by a remote facilitator.

Telesimulation: Telesimulation is a process by which telecommunication and simulation resources are utilized to provide education, training, and/or assessment to learners at an off-site location.

Video-Assisted Debriefing: The practice of using video captured during simulation sessions for reflective discussions on learner and team performance.

Virtual Environment: 3D computer generated objects that can be viewed on a screen or in a head-mounted display.

Virtual Reality: Computer generated 3D images viewed by a learner in a virtual environment using a low-cost or high-end head mounted display.

Chapter 3
Approach to Scenario Development for Manikin-Based Simulation

ABSTRACT

Simulation education is used in a variety of health professions for training and continuing education. To accomplish this, instructors must identify learning objectives and suitable equipment and locations for simulation training. In addition, simulation educators may develop or adapt simulation scenarios to meet these objectives. Manikin-based simulation is the use of dolls or humanoid figures called manikins (mannequins) to practice procedures that would typically be performed on a human patient. This chapter describes the types of manikin-based simulation—low-fidelity and high-fidelity manikins—and explores various use-cases for manikin-based simulation in healthcare. Finally, this chapter outlines the approach to basic simulation scenario development for manikin-based simulation.

INTRODUCTION

Simulation has been widely used as a training and evaluation modality in health professional education. Simulation educators support simulation education and implementation at their institution through careful planning in identifying opportunities to integrate simulation into the training curriculum, developing simulation scenarios, identifying necessary resources (location,

DOI: 10.4018/978-1-7998-4378-8.ch003

staff and equipment), organizing the simulation environment and identifying challenges and requirements for simulation education at their institution. Simulation centers have been established as dedicated locations for simulation education in hospitals and training institutions such as medical and nursing schools. In contrast to clinical experience, errors can safely occur in the simulated environment. In this way practice can occur safely in simulated settings decreasing the risk of errors in clinical settings. The history of manikin development has been traced in Chapter 1 on "Introduction to Simulation in the Healthcare Professions". Manikin-based simulation involves the use of humanoid simulators, often referred to as "manikins" or "mannequins", as educational tools to support the delivery of realistic clinical scenarios guided by specified learning objectives. Over the years, a wide array of humanoid simulators, often referred to as manikins, have been developed and used to support healthcare training in various specialties including emergency medicine, anesthesia, nursing and pediatrics (Lopreiato & Sawyer, 2015; Padilha, Machado, Ribeiro, Ramos, & Costa, 2019; Wang et al., 2008; Weinger et al., 2017). Simulation is recognized worldwide as an effective method of learning clinical skills and is a mandatory part of the modern healthcare professional training curriculum. Manikins are used in many medical and nursing schools, hospitals and other higher education institutions in the United States, Europe and around the world.

BACKGROUND

Manikins come in various sizes with varying features to represent adult, juvenile and even newborn patients. The manikin's appearance can be customized by the manufacturer with different skin colors and tones which are then matched to the appropriate patient characteristics in the scenario. In addition, the manikin must be dressed appropriately for the case to create a sense of realism for the learner. For example, the manikin is dressed in a hospital gown and placed on a hospital bed for a hospital-based scenario or in street attire on a stretcher for a trauma or emergency room scenario.

Manikins are equipped with a range of features that include the ability to portray realistic vital signs and physiologic responses and to allow learners to perform procedures such as obtaining vascular access or performing chest tube placement. Ultrasound simulators have been used for training in ultrasound techniques (Tolsgaard et al., 2015). Birthing simulators have the appearance of female pregnant manikins and can be used to conduct obstetrical procedures and delivery of newborns. Surgical manikins are used to perform various types of surgical and trauma procedures (C. H. Evans & Schenarts, 2016; Naur, Nilsson, Pietersen, Clementsen, & Konge, 2017; See, Chui, Chan, Wong, & Chan, 2016; Valdis, Chu, Schlachta, & Kiaii, 2016).

In the context of a simulation scenario, manikins can be broadly arranged into two categories: low-fidelity simulators and high-fidelity simulators. The distinction between the two types of simulators is based on the degree to which they can represent vital signs and clinical features like heart and lung sounds. High-fidelity simulators typically have considerable technological components, such as physiology engines, in addition to other features, such as Bluetooth wireless communication to vital sign monitors and control devices (Hunziker et al., 2010; Wetzel, Lang, Pendergrass, Taylor, & Geis, 2013). However, the presence of technology is not necessary in order for the learner to have a high-fidelity experience (L. Evans & Taubert, 2019).

While obtaining the requisite equipment for use in simulation education is a significant first step, it is insufficient for institutions to simply purchase the manikins alone. Identifying and selecting manikins for use by learners in a simulation setting can be challenging for simulation facility directors. There are a wide range of manikins available from different suppliers and at costs that range from hundreds to tens of thousands of dollars. SimMan is an example of an adult manikin that provides simulation training in realistic patient care scenarios. Manikins which are often whole-body patient simulators, which allow for safe real-time simulation of a patient's anatomy, physiology and medical history. SimMan enables learners to practice patient emergency care in advanced patient simulation teams. SimMan is now one of the most popular and proven software on the market, with over 1.5 million downloads last year alone.

When it comes to simulation training, infrastructure and environmental considerations are also crucial factors to take into account because certain high-fidelity manikins require a specific temperature range in order to function properly. They also need to be protected from dust and humidity while they are being stored because some of them may grow mold. Additionally, in order for the internal air pumps and compressors that mimic breathing movements to function, they require either a constant supply of electricity or, at the very least, occasional charging of the batteries. When moving from one training venue to another, smaller manikins are easier to relocate than bigger manikins, which either need to be transported in vehicles or on carts.

In order to make effective use of manikins in educational contexts, the instructor needs to be able to develop and/or provide simulation experiences that assist students in achieving certain learning goals while making use of the manikins, personnel, and training supplies that are at their disposal. It is the responsibility of simulation educators to set appropriate learning objectives and then use those learning objectives to locate or create a simulation scenario that satisfies those learning objectives. The delivery of simulation experiences is the responsibility of facilitators, who are tasked with delivering those experiences by presenting the learning material, guiding learners through the case, and examining the lessons acquired through debriefing. Emerging within the field of simulation specialists is the role of the simulation technologist, whose responsibilities include the initial setup of manikins, the pre-programming of simulator responses, the assistance of simulation educators during simulation sessions by modifying the manikin's response or vital signs, the cleaning and resetting of manikins after each case, and the proper storage and maintenance of simulation equipment (Akaike et al., 2012; Roussin & Weinstock, 2017; Ziv et al., 2006).

APPROACH TO MANIKIN-BASED SIMULATION DEVELOPMENT

The objectives of this chapter are to describe the types of manikin simulators, considerations and use-cases for manikin-based simulation in healthcare, the processes and procedures for manikin-based simulation, and an overview of the approach to simulation case development for manikin-based simulation.

Types of Manikin-based Simulation

Low-Fidelity Manikin-Based Simulation

Low Fidelity manikin-based simulation uses simple manikins with few or no technological enhancements. Learners are able to interact with these manikins in a variety of predetermined ways under the direction of the simulation facilitator in order to accomplish their educational objectives. However, these manikins can only provide a limited clinical response, or in some circumstances, no reaction at all. For instance, low fidelity manikins can be utilized for the purpose of practicing a single component of cardiopulmonary resuscitation

(CPR) or a series of CPR operations, such as chest compressions or endotracheal intubation. A manikin equipped with a mouth, an oral cavity with a tube leading to inflatable lungs, and a mobile chest wall that demonstrates chest rise with lung inflation while using the bag and mask device can be used to perform bag and mask ventilation. This can be done by using a bag and mask device in conjunction with the manikin. Nevertheless, the manikin is not capable of representing spontaneous respiratory movements, lung noises, heart sounds, or vocalizations in any way. The educator is responsible for relaying to the student at the right moment during the scenario information regarding whether the clinical status of the manikin is getting better or getting worse. It takes ability to be able to introduce the knowledge without interrupting the flow of the situation, which would make the learning experience less beneficial. To provide this information, the facilitator may use a variety of low-tech or high-tech tools, such as verbal callouts of the heart rate and flash cards that indicate the level of cyanosis of the infant. Additionally, the facilitator may use monitor applications on stand-alone or paired smartphones or tablet devices to indicate the heart rate and rhythm, blood pressure, respiratory rate, and oxygen saturations.

Low fidelity manikins can also be used as substitutes for tethered high-fidelity manikins. For example, a birthing simulator often comes with a low fidelity newborn manikin that is delivered and then substituted for a high-fidelity manikin which is then used for a simulation scenario on advanced newborn resuscitation and procedures. While the low fidelity manikin may not have the same technological capabilities as the substituted high-fidelity manikin, its flexibility means that it can be used to carry out birthing maneuvers and its light weight and mobility make it suitable to the purpose of demonstrating placement on mother's abdomen immediately after delivery, then movement to the resuscitation area. In some cases where there are no obstetric learning objectives, the low fidelity manikin is simply used to indicate that the baby has been born, has received delayed cord clamping and has been moved to the resuscitation area.

In order to enhance the effectiveness of training using other, more high-tech modalities, low fidelity manikins can be utilized. For instance, a low fidelity manikin could be utilized in ultrasound training, in which the student would place an ultrasound probe on the low fidelity manikin's chest or abdomen in order to practice scanning in order to identify a clinical abnormality. Due to the absence of any mechanical hardware that could potentially interfere with ultrasound waves, low fidelity manikins are ideal for this type of application. More recently, they have been utilized in the context of simulations involving virtual reality (VR) and augmented reality (AR). The user participates in virtual reality simulations by donning a head-mounted display that depicts a clinical setting in which the patient requires a procedure, such as chest compressions. The user then gives chest compressions to the low fidelity manikin while wearing the VR headset to receive visual and audible feedback on their performance. If the user puts on the headset for augmented reality, they will be able to see the low fidelity manikin with additional information like as vital signs or cyanosis superimposed over it. This will make the learning experience more enjoyable for the user. In Chapter 4 on "Approach to Scenario Development for Virtual Simulation," you will find further information on the types of learning tools that are described above.

Low fidelity manikins have basic features which may require learners and facilitators to use their imagination in interpreting responses. As simulation education largely relies on the authenticity of the learner experience, many facilitators who use low fidelity manikins find them less desirable because of their lack of responsiveness to interventions. However, there are a few exceptions. Manikins that are used for practicing bag and mask ventilation include "lungs" which will inflate with appropriate ventilation causing chest rise that can be noted by the learner as proof of their success in maintaining an open airway and good mask seal and providing adequate pressure with the bag and mask ventilation breaths. However, sometimes the teaching point is that strategies to improve ventilation such as repositioning the head or adjusting the mask. In this case, the facilitator must say "there is no chest rise" when there is chest rise to prompt the learner to attempt to improve ventilation. This means learners must further "suspend disbelief" and can detract from their experience. Additionally, there is no way for the facilitator to demonstrate spontaneous breathing.

Some low fidelity manikins such as the Neonatalie manikin (Laerdal) have creatively addressed these issues by including manual elements such as a bulb inflator with tubing connected to the manikin lungs so that the facilitator can manually inflate the lungs or inhibit chest rise even when bag and mask ventilation is being properly performed. However, in most instances, the facilitator must indicate to the learner the physiologic state of the patient. This can be done using color-coded cards to represent cyanosis and by tapping out the heart rate to indicate bradycardia. The facilitator can also use a standalone or paired set of tablet or mobile devices to simulate a cardiopulmonary monitor. The cardiopulmonary monitor in a clinical setting represents the heart rate, respiratory rate, oxygenation, blood pressure, temperature, end-tidal carbon dioxide and other measures. Mobile apps which may be free (Neonatal Resuscitation Program Monitor app) or low cost (Sim Mon), can be manually set or adjusted using a paired app to show an increasing or decreasing heart rate, respiratory rate or oxygenation status. See Figure 1.

Figure 1. Schematic diagram showing low-fidelity manikin with stand-alone device(s) and facilitator

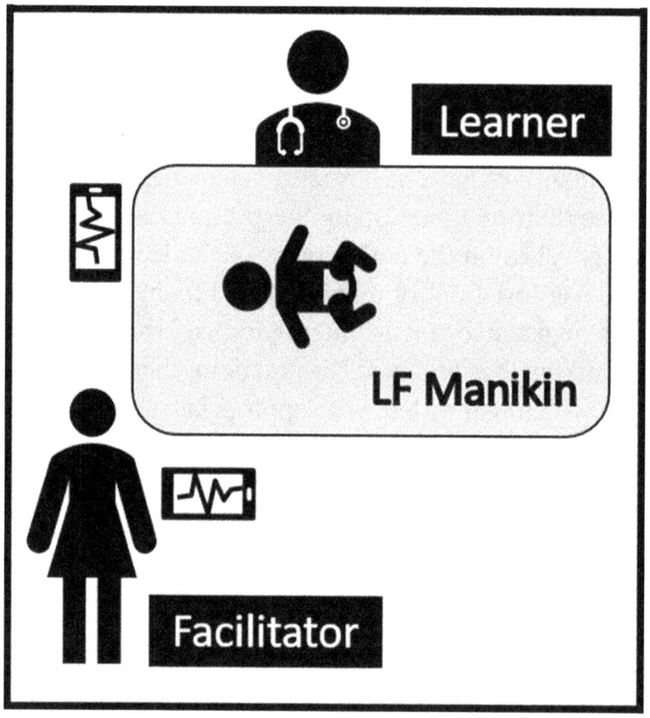

These applications can also display a variety of abnormal heart rhythms such as bradycardia, tachycardia, heart block or ventricular fibrillation.

For the practice of fundamental as well as more sophisticated operations and skills, including as bag-and-mask breathing, cardiac resuscitation, and needle aspiration, low fidelity manikins are helpful instruments that are also quite inexpensive. It's possible that the limited responses offered by low fidelity manikins are really advantageous for certain types of learners or in specific settings. The cognitive load of the learner can be lightened and the risk of being inundated with an excessive amount of information can be mitigated by reducing the number and diversity of sensory inputs that are received by the learner while the scenario is being played out. Because the functions of low fidelity manikins do not depend on wifi or Bluetooth signals, which could cause interference with the activities of other manikins in the same location, they may be preferable for use in big groups that make use of a shared environment.

High-Fidelity Manikin-Based Simulation

High-fidelity manikins are designed to closely mimic humanoid features. They are manufactured in various sizes to represent adult, juvenile, infant, and newborn age ranges. For example, Pediasim and Pediatrics (HPS) are advanced child and infant-sized manikins that support a variety of medical training activities such as CPR, emergency medicine and emergency medicine. These simulators feature advanced physiology and additional features such as the ability to change skin color, mechanical breathing and heart rate and software on a laptop or tablet device. This software can be used to control the manikin's appearance and responses including, but not limited to lung compliance, bronchial resistance, respiratory effort, appearance of capillary refill time, and oxygenation and end-tidal carbon dioxide monitoring can be done using real sensors.

Recent research has demonstrated that there are flaws in the way that some of the features are portrayed, which may be detrimental to learning goals. This is the case even though all high-fidelity manikins make an attempt to depict humanoid features with some anatomic accuracy. Developers have been able to more accurately replicate anatomical features and create advanced high-fidelity manikins with structures that are anatomically accurate as a result of advancements in technology such as magnetic resonance imaging and computed tomography scans that can be converted into 3D models. These scans are examples of technologies that have advanced in recent years. For instance, manikins designed for endotracheal intubation need to have an anatomically accurate representation of the relationships between the oral cavity, esophagus, trachea, bronchi, and lungs. Additionally, these manikins need to be compatible with standard mechanical ventilators, patient circuits, and different modes of ventilation.

High fidelity manikins have features that support wireless communication and real-time feedback on learner performance. High fidelity manikins may be connected using a wired or wireless connection to a compressor and monitor. Wireless "untethered" models rely on Bluetooth signals to communicate with the software and monitor. This gives an element of portability and flexibility to their use as they can more easily be transported from one location to another and used in both simulation and clinical spaces. Programmable features include heart rate and breathing responses such as retractions, "see-saw" breathing and abdominal distension. These responses are displayed along with other vital signs on a simulated cardiopulmonary monitor. Some models also provide real-time feedback on the quality of chest compressions provided during cardiopulmonary resuscitation. Feedback from manikins can be used during simulation and patches such as the Zoll defibrillator patch can be used in actual clinical situations to provide "CPR coaching" to improve the depth and rate of chest compressions leading to a greater likelihood of return of spontaneous circulation (ROSC)(Abella et al., 2007; Kim, Lee, Kim, & Park, 2015). In using these kinds of simulators, learners can transition to

Figure 2. Schematic diagram showing high-fidelity manikin connected to monitor and facilitator controlling the manikin's responses and vital signs

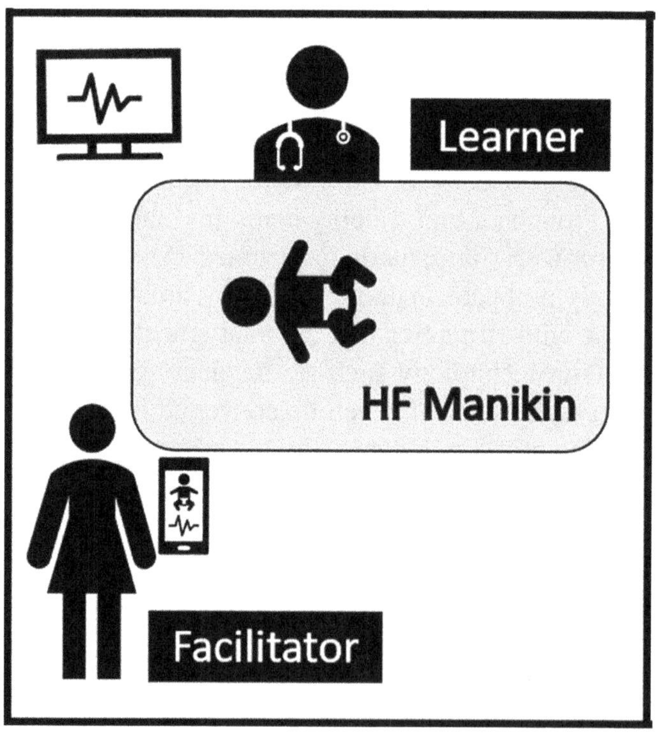

the clinical settings smoothly and successfully, and they are equipped with skills and self-confidence when they encounter real patients.

The employment of high-fidelity manikins could be beneficial in some settings involving teams. In contrast to the more common practice of using low fidelity manikins for the purpose of training individual aspects of cardiopulmonary resuscitation (CPR), high-fidelity manikins are often utilized for team-based simulation situations. When taking part in these activities, which are frequently referred to as integrated skills stations, the learner or learners demonstrate their level of competency by sequentially completing a number of tests or processes. The use of high-fidelity manikins is used in scenario-based training in which individuals and teams are put through a series of resuscitation stages. The reactions of the manikins are managed by the facilitators through the use of a pre-defined sequence of steps that are linked to the goals of the scenario. These steps can also be programmed into the software so that when an appropriate action is carried out by the learner, the facilitator only needs to note that it was done in order to prompt the software to change the vital signs. When these steps are programmed into the software, the facilitator only needs to make a note that the action was carried out. The only thing that the learners interact with is the manikin and its replies, while the only thing that the facilitator interacts with is the software. There are some simulation facilities in which the facilitator does not even need to be present in the room in order to observe the students because they can view them remotely through a one-way mirror or with cameras and microphones installed in the room. Learners are able to continue the simulation without being interrupted or having the overpowering impression that they are being watched by a facilitator who is present in the room thanks to this. The learner may be able to interact with the manikin and team more successfully in order to achieve the objectives of the scenario if the facilitator has the capacity to limit interaction between themselves and the learner. This ability strengthens the realism of the scenario. This results in an increase in the number of possibilities for learners to gain experience through experiential learning since learners are given the chance to try out new strategies and observe the results without the facilitator interfering or interrupting them.

The acquisition of training manikins is one of the most significant factors that contributes to the overall cost of simulation education. The price of high-fidelity manikins is typically in the tens of thousands of dollars, which is a huge increase from the price of low fidelity manikins. Because of this, simulation programs will typically have a large number of low fidelity manikins but only a small number of high-fidelity manikins. Due to the fact that this cost is passed on to replacement components, facilitators will frequently reserve the usage of high-fidelity manikins for scenario-based training even if these manikins may assist basic process training. The use of high-fidelity manikins makes it possible for learners and teams to act out complicated scenarios that involve interaction among team members and different procedures. The variety of answers that high-fidelity manikins are capable of providing enhances the learning experience for experienced students by simulating the difficulty of real-life clinical situations more accurately (Mills et al., 2016). When setting up wireless manikins in a confined area, care must be taken to minimize "cross-talk" or interference with the peripheral devices linked to other manikins. This can be accomplished by taking certain precautions during the setup process. When this occurs, it is possible that signals intended for one manikin will be intercepted and used by another manikin, resulting in a response that was not anticipated.

Use Cases for Manikin-Based Simulation

There is a strong interest in the application of manikin simulations in medical research and clinical practice. Historically manikin-based simulation has been used primarily for procedural training. Use cases for procedural training under emergent and non-emergent conditions. These include but are not limited to:

Airway Procedures

Clinical practice in critical care settings requires proficiency at procedures to stabilize and maintain the patient's airway. Use cases that are typical for training in emergency medicine, adult, pediatric, and newborn intensive care include tracheal tube adjustments, endotracheal intubation, oral and laryngeal mask airway placements, and endotracheal intubation. Many low fidelity and high-fidelity manikins enable the installation of oral airways and endotracheal tubes of the right size. However, only a small percentage of manikins have airways that are anatomically accurate in terms of their structure, texture, and appearance. This lack of accuracy has been described in various papers (Klock Jr., 2012; Sawyer, Strandjord, Johnson, & Low, 2016), which has led to the development of manikins that are more anatomically correct in order to facilitate learning. A significant obstacle is that it is impossible to replicate the feel and fragility of human flesh using a manikin that is designed for repeated practice sessions. This is a challenge for medical professionals. Confirming that the emergency airway is situated in the suitable location is another factor to take into account. In high-fidelity manikins, software displays show accurate placement. In low fidelity manikins, on the other hand, chest rise and auscultation are required in order to detect whether the laryngeal mask airway or endotracheal tube is in the correct position.

Enteral Nutrition Procedures

Simulation can be used as a method for instructing nurses and other hospital staff on standard processes for ensuring patients receive adequate nourishment. Procedures for enteral nutrition include the insertion of a nasogastric or orogastric feeding tube, as well as the replacement of a g-tube. Enteral feeding is a highly common process, and the insertion of feeding tubes in medical institutions such as hospitals and nursing homes, as well as in private homes, can be carried out by caregivers and nurses with varying degrees of education and training.

Intravenous Access Procedures

A wide range of clinical and laboratory staff perform intravenous access procedures in clinical settings. While trial and error on actual patients has been a long-standing approach, simulation using intravenous access trainers can reduce the learning curve and decrease patient complications with these procedures. Intravenous access procedures such as peripheral IV (PIV), peripherally placed central catheter (PICC), peripheral arterial line, central (subclavian or femoral) line, and umbilical arterial and venous catheter placement are procedures that can be practiced on a manikin. Newborn and adult manikins have features that allow for various peripheral and central lines to be placed. This allows for sterile technique to be practiced as appropriate and for potential complications such as pneumothorax, bleeding and air embolism to be avoided or managed proactively during the simulation.

Diagnostic and Therapeutic Procedures

It is possible to imitate diagnostic and therapeutic operations such as needle thoracocentesis, chest tube placement, pericardiocentesis, and the placement of pericardial drains; abdominal paracentesis; lumbar puncture; bladder tap; and ventricular tap. Learners are able to go through the steps of obtaining informed consent, preparing the patient, using safety checklists, performing the procedure, addressing complications, and documenting the procedure by simulating medical procedures that are typically carried out by specialists in emergency medicine, pediatrics, internal medicine, adult, pediatric, and newborn intensive care. These procedures are commonly carried out. Because of the rarity of certain of these processes, simulation is necessary not only for initial training but also for ongoing skill maintenance. In the event of an emergency, such as a heart attack or pulmonary embolism, tension pneumothorax, or pericardial tamponade, further procedures may be required to be carried out as rapidly as possible. As a result, it is vital to have the opportunity to rehearse the steps for conducting the process in a timely and safe manner in order to guarantee both the quality and safety of patient care.

Surgical Procedures

Surgical procedures including laparoscopic surgery, robotic surgery and obstetric procedures can be performed using simulators. Some manikins are designed to recreate the experience of doing open surgical procedures. Practice for laparoscopic surgeries can be done on "task trainers," which can take the form of either physical simulators or virtual reality simulators (Clements, Morrison, & Schenkman, 2016; Lin et al., 2009; Vaccaro et al., 2013; Valdis et al., 2016). The value of using manikins in surgery extends beyond the technical skills to the interactions between the various members of the surgical team, which includes the surgeon, the anesthetist, surgical assistants, and surgical nursing staff. In other words, the value of using manikins in surgery goes well beyond the technical skills (Stevens, Galloway, & Willemsen-Dunlap, 2019). Obstetric procedures such as labor and delivery maneuvers can be practiced on purpose-built obstetric simulators such as Lucy's Maternal and Newborn Birth Simulator, which is a simulation system designed to provide learners caring for pregnant women and babies with a realistic experience. Other obstetric simulators include Lucy's Maternal and Newborn Birth Simulator and Lucy's Maternal and Newborn Birth Simulator. The use of these types of simulators allows for the possibility of realistic practice in obstetric procedures for the delivery of infants in emergency situations.

Patient Communication

The ability to communicate effectively is essential to establishing a trusting relationship between a doctor and patient, which in turn paves the way for more expeditious diagnosis and treatment. The role of standardized patients can be played by manikins with speakers already constructed into them. The learner who are conducting a speedy evaluation will ask questions, and the facilitator, who is located in a different room, will answer to those questions. While the absence of emotional cues could be considered a limitation of this use case, it does provide the facilitator with the opportunity to integrate pertinent historical information such as drugs and allergies in a seamless manner into the experience of participating in the simulation.

Manikin-Based Scenario Development

In this section, we will cover approaches to manikin-based scenario development. There are a lot of different approaches to making a solid scenario. In point of fact, simulation scenarios for common scenarios involving basic life support, adult and pediatric advanced life support, and neonatal resuscitation have already been developed and are available for facilitators to use. These scenarios cover basic life support, advanced life support for adults and children, and neonatal resuscitation. However, as a simulation facilitator, you may need to modify these situations to fit the atmosphere of your particular hospital or clinic, or if your learners are emergency medical technicians, you may need to adapt them to the pre-hospital setting. In other instances, the circumstance is extremely uncommon, and there is no publicly available simulation case that can be modified and used. Each simulation case must have clearly defined objectives, a description of the patient, the expected actions of the learners, and the physiologic response of the patient to those actions, which may be positive or negative. These requirements must be met regardless of whether the facilitator is adapting an existing scenario or developing a new scenario.

Adapting an Existing Scenario

Adapting an existing scenario is a way to quickly get started with simulation education. When customizing a scenario, the first step is to analyze the objectives of the scenario to see whether or not they align with your educational goals. In the event that they do not, you will have to determine which aspects of the scenario require revision in order to bring them into line with the goals you have set. The target demographic should be the next thing you think about. Does the audience (or learner group) of the scenario that you are using match the audience (or learner group) that you are using? In the event that this is not the case, it may be necessary to make some modifications or edits in order to guarantee that the actions and behaviors of the predicted learner adhere to those of your learners. Thirdly, how challenging of a situation are we dealing with here? Does it correspond to the standards you have set for your learner's performance? If some of your students are more experienced than others, you may need to make the situation more challenging by including more challenging components. Last but not least, check to see that the original author is given credit.

Creating a New Scenario

Simulations are powerful ways to teach and learn. The process of creating a new scenario combines content expertise with creative thinking in an effort to capture a wide range of possible learner actions within the limitations of equipment, supplies and staff. Scenario writers should keep an open mindset while engaged in scenario development as this supports the exploration of these alternatives. Allowing for a range of possible learner actions and manikin responses allows learners to gain new insights into the range of options and risks involved in making decisions about care that would have major consequences for the patient safety and outcomes.

The lessons learned during simulation are readily transferred to clinical practice. For this reason, scenario development requires adequate preparation and an in-depth knowledge of the subject to avoid teaching inaccuracies. If you are not an expert in the area, you may need to consult references or invite the opinion of experts on your scenario. If the scenario is meant to be used across different institutions or internationally, it is important to have collective discussions on elements that may need to be featured in various settings to meet the scenario objectives. This will ensure the scenario captures the specifics of each context and remains relevant for training learners in different settings.

It is essential to first define the learning objectives before moving on. After you have gathered information on the topic, the next step is to identify your learning goals. In an ideal world, two or three learning objectives should be explicitly articulated for each scenario, using terminology that are measurable. Choose learning goals that can be witnessed during the scenario so that you can gauge how well students are doing with them. Simulations offer students the chance to demonstrate what they've learned through observable action.

Figure 3. Learning objectives

Knowledge	Comprehension	Application	Analysis	Synthesis	Evaluation
define	classify	apply	analyze	arrange	assess
identify	compile	calculate	calculate	assemble	compare
label	conclude	demonstrate	categorize	compose	critique
list	discuss	develop	classify	construct	decide
match	describe	interpret	criticize	design	determine
name	explain	locate	compare	develop	establish
recall	express	operate	contrast	diagnose	evaluate
recognize	give examples	perform	determine	manage	judge
record	identify	practice	differentiate	organize	justify
relate	interpret	predict	distinguish	plan	measure
repeat	recognize	present	examine	propose	rate
select	summarize	report	outline	relate	recommend
state	translate	use	test	summarize	select

The following illustration, Figure 3, provides some instances of phrases that might be utilized while developing learning objectives.

After defining your learning objectives, define the clinical setting and patient characteristics for the facilitator. Include a list of equipment needed for the scenario. Provide a short script for the facilitator to read to the learner introducing the scenario. Then list expected participant actions and the manikin's response including color, tone, and vital signs in stages. Most simple scenarios will have three stages: Initial, Middle, and End.

Initial Stage

The initial stage, often known as the beginning of the scenario, depicts the patient in his or her baseline state. The starting vital signs and state of the manikin in the beginning stage of a scenario may be at a normal baseline and begin to deteriorate in a hospitalized patient, or they may be at a low baseline with the potential for further deterioration in a depressed newborn. Either way, the patient's condition is expected to worsen.

Middle Stage

The stage of the scenario that takes place roughly in the middle is the portion of the simulation in which the majority of the learner actions are carried out. At this point, the clinical symptoms and signs that the patient is exhibiting are modified so that they better reflect the patient condition for which the scenario is being done. For instance, a patient who has a right tension pneumothorax will show indicators of respiratory distress such as attenuated breath sounds on the right side, tachypnea (increased respiratory rate), tachycardia (increased heart rate), cyanosis, and decreased oxygen saturation. The learner is responsible for making a diagnosis of the ailment and carrying out certain procedures in order to stabilize the patient. If these actions are not carried out in a timely manner, the patient's condition may worsen further. For instance, the patient's heart rate may drop, their respiratory effort may decrease, and their cyanosis and oxygenation may become more severe. If these actions are not carried out, the patient's condition may worsen.

End Stage

The learning process is finished when the last stage of the scenario is reached. If all goes according to plan, a scenario's end point will occur when the patient's health has improved as a direct result of the proper diagnosis and the activities that were taken in response to that diagnosis, bringing the scenario to its conclusion. If the student is unable to make the accurate diagnosis or take the appropriate procedures to resuscitate the patient, the facilitator may cut short the scenario and move on to debriefing or discussing the case. The learning process is finished when the last stage of the scenario is reached. If all goes according to plan, a scenario's end point will occur when the patient's health has improved as a direct result of the proper diagnosis and the activities that were taken in response to that diagnosis, bringing the scenario to its conclusion. If the student is unable to make the accurate diagnosis or take the appropriate procedures to resuscitate the patient, the facilitator may cut short the scenario and move on to debriefing or discussing the case. At the end of your scenario, you may provide standard debriefing questions such as:

What was the condition of the patient
What went well?
What didn't go well?
What will you do differently next time

Other questions that are tied to scenario objectives may be helpful to drive home the objectives of the scenario. For example, in the scenario on tension pneumothorax, the scenario debriefer might ask:

What made you suspect a pneumothorax? or
How would you diagnose a tension pneumothorax?

Table 1. Simple scenario template

Stage	Learner Action	Manikin Response	Facilitator notes
Initial			
Middle			
End			

Table 2. Simple scenario example

Stage	Learner action	Manikin response	Facilitator notes
Initial Delivery of a full-term newborn without respiratory effort, floppy with poor tone and no cry.	Place on warmer, dry and stimulate the baby using cloth	No change in respiratory effort and tone with stimulation. Heart rate 80bpm.	
Middle Initiation of positive pressure ventilation	Starts positive pressure ventilation (PPV) with a bag and mask device by 60 seconds of life. Continues PPV for at least 30 seconds.	Breath sounds heard bilaterally. Spontaneous breathing and crying after 30 seconds of PPV. Heart rate 120 bpm.	Monitor for effective PPV by noting chest rise on manikin.
End Assessment of response to PPV and ongoing supportive care.	Transition from PPV to room air while monitoring oxygen saturations. Keep warm. Monitor closely.	Heart rate 140bpm. Good spontaneous breathing and crying.	

Performance Reporting

A reporting checklist that consists of the learning objectives should be developed as a resource for the facilitator. This checklist can be used to systematically collect data on learner performance as well as any issues encountered during the scenario. Frequently encountered errors can be addressed through didactic training and additional simulation practice. The majority of the assessments carried out during simulations are formative. This indicates that the information received from the assessment is used to improve performance and rectify flaws prior to a summative performance review being carried out. Formative evaluations may include straightforward checklists or more complicated formats such as objective structured clinical examinations (OSCE) in order to investigate knowledge gaps and stimulate practice (Mangold et al., 2015). This method is suitable for assessing a wide variety of performance measures, including clinical decision-making, procedural skills, as well as communication with patients and other team members. The majority of the assessments carried out during simulations are formative. This indicates that the information received from the assessment is used to improve performance and rectify flaws prior to a summative performance review being carried out. Formative evaluations may include straightforward checklists or more complicated formats such as objective structured clinical examinations (OSCE) in order to investigate knowledge gaps and stimulate practice (Mangold et al., 2015). This method is suitable for assessing a wide variety of performance measures, including clinical decision-making, procedural skills, as well as communication with patients and other team members. The majority of the assessments carried out during simulations are formative. This indicates that the information received from the assessment is used to improve performance and rectify flaws prior to a summative performance review being carried out. Formative evaluations may include straightforward checklists or more complicated formats such as objective structured clinical examinations (OSCE) in order to investigate knowledge gaps and stimulate practice (Mangold et al., 2015). This method is suitable for assessing a wide variety of performance measures, including clinical decision-making, procedural skills, as well as communication with patients and other team members. Evaluation of learner performance during simulations is covered in more detail in Chapter 6 on "Evaluation of Simulation Performance".

SOLUTIONS AND RECOMMENDATIONS

Simulation education is useful for any public or private healthcare organization that wishes to support an environment of inquiry and life-long learning for patient safety. Scenario development is a useful tool for healthcare educators and simulation facilitators and should be conducted with input from stakeholders who can provide local information on context and learner preferences. Simulation scenarios enable learners to practice their skills, learn from mistakes, anticipate events that they may encounter in the clinical setting, understand risk, and break out of their established mental models as they become aware of alternative approaches. Organizations can use the outcomes of simulation to identify safety risks and generate ideas for preemptive organizational action to mitigate these risks.

Simulation development should involve both content and educational specialists. Include content experts. If you are running a scenario that will require a blood transfusion, seek the input of a hematologist or other laboratory specialist. If you are building scenarios on a specific area such as pediatric or newborn care, you should involve pediatricians or newborn specialists. A session for brainstorming and sharing of ideas is important for developing a robust scenario. Consider beginning scenario development in a workshop setting to allow for free flow of ideas leading to the creation of outlines for various learner actions and potential outcomes in each scenario. Once these outlines have been generated, a small core team can be tasked with completing the scenario.

Test the new scenario you have created with a small group of experienced learners and incorporate their feedback to improve any areas that are unclear before using it more broadly. Your scenario should be adaptable for use with both low fidelity and high-fidelity manikins. When your scenario is complete, consider making it available to others through publication on sites like MedED Portal (mededportal.org) or other online repositories.

FUTURE RESEARCH DIRECTIONS

A simulation educator supports simulation education and implementation at their institution by identifying opportunities for simulation to be integrated into the training curriculum, developing simulation scenarios, identifying necessary resources (location, staff & equipment), organizing the simulation environment, and identifying challenges and requirements for simulation education at the institution. Hospitals and medical and nursing schools have built simulation centers for the purpose of providing students with hands-on training in the use of simulations. However, the use of in-situ simulation may increase the fidelity of the experience and the degree to which in-situ vs. facility-based simulation supports learning may vary by the goals of the scenario and is an area of ongoing study.

Errors can be made in the simulated environment without risk of harming the patient, unlike in the real world. As a result, the risk of errors in clinical settings can be reduced through safe practice in a simulated environment. Areas for future research in scenario development include testing scenario adaptability to various learners, settings and simulation tools including low fidelity and high-fidelity manikins. Even though purchasing manikins is an important first step in the simulation education process, it is not sufficient on its own. For simulation facility directors, identifying and selecting manikins for usage by learners can be a challenge. More research on the features of manikins that increase their educational efficacy is needed.

CONCLUSION

In conclusion, manikin-based simulation can be performed with a range of low or high-fidelity manikins. The choice of what type of manikin to use depends on the learning objectives and learner characteristics as well as the experience and comfort level of the facilitator. Scenarios can be adapted or created to meet learning objectives. It is possible to divide manikins into low and high-fidelity simulators by their ability to accurately portray clinical aspects like heart and lung sounds in a simulation scenario. Physiology engines and wireless communication to vital sign monitors and control devices are common in high-technology simulators. Technology isn't always necessary for a high-quality learning experience. However, new scenarios must be evidence-based with clear learning objectives and attention must be given to testing newly created scenarios to ensure that they are easy to use and effective for the intended learner group.

REFERENCES

Abella, B. S., Edelson, D. P., Kim, S., Retzer, E., Myklebust, H., Barry, A. M., O'Hearn, N., Hoek, T. L. V., & Becker, L. B. (2007). CPR quality improvement during in-hospital cardiac arrest using a real-time audiovisual feedback system. *Resuscitation*, *73*(1), 54–61. doi:10.1016/j.resuscitation.2006.10.027 PMID:17258853

Akaike, M., Fukutomi, M., Nagamune, M., Fujimoto, A., Tsuji, A., Ishida, K., & Iwata, T. (2012). Simulation-based medical education in clinical skills laboratory. *The Journal of Medical Investigation*, *59*(1-2), 28–35. doi:10.2152/jmi.59.28 PMID:22449990

Clements, M. B., Morrison, K. Y., & Schenkman, N. S. (2016). Evaluation of Laparoscopic Curricula in American Urology Residency Training: A 5-Year Update. *Journal of Endourology*, *30*(3), 347–353. doi:10.1089/end.2015.0561 PMID:26731240

Evans, C. H., & Schenarts, K. D. (2016). Evolving Educational Techniques in Surgical Training. *The Surgical Clinics of North America*, *96*(1), 71–88. doi:10.1016/j.suc.2015.09.005 PMID:26612021

Evans, L., & Taubert, M. (2019). State of the science: the doll is dead: simulation in palliative care education. *BMJ Supportive & Palliative Care*, *9*(2), 117–119. doi:10.1136/bmjspcare-2018-001595 PMID:30254018

Hunziker, S., Buhlmann, C., Tschan, F., Balestra, G., Legeret, C., Schumacher, C., Semmer, N. K., Hunziker, P., & Marsch, S. (2010). Brief leadership instructions improve cardiopulmonary resuscitation in a high-fidelity simulation: A randomized controlled trial. *Critical Care Medicine*, *38*(4), 1086–1091. Advance online publication. doi:10.1097/CCM.0b013e3181cf7383 PMID:20124886

Kim, M. J., Lee, H. S., Kim, S., & Park, Y. S. (2015). Optimal chest compression technique for paediatric cardiac arrest victims. *Scandinavian Journal of Trauma, Resuscitation and Emergency Medicine*, *23*(1), 36–36. doi:10.118613049-015-0118-y PMID:25896601

Klock, P. A. Jr. (2012). Airway simulators and mannequins: A case of high infidelity? *Anesthesiology*, *116*(6), 1179–1180. doi:10.1097/ALN.0b013e318254d0b2 PMID:22487862

Lin, D. W., Romanelli, J. R., Kuhn, J. N., Thompson, R. E., Bush, R. W., & Seymour, N. E. (2009). Computer-based laparoscopic and robotic surgical simulators: Performance characteristics and perceptions of new users. *Surgical Endoscopy*, *23*(1), 209–214. doi:10.100700464-008-9805-3 PMID:18297349

Lopreiato, J. O., & Sawyer, T. (2015). Simulation-based medical education in pediatrics. *Academic Pediatrics*, *15*(2), 134–142. doi:10.1016/j.acap.2014.10.010 PMID:25748973

Mills, B. W., Carter, O. B. J., Rudd, C. J., Claxton, L. A., Ross, N. P., & Strobel, N. A. (2016). Effects of Low- Versus High-Fidelity Simulations on the Cognitive Burden and Performance of Entry-Level Paramedicine Students: A Mixed-Methods Comparison Trial Using Eye-Tracking, Continuous Heart Rate, Difficulty Rating Scales, Video Observation and Interviews. *Simulation in Healthcare: Journal of the Society for Simulation in Healthcare, 11*(1), 10-18. doi:10.1097/SIH.0000000000000119

Naur, T. M. H., Nilsson, P. M., Pietersen, P. I., Clementsen, P. F., & Konge, L. (2017). Simulation-Based Training in Flexible Bronchoscopy and Endobronchial Ultrasound-Guided Transbronchial Needle Aspiration (EBUS-TBNA): A Systematic Review. *Respiration: International Review of Thoracic Diseases, 93*(5), 355-362. doi:10.1159/000464331

Padilha, J. M., Machado, P. P., Ribeiro, A., Ramos, J., & Costa, P. (2019). Clinical Virtual Simulation in Nursing Education: Randomized Controlled Trial. *Journal of Medical Internet Research, 21*(3), e11529–e11529. doi:10.2196/11529 PMID:30882355

Roussin, C. J., & Weinstock, P. (2017). SimZones: An Organizational Innovation for Simulation Programs and Centers. *Academic Medicine, 92*(8), 1114–1120. doi:10.1097/ACM.0000000000001746 PMID:28562455

Sawyer, T., Strandjord, T. P., Johnson, K., & Low, D. (2016). Neonatal airway simulators, how good are they? A comparative study of physical and functional fidelity.(ORIGINAL ARTICLE)(Report). *Journal of Perinatology, 36*(2), 151–156. doi:10.1038/jp.2015.161 PMID:26583944

See, K. W. M., Chui, K. H., Chan, W. H., Wong, K. C., & Chan, Y. C. (2016). Evidence for Endovascular Simulation Training: A Systematic Review. *European Journal of Vascular and Endovascular Surgery: The Official Journal of the European Society for Vascular Surgery, 51*(3), 441-451. doi:10.1016/j.ejvs.2015.10.011

Stevens, R., Galloway, T., & Willemsen-Dunlap, A. (2019). Advancing Our Understandings of Healthcare Team Dynamics From the Simulation Room to the Operating Room: A Neurodynamic Perspective. *Frontiers in Psychology, 10*, 1660. doi:10.3389/fpsyg.2019.01660 PMID:31456706

Tolsgaard, M. G., Ringsted, C., Dreisler, E., Nørgaard, L. N., Petersen, J. H., Madsen, M. E., Freiesleben, N. L. C., Sørensen, J. L., & Tabor, A. (2015). Sustained effect of simulation-based ultrasound training on clinical performance: A randomized trial. *Ultrasound in Obstetrics & Gynecology, 46*(3), 312–318. doi:10.1002/uog.14780 PMID:25580809

Vaccaro, C. M., Crisp, C. C., Fellner, A. N., Jackson, C., Kleeman, S. D., & Pavelka, J. (2013). Robotic virtual reality simulation plus standard robotic orientation versus standard robotic orientation alone: A randomized controlled trial. *Female Pelvic Medicine & Reconstructive Surgery, 19*(5), 266–270. doi:10.1097/SPV.0b013e3182a09101 PMID:23982574

Valdis, M., Chu, M. W. A., Schlachta, C., & Kiaii, B. (2016). Evaluation of robotic cardiac surgery simulation training: A randomized controlled trial. *The Journal of Thoracic and Cardiovascular Surgery*, *151*(6), 1498–1505. e1492. doi:10.1016/j.jtcvs.2016.02.016 PMID:26964911

Wang, E. E., Quinones, J., Fitch, M. T., Dooley-Hash, S., Griswold-Theodorson, S., Medzon, R., Korley, F., Laack, T., Robinett, A., & Clay, L. (2008). Developing technical expertise in emergency medicine—The role of simulation in procedural skill acquisition. *Academic Emergency Medicine*, *15*(11), 1046–1057. doi:10.1111/j.1553-2712.2008.00218.x PMID:18785939

Weinger, M. B., Banerjee, A., Burden, A. R., McIvor, W. R., Boulet, J., Cooper, J. B., Steadman, R., Shotwell, M. S., Slagle, J. M., DeMaria, S. Jr, Torsher, L., Sinz, E., Levine, A. I., Rask, J., Davis, F., Park, C., & Gaba, D. M. (2017). Simulation-based Assessment of the Management of Critical Events by Board-certified Anesthesiologists. *Anesthesiology*, *127*(3), 475–489. doi:10.1097/ALN.0000000000001739 PMID:28671903

Wetzel, E. A., Lang, T. R., Pendergrass, T. L., Taylor, R. G., & Geis, G. L. (2013). Identification of latent safety threats using high-fidelity simulation-based training with multidisciplinary neonatology teams. *Joint Commission Journal on Quality and Patient Safety*, *39*(6), 268–268. doi:10.1016/S1553-7250(13)39037-0 PMID:23789165

Ziv, A., Erez, D., Munz, Y., Vardi, A., Barsuk, D., Levine, I., . . . Berkenstadt, H. (2006). The Israel Center for Medical Simulation: a paradigm for cultural change in medical education. Acad Med, 81(12), 1091-1097. 00001888-200612000-00014 doi:10.1097/01.ACM.0000246756.55626.1b

KEY TERMS AND DEFINITIONS

Augmented Reality: Computer generated holographic images can be viewed by the learner in the physical environment using a mobile device or specially designed headset.

High-Fidelity Manikin: This term refers to a technology-enabled manikin with features such as mechanical respiration and heart rate.

Low-Fidelity Manikin: This is typically a low cost, low technology manikin with minimal features.

Objective Structured Clinical Examination (OSCE): An approach to assessment that involves defined objectives and anticipated actions, often with an accompanying checklist for assessment.

Simulation Debriefer: A simulation instructor who leads the learners through a reflective analysis of simulation events.

Simulation Facilitator: A simulation instructor who guides the learners through the scenario with the goal of meeting learning objectives.

Simulation Technician/Specialist: An individual who supports the practice of simulation through setting up and managing simulation manikins and supplies.

Teledebriefing: Teledebriefing describes a process in which learners who are participating in a simulation scenario undergo debriefing with a facilitator located at an off-site location.

Telefacilitation: The conduct of a telesimulation by a remote facilitator.

Telesimulation: Telesimulation is a process by which telecommunication and simulation resources are utilized to provide education, training, and/or assessment to learners at an off-site location.

Video-Assisted Debriefing: The practice of using video captured during simulation sessions for reflective discussions on learner and team performance.

Virtual Environment: 3D computer generated objects that can be viewed on a screen or in a head-mounted display.

Virtual Reality: Computer generated 3D images viewed by a learner in a virtual environment using a low-cost or high-end head mounted display.

Chapter 4
Approach to Scenario Development for Virtual Simulation

ABSTRACT

Virtual simulation is the use of 3D models and environments to practice activities that would typically be performed in a healthcare setting. This chapter describes two types of virtual simulation: virtual reality and augmented reality. The types and use-cases for virtual simulation in healthcare are explored including teamwork training, standardized virtual patients, and procedure-based training. The chapter discusses approaches to basic simulation scenario development for virtual simulation and introduces best practices for debriefing and feedback in virtual simulation.

INTRODUCTION

Virtual simulation engages the learner in using 3D computer generated models representing patients, hospital settings or other healthcare providers as educational tools to support the delivery of realistic clinical scenarios guided by specified learning objectives. Over the years, computer-generated environments have evolved, becoming more accessible through the advances of technology and have been intensely evaluated for effectiveness (Kaplan et al., 2020). Virtual simulations are now used to support healthcare training in a wide range of specialties including emergency medicine, anesthesia, nursing

DOI: 10.4018/978-1-7998-4378-8.ch004

and pediatrics (Lopreiato & Sawyer, 2015; Padilha, Machado, Ribeiro, Ramos, & Costa, 2019; Wang et al., 2008; Weinger et al., 2017). The history of virtual simulation has been traced in Chapter 1 titled “Introduction to simulation in the healthcare professions”.

Standardized virtual patients have been developed with various features to represent adult, juvenile and even newborn patients (Combs & Combs, 2019; Isaza-Restrepo, Gómez, Cifuentes, & Argüello, 2018; Kononowicz et al., 2019; Peddle, McKenna, Bearman, & Nestel, 2019). In the same way that actual manikins can have their appearances altered, the appearance of the virtual patient can be altered by the designer to have a variety of skin hues and tones, which are then matched to the proper patient attributes in the scenario. In addition, the virtual patient may be easily adjusted to display a range of emotions, and its look can be modified to depict someone who is elderly or fat, and it can be dressed in a manner that is appropriate for the scenario to give the learner a sense of realism (Motz et al., 2018; Sweigart & Hodson-Carlton, 2013). Additionally, members of the family can be inserted into the scenario with relative ease. For instance, a woman of mixed race and middle age may be seen accompanying a young Hispanic man who is either clad in a hospital gown and positioned on a hospital bed for a scenario set in a hospital or dressed in street clothes and placed on a stretcher for a scenario set in a trauma center or emergency room.

Monitors that provide realistic vital signs and physiologic responses are something that can be included in virtual simulations. Learners have the opportunity to study the steps of procedures such as conducting chest tube installation, acquiring vascular access, and neonatal resuscitation. Those learning ultrasound procedures have been able to benefit from the usage of augmented reality ultrasound simulators (Tolsgaard et al., 2015). Augmented reality capabilities have been added to birthing simulators, allowing the unborn child to be observed while still inside the mother’s uterus. Learners can be guided through the performance of a variety of surgical and trauma operations with the help of telescopy, which can be utilized in conjunction with augmented reality on operating tables (Evans & Schenarts, 2016; Naur, Nilsson, Pietersen, Clementsen, & Konge, 2017; See, Chui, Chan, Wong, & Chan, 2016; Valdis, Chu, Schlachta, & Kiaii, 2016).

BACKGROUND

Virtual simulations can have varying degrees of fidelity. In the same way that instructors must consider the degree to which manikin-based simulators can represent the physical environment, the degree to which virtual simulations represent the physical environment, patient vital signs, and clinical features that are required for the simulation scenario must be considered. Head-mounted displays make high-fidelity virtual simulations possible to experience in a way that is similar to the real thing. Additional technological components, such as gaze tracking, stress monitoring, and physiology engines, may be incorporated into the simulations to enable the activity to track and adapt to the learner's responses. These components may be present in the simulations. The learner engages in interaction with their surroundings through the use of hand controller devices or specialized gloves equipped with tactile feedback (Hunziker et al., 2010; Wetzel, Lang, Pendergrass, Taylor, & Geis, 2013). It is not necessary for the virtual environment to be an exact replica of the actual setting in which the learners work to provide a high-quality learning experience; nonetheless, significant components should be represented to increase training fidelity (Stone, 2011).

Although it is essential for students to have access to the necessary hardware for use in virtual simulation education, it is not sufficient for educational institutions to simply purchase the devices; in addition, they are required to point students in the direction of content that is pertinent to their studies. It can be difficult for directors of simulation facilities to locate and choose appropriate virtual training modules. There is a vast selection of virtual simulations available from a variety of vendors, and the prices for these simulations range from cheap to no cost to thousands of dollars for software that is designed just for the user. In certain training scenarios, however, recent reports have revealed that the cost of conducting the training using virtual simulation can be lower than the cost of conducting the training using manikin-based simulation or live exercises (S. L. Farra et al., 2019; Haerling, 2018). Infrastructure considerations are also significant because certain head-mounted displays call for high-end gaming computers that have a short battery life and an appropriate temperature range to function properly. The use of mobile or tablet devices for running virtual simulations makes them far more portable and suitable for environments with limited resources (Mairami et al., 2019; Vishwanath, Kam, & Kumar, 2017). Virtual simulations, on the other hand, can be easily relocated from one training location to another for in-person instruction, or they can be accessed by learners individually or collectively over the internet from remote geographic locations. In general, virtual simulations offer a number of advantages over manikin-based simulations (Umoren et al., 2014).

To be able to use virtual simulations effectively in educational contexts, the instructor needs to be able to develop and/or offer simulation experiences that assist learners in achieving certain learning goals. This is similar to the situation that exists when using manikin-based simulations. It is the responsibility of simulation educators to establish appropriate learning objectives that can be accomplished in a virtual simulation environment, and then to use these learning objectives to either find or create a simulation scenario that accomplishes these learning objectives. The amount of responsibility that falls on simulation facilitators is significantly reduced when using virtual simulations. This is because the simulation itself can be programmed to independently carry out tasks such as providing an introduction to the activity, monitoring learner responses, and offering standardized feedback. However, it is still vital for instructors to orient learners to virtual simulations as a training modality and to the relevance of the topic that is going to be addressed as well as the learning objectives along with giving them with information on how to access the simulation. Information technology specialists are responsible for the device setup process as well as providing support to simulation educators during simulation sessions. This support includes troubleshooting device issues, cleaning and resetting head-mounted devices after each case, and ensuring proper storage and maintenance (Akaike et al., 2012; Roussin & Weinstock, 2017; Ziv et al., 2006). In this sense, their position is crucial, and it is analogous to the role of simulation technologists when it comes to dealing with manikin-based simulation.

APPROACH TO VIRTUAL SIMULATION DEVELOPMENT

The objectives of this chapter are to describe the types of virtual simulations, considerations and use-cases for virtual simulations in healthcare, the processes and procedures for the use of virtual simulation, and a brief overview to the approach to virtual simulation case development for healthcare professionals. While technical descriptions of 3D graphics modeling and programming of virtual simulations are out of scope for this book, this information is widely available for software platforms such as Unity [Unity Technologies] and

Unreal Engine [Epic Games] used by technical teams for virtual simulation development.

Types of Virtual Reality Simulation

Low-Cost Virtual Reality Simulation

Low-cost virtual reality simulations use mobile devices which the learner may already possess, with few or no additional equipment. Learners can interact with these simulations in specific ways to meet their learning goals, for as by touch or gaze selection. However, these simulations can only present a limited number of alternatives for interactive participation. For instance, low-cost virtual reality simulations can be utilized for rehearsing the processes of neonatal resuscitation; however, these simulations cannot be used for learning the manual components of treatments like as endotracheal intubation or bag and mask breathing. It is possible for represented items and virtual patients to have a high level of fidelity, depending on the level of sophistication of the virtual simulation. This could include the ability to portray spontaneous breathing movements, lung noises, heart sounds, or vocalizations. As a result, the teacher is not required to present the material or explain the context of the healthcare setting to the student because the learner is able to observe the setting on their own. Instructional designers have a responsibility to provide information that indicates the heart rate and rhythm, blood pressure, respiratory rate, and oxygen saturations wherever it is relevant to the scenario. However, they must do so in a way that does not detract from the learning experience.

Low-cost VR training can be used to augment other more high-tech training modalities. For instance, a low-cost virtual reality (VR) simulation might be utilized to reinforce the cognitive phases of cardiopulmonary resuscitation (CPR) and serve as an auxiliary for in-person simulation training. Low-cost VR training has been described for diagnostic skills (Gutiérrez-Maldonado, Ferrer-García, Plasanjuanelo, Andrés-Pueyo, & Talarn-Caparrós, 2015; Riva & Wiederhold, 2015). Simulations of neonatal resuscitation have been carried out with their use becoming more common in recent years (Mairami et al., 2019). Mobile virtual reality simulations involve the user wearing a low-cost head-mounted display in conjunction with a mobile phone that contains a clinical scenario in which the patient requires a procedure. For instance, the patient may require bag and mask ventilation. The user navigates the virtual world by looking about, and selects items by either tapping on the display or pressing a button on the viewer. The user then gives the virtual newborn bag and mask ventilation while receiving visual feedback on chest rise and auditory feedback with ventilation sounds and the babies cry indicating successful resuscitation. The user is given visual feedback on chest rise and auditory feedback with ventilation sounds. The simulation has built-in processes for performance-based feedback and debriefing after each step. In Chapter 6, which is titled "Evaluation of Simulation Performance," additional information on evaluating performance during virtual simulations is offered.

Because simulation education relies heavily on the authenticity of the learner experience, many facilitators who use low-cost virtual simulations find them less desirable due to their lack of interactivity and utility for complex interventions. In addition, low-cost virtual simulations are typically not as realistic as their high-cost counterparts (Chen, Grierson, & Norman, 2015; Nippita et al., 2018; Scholz et al., 2012). Mobile virtual simulations that are used for practicing bag and mask ventilation include animations of virtual "chest rise" with feedback on the rate of ventilation that can be used for just-in-time proof of their success in providing the bag and mask ventilation breaths. This feedback can be used for just-in-time proof that they are successfully providing the bag and mask ventilation breaths. The process of recreating maneuvers that are typically physical actions, such as the steps to improve ventilation, such as repositioning the head or adjusting the mask, is particularly challenging in low-cost virtual simulations. This is because the learner may need to be prompted to perform specific actions to trigger an animation, such as clicking on the forehead or mask, rather than performing the action directly. For example, the steps to improve ventilation include repositioning the head. Another step includes adjusting the mask. It is not known what the influence of this strategy is on learning or how it translates into practice.

However, low-cost VR simulations such as the eHBB VR mobile simulation (UW) have creatively incorporated elements like random changes in room color, receiving blanket, and presence of sink or bucket for hand washing. Infant tone and activity can be realistically simulated through animations and spontaneous breathing and crying. These elements can help to increase immersion in the activity.

Figure 1. eHBB mobile virtual reality simulation

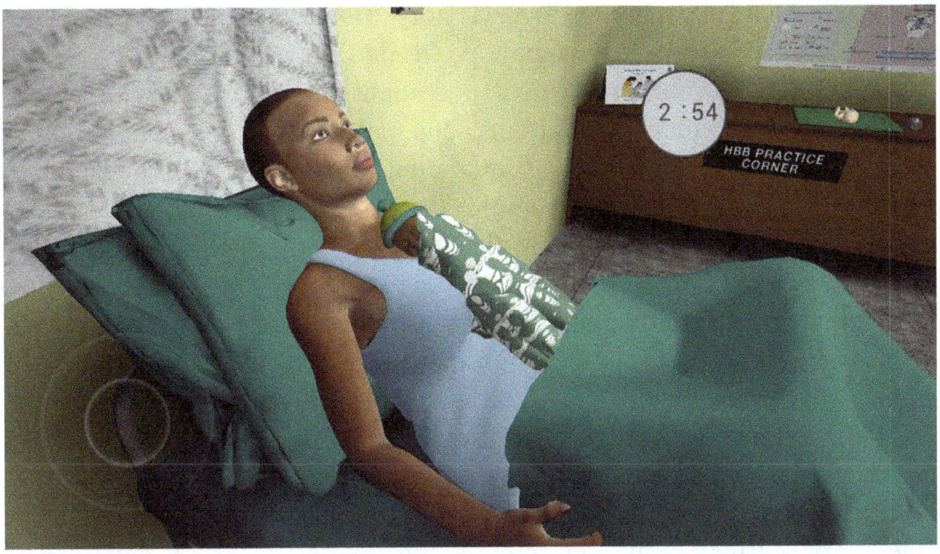

Mobile devices are affordable tools for practicing basic skills and procedures such as bag-and-mask ventilation, cardiopulmonary resuscitation and needle aspiration. Touch Surgery is an example of a mobile virtual simulation which enables learners to practice procedural steps. The limited number of options for interactivity provided by low-cost VR and AR may actually be beneficial for certain learner types and contexts, particularly in low-resource settings and for learners who are unfamiliar with technology. Decreasing the orientation needed for a learner to participate in a training scenario reduces cognitive load(S. A. W. Andersen, Mikkelsen, Konge, Cayé-Thomasen, & Sørensen, 2016; Fraser et al., 2012; Marei, Donkers, Al-Eraky, & Van Merrienboer, 2019). In large, distributed groups, low-cost VR and AR simulations may be preferred as learners can use their own devices with little or no need for instructor assistance (S. A. W. Andersen et al., 2016).

Head Mounted Display Virtual Reality Simulation

Head Mounted Display (HMD) virtual reality (VR) devices offer a greater variety of functions and ways to interact with the environment than cheaper VR devices. The improved graphic options both raise the level of realism of the computer-generated characters and deepen the sense of immersion provided by the encounter. This piece of software can be used to create a representation of the patient or their family's appearance as well as their responses, which may include but are not limited to respiratory effort, perfusion, heart and lung sounds, and cardiorespiratory monitors. In addition, it is possible to recreate the environment for use in inpatient, outpatient, or prehospital settings.

Although all patient simulations, and particularly those representing procedures such as endotracheal intubation, make an effort to accurately represent anatomic features and animated actions, concerns have been raised that these simulations are not realistic enough to support learning goals due to inaccuracies in how the features are represented. Nevertheless, magnetic resonance imaging and computed tomography scans may now be translated to 3D models, which enables an extraordinarily exact recreation of anatomical features in some circumstances (Ammanuel, Brown, Uribe, & Rehani, 2019; Ceccaldi et al., 2019). These have been utilized well for pre-operative preparation as well as educational purposes for parents..

One further thing to think about when it comes to virtual simulations is whether or not they require an internet connection for certain functions or all of them. Connectivity to the internet is necessary for playing any multi-player virtual simulation. On the other hand, some single-player activities and virtual patients that are enabled with artificial intelligence might not. If a simulation includes services such as automatic conversation and feedback that need "server-side" processing, then the simulation will need to be connected to the internet in order for these functions to work properly.

When it comes to the amount of space that is needed, the majority of VR activities require a certain location for each student. This location is decided by whether the activity must be completed while seated or standing, and whether or not there is room for movement inside the activity. The question of whether or not the virtual reality head-mounted display (VR HMD) is tethered is also relevant. Virtual reality head-mounted displays (HMDs) can be cordless or tethered to a laptop with VR capabilities. Models that are more recent that are wireless and "untethered" allow for greater flexibility of movement and lessen the risk of tripping, but also have restrictions on the kinds of activities that can be done and the duration of battery life. However, they are more portable and can be utilized in a variety of settings, including at home, in classrooms, and during simulations. They can also be carried from one location to another. A number of the tools also offer feedback on the user's performance in real time.

Figure 2. Diagram showing (a) Wireless VR Head-mounted display (HMD) and (b) tethered VR HMD connected to VR-capable laptop

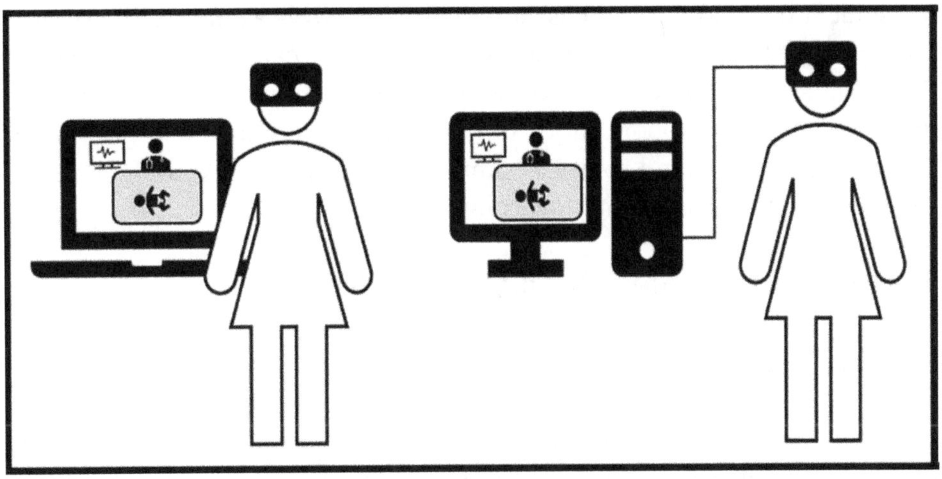

While manikin-based simulations are often used for procedural skills practice, virtual simulations are frequently utilized for gathering patient histories, communicating with patients, and simulating team-based scenarios (Peddle et al., 2019; Umoren RA, 2017). In these situations, the students exhibit their mastery of the material by posing questions or offering comments that reflect empathy (Motz et al., 2018). The use of virtual simulations in scenario-based training that places individuals within the framework of a simulated patient care team has become increasingly common in recent years. An additional option is for a group of students to participate together in a scenario that is hosted on a multiplayer website. The evolution of virtual reality platforms has resulted in an increase in the level of realism achieved by the platforms' avatars, who now exhibit facial expressions and hand movements that are eerily similar to those of the user. Hand-held controls allow facilitators to exercise control over the replies of their avatars. These steps can be driven by the participant, or they can be pre-programmed into the software, so that when an appropriate action is carried out by the learner, the activity automatically provides feedback or advances the scenario. Alternatively, these steps can be driven by a combination of both the participant and the software. The facilitator has the option of taking part in synchronous multiplayer activities or conducting post-event debriefing with the students who are using the virtual simulation to attain certain learning goals (Umoren et al., 2018; Umoren et al., 2014). The access granted to the facilitator in certain virtual simulations may include additional controls that, when activated, might cause changes to the simulation that either make it easier or more difficult to complete. Since the student does not have access to the same controls as the facilitator, it is possible that this will not be clear to the learner. Learners can take part in these kinds of simulations with or without the constraint of a time limit, and they have multiple opportunities to improve their abilities and get further experience. As in manikin-based simulation, virtual simulation debriefing and reflection aid experiential learning.

Types of Augmented Reality Simulation

Mobile Augmented Reality

Low-cost augmented reality simulations can be experienced on mobile phones and tablets and can also be used along with standardized patients and manikins (D. Andersen et al., 2017; Cao & Cerfolio, 2019; Gerup, Soerensen, & Dieckmann, 2020; Kaplan et al., 2020). A mobile augmented reality simulation can, for instance, be used in conjunction with a low-fidelity manikin to convey extra information such as changes in vital signs and depict physical responses such as cyanosis to advanced resuscitation and operations. Simulation in medicine and surgery has produced use cases that have been described (D. Andersen et al., 2016; D. Andersen et al., 2017; Nifakos & Zary, 2014). Even though the low-cost AR simulation and manikin combination might not have the same technological capabilities as the high-fidelity manikin, the fact that mobile phones are available at a lower cost than augmented reality headsets means that mobile AR can be employed in settings with fewer resources.

Figure 3. Diagram showing (a) Mobile augmented reality and (b) Augmented reality headset

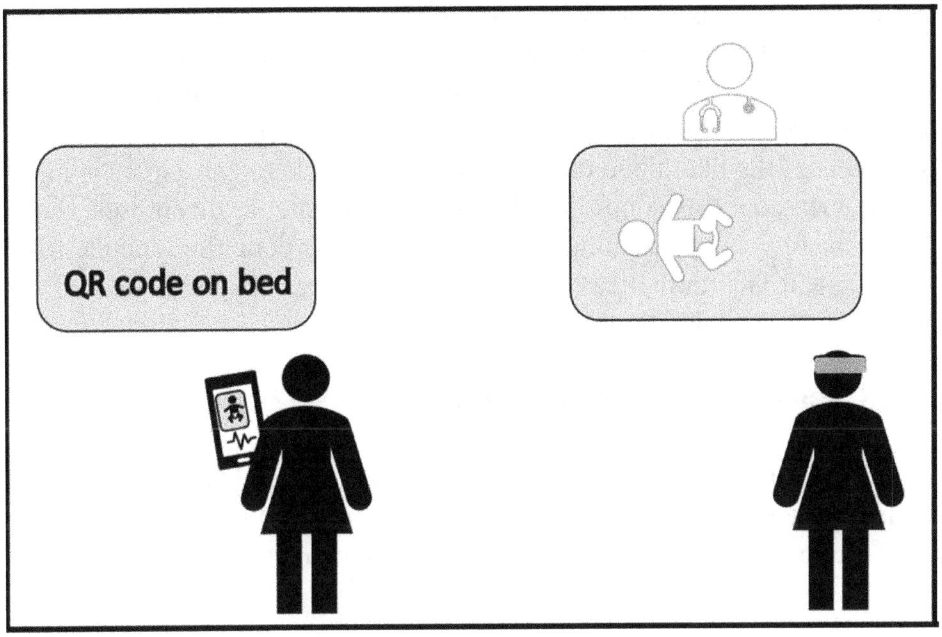

Augmented Reality Headsets

Augmented Reality (AR) headsets differ from VR HMDs in that rather than being placed in a computer-generated environment through the headset, the learner can see computer-generated objects in their actual environment. Because the simulations take place in the same clinical setting as the learners' actual practice, the ability to visualize the surroundings allows for a higher level of realism to be achieved in these exercises. In addition, some augmented reality headsets include features that allow remote instructors to monitor what their students are viewing and annotate on their field of view. Although augmented reality headsets can cost up to three times as much as high-end mobile phones, they have substantial advantages over mobile augmented reality in that they do not require the user to have their hands free to carry out the procedures that are being simulated. In addition, they have been used in conjunction with training that is based on manikins to show internal organs and functions such as the activity of the heart and lungs, as well as the position of the fetus within the uterus of the mother in cases involving obstetrics. This is accomplished by superimposing computer-generated images and objects onto the manikin in question. For instance, the Lucina AR (CAE Healthcare) manikin is an obstetric manikin that, when combined with the Microsoft HoloLens AR headset, enables a learner or group of learners to observe the process of birth. This manikin is manufactured by CAE Healthcare. However, these activity possibilities are restricted, and because of this, simulation programs frequently have access to only a few augmented reality headsets. This reduces the likelihood that students will be able to participate in high-end augmented reality simulation. However, augmented reality presents huge prospects for communication, remote assistance, depicting standardized patients, and facilitating team-based learning. These are only a few of the many potential applications of AR.

Use Cases for Virtual Simulation

Virtual simulation has been used for training in technical and non-technical skills. While many virtual simulation use cases support individual learning, there are some group learning options. These include but are not limited to:

Procedural Skills

Virtual simulations have been used for training on airway procedures such as endotracheal intubation which is important for emergency medicine, adult, pediatric and newborn intensive care. Both low-cost mobile phone-base simulations and HMD devices with controllers have been used (De Oliveira, Glassenberg, Chang, Fitzgerald, & McCarthy, 2013; Walker, Underwood, Bernhagen, Markin, & Boedeker, 2012; Wong et al., 2019). It is thought that these simulations increase the learners' knowledge of anatomical landmarks which can contribute to clinical success. However, the motor skills are difficult to teach in this way without significant enhancements for tactile feedback (Kuchenbecker, Parajon, & Maggio, 2017; Patel et al., 2014). In general, the steps of procedures and complications can be readily taught through virtual simulations (both AR and VR). However, manikin-based training is generally considered to be essential for supplementing virtual training in activities with a significant procedural component like endotracheal intubation and intravenous access (Andreatta et al., 2015; Garner, Prater, Raj, Leena, & Anitha, 2018; Günay İsmailoğlu & Zaybak, 2018; Keleekai et al., 2016; Loukas, Nikiteas, Kanakis, & Georgiou, 2011; Loukas et al., 2010; Yousif, Machan, Alaska, & Suner, 2017).

Diagnostic and Therapeutic Procedures

Diagnostic and therapeutic procedures such as thoracocentesis and laparoscopic surgery can be practiced on virtual reality simulators (Clements, Morrison, & Schenkman, 2016; Lin et al., 2009; Vaccaro et al., 2013; Valdis et al., 2016). Learners are able to go through the steps of performing the procedure thanks to simulations of these procedures performed by professionals in surgical disciplines such as urology and gastrointestinal surgery. It is the responsibility of the instructors to make sure that important tasks including obtaining the patient's informed consent, preparing the patient for surgery, managing difficulties, and dealing with the surgical team are emphasized (Stevens, Galloway, & Willemsen-Dunlap, 2019). In situations in which operations are only carried out infrequently, simulation can be used for both initial training and ongoing skill maintenance. It is vital to provide learners with the opportunity to practice the steps to guarantee both the quality and safety of patient care. This is also true in simulations that use manikins. Learners are able to go through the steps of performing the procedure thanks to simulations of these procedures performed by professionals in surgical disciplines such as urology and gastrointestinal surgery. It is the responsibility of the instructors to make sure that important tasks including obtaining the patient's informed consent, preparing the patient for surgery, managing difficulties, and dealing with the surgical team are emphasized (Stevens, Galloway, & Willemsen-Dunlap, 2019). In situations in which operations are only carried out infrequently, simulation can be used for both initial training and ongoing skill maintenance. It is vital to provide learners with the opportunity to practice the steps to guarantee both the quality and safety of patient care. This is also true in simulations that use manikins.

Communication and Teamwork

Virtual simulations have been extensively used for communication and teamwork training(Caylor, Aebersold, Lapham, & Carlson, 2015; Sweigart L, 2015; Umoren RA, 2017; R. A. Umoren et al., 2018). For the purpose of providing a framework for communication and team training in virtual scenarios ("Agency for Healthcare Research and Quality TeamSTEPPS® 2.0," 2016; Harvey, Wright, Taylor, Bath, & Collier, 2013), structured communication tools and strategies have been utilized. One example of this is the TEAMSTEPPS program, which stands for "Team Strategies and Tools for

Enhancing Patient Safety." These situations can be played by a single player or by multiple players simultaneously. The learner could be put in a situation where they have to interact with a virtual team or with other learners who are in different locations all over the world. The use of virtual simulations that feature avatars can have the benefit of either portraying roles that learners may not generally play in clinical settings or depicting locations and clinical settings to boost the level of realism experienced during the learning process.

Disaster Simulations

Virtual simulations have found practice use in disaster simulations and emergency triage training. Hospitals have been forced to evacuate patients due to a variety of natural disasters, including fires, floods, earthquakes, and hurricanes. The staff members of the hospital need to receive training on what to do in the event of an emergency. However, the organization of live simulations of this nature is notoriously challenging and expensive. It has been suggested that emergency room and newborn intensive care evacuation training could benefit from the use of virtual simulations. This would be a simple way to train healthcare staff (S. Farra et al., 2019; Farra, Miller, & Hodgson, 2015; Sharon Lee Farra et al., 2015; Gray, Thomas, Burns, & Umoren, 2019).

Virtual Scenario Development

The purpose of a simulation scenario is to help healthcare professionals acquire the knowledge and understanding to anticipate actions that they may need to carry out in a clinical context. Nevertheless, to make the most out of the employment of virtual scenarios, it is necessary for both the learner and the instructor to have faith in the legitimacy, significance, and worth of the procedure. The direct participation of stakeholders in the creation of scenarios as usability testers will ensure that they truly understand, own, and are therefore more likely to utilize or assist with the deployment of the scenarios. While a team of scenario developers is required to develop an appropriate and immersive scenario that provides the necessary context for learner actions and decisions, the direct participation of stakeholders in the creation of scenarios will ensure this. This section explains the essential steps of the process of developing a virtual scenario and gives a guide to what is involved in the creation of virtual healthcare simulations. Creating virtual healthcare simulations requires a lot of work.

While commercial and institutional groups have developed virtual simulation scenarios for basic life support, adult and pediatric advanced life support and neonatal resuscitation, there are relatively fewer specialized scenarios available. Some virtual simulation systems include customization options for facilitators. These features are useful for facilitators who may need to adapt the situations to the hospital or clinic in which they work. However, these possibilities are typically quite pricey; therefore, locating virtual simulations that are customizable "out of the box" is essential in the event that simulation teachers do not possess the expertise necessary to construct their own. This is especially the case when the situation at hand is unusual or requires a high level of expertise, both of which make it doubtful that a customization would be financially viable. It does not matter if the facilitator is tailoring an existing scenario or if they are creating a brand-new scenario; having clearly stated goals is an absolute necessity in either case. Since the implementation of the scenario is often dependent on non-clinical developers, clinical expertise must be provided together with vigilant oversight to guarantee that inaccuracies are avoided. This is necessary to ensure that the scenario is carried out correctly. Therefore, it is the responsibility of the clinical expert (the simulation instructor or the internal consultant) to provide a description of the patient as well as the patient's response to the activities that are anticipated from the learners. During the process of designing and evaluating brand-new virtual scenarios, it is essential to incorporate a wide variety of stakeholders, including experts in information technology as well as the end-users themselves.

Customizing an Existing Scenario

The process of customizing an existing scenario enables facilitators experienced in simulation scenario development and execution to take advantage of existing commercial simulations in an effective manner and deploy new scenarios quickly to learners. In accordance with what is presented in Chapter 3, "Approach to scenario development for manikin-based simulation", the process of customizing a scenario starts with an assessment of the scenario objectives to determine whether they coincide with your educational goals. If they do not, then you may be able to personalize the scenario to coincide with your goals if the overall environment (inpatient or outpatient) and the characters (physicians, nurses, parents) are comparable or the same. This is the case if the scenario involves a medical setting. Additionally, the addition of new characters is a possibility; however, doing so will necessitate the involvement of the development team. Depending on the extent to which the design of the original simulation permits customization, the addition of new objects and characters into the environment may either be highly feasible or expensive. This will depend on the degree to which the design of the original simulation permits customization. The target demographic should be the next thing you think about. It may be reasonably easy to employ the same environment for a new scenario, even if the audience (or learner group) of the original scenario does not match the learner group that you are teaching. The level of difficulty of the situation is the final factor to take into consideration. A common feature of simulation games is the gradual increase in challenge that players experience as they move through the game. Because of this, you might be able to provide support for learners of varying levels using the same virtual simulation. It is essential to run the modified scenario past individuals who were not involved in the construction of the scenario to assess the scenario's level of clarity and calculate the typical amount of time required to finish the scenario.

Creating a New Scenario

The process of creating a new scenario has two major parts: first, choosing learning objectives, a task that comprises identifying the learner type and need; and second, describing the events that will occur within the simulation and their implications. While the initial work of identifying learning objectives and goals can be performed by content experts, significant input is needed from computer programmers and game designers on the second major task of scenario planning - implementing the design in a way that tells the story and engages the learner. When planning your scenario, consider different levels of learner and the potential for use across different health professions.

When it comes to supporting simulation-based education that can be transferred to clinical practice, immersive virtual simulations have the potential to be highly powerful tools. To avoid inaccurate teaching and the tremendous effect that imagery may have on learning and memory, developing virtual scenarios demands an in-depth knowledge of the subject. It is possible that you will need to contact references or subject-matter experts, just as you did with the manikin-based situations. After you have gathered information on the topic, the next step is to identify your learning goals. In an ideal world, two or three learning objectives should be explicitly articulated for each scenario, using terminology that are measurable. Choose learning goals that can be witnessed during the scenario so that you can gauge how well students are doing with them. Simulations offer students the chance to demonstrate what they've learned through observable action. When defining learning objectives, the terms shown in the following graphic are some examples of those that should be avoided.

Table 1. Words to avoid when defining learning objectives

appreciate	believe	improve	learn
approach	grasp	increase	think
become	grow	know	understand

After defining your learning objectives, define the clinical setting and patient characteristics for the facilitator. Include a list of items or "objects" needed for the scenario. Provide a short introduction to orient the learner to the scenario. Then list expected participant actions and the manikin's response including appearance and vital signs. Like manikin-based scenarios, virtual scenarios will have three main stages: Initial, Middle, and End. See Tables 2 and 3 for a simple scenario template and sample scenario.

Table 2. Simple scenario template

Stage	Learner Action	Object Response	Standardized Feedback
Initial			
Middle			
End			

Initial Stage

The Initial stage or beginning of a scenario features the introduction which may include the baseline state or vital signs. If the scenario includes a virtual patient, the patient may start with a normal or abnormal baseline with potential for further deterioration.

Middle Stage

In the middle stage, there can be an automatic change from baseline, or the user actions may trigger a change in the patient's clinical symptoms and signs. For example, a patient with a pericardial effusion will have diminished cardiac sounds, tachycardia (increased heart rate), and widened pulse pressures. The learner must recognize this rare condition and specific actions including positioning the patient and performing pericardial tap are needed stabilize the patient. If these actions are not performed quickly, the patient's condition continues to deteriorate with bradycardia (low heart rate) cyanosis, and decreased oxygen saturations.

End Stage

For virtual patient scenarios, the endpoint occurs after appropriate actions have been performed and the patient's condition improved bringing the scenario to the End stage. However, in some cases, the learner fails to perform the correct actions. While in manikin-based scenarios, the facilitator may truncate the scenario and move to debrief or discuss the case, asynchronous virtual scenarios may offer "help" options or may time-out and allow the learner to try again by restarting the scenario. This is one of the advantages of virtual simulations – the opportunity to have an unlimited number of attempts.

Table 3. Simple scenario example

Stage	Learner Action	Object Response	Standardized Feedback
Initial Delivery of a full-term newborn without respiratory effort, floppy with poor tone and no cry.	Select warmer to place infant. Select cloth to dry and stimulate the baby using cloth drying animation. Select virtual stethoscope to hear heartbeat.	No change in respiratory effort and tone with stimulation. Heart rate 80bpm (heard with use of virtual stethoscope)	Text-based or audible feedback or points for each correct step. Low heart rate.
Middle Initiation of positive pressure ventilation	Select bag and mask device to start positive pressure ventilation (PPV) by 60 seconds of life. Select bag to give breaths and continues PPV for at least 30 seconds. Select stethoscope to hear breath sounds and heartbeat.	Chest movement with PPV. Spontaneous breathing and crying animation triggers after 30 seconds of PPV. Breath sounds heard bilaterally with use of stethoscope. Heart rate 120 bpm with use of stethoscope.	Text-based or audible feedback or points for each correct step. Spontaneous breathing and crying animation Increasing heart rate.
End Assessment of response to PPV and ongoing supportive care.	Select bag and mask device to stop PPV. Select hat to place on baby's head to keep warm. Select stethoscope to hear heartbeat.	Continues spontaneous breathing and crying animation. Heart rate 140bpm.	Text-based or audible feedback or points for each correct step. Spontaneous breathing and crying animation. Normal heart rate.

Storyboarding Techniques

A good scenario is very much a story, and a good simulation should feel like a game to the learner - a serious game. A "storyboard" can be used to plan the initial, middle and end stages using text and graphics that will be represented along with the virtual environment for virtual reality simulations or the physical environment for augmented reality simulations. The storyboard illustrates the various characters, objects, and settings, as well as the order in which they will appear in each scene, as well as how the learner and the facilitators will influence the progression of the story. Instead of focusing on only one learner group, it might be more beneficial to build a scenario that is applicable to a variety of learners; in this case, the "avatar" that represents the learner should probably have a variety of customizable options and an appearance that reflects this. There are many different ways to depict storyboards, ranging from hand-drawn illustrations to computer-generated imagery. During the process of scenario development, the simulation development team, which consists of a simulation expert, a scenario programmer, and a graphics designer/animator, uses this form to interact with one another. It is possible that using specialized software will help to support the process of storyboarding a more complex series of events in situations in which there are branching aspects in the scenarios.

To get started, you should design a prototype that has all of the important game features and interactions, including feedback. Put this prototype through its paces with a few end-users, including some learners and facilitators, to ascertain whether or not they find it easy to use and to get their initial thoughts on the product. It's possible that the next step will require going back to the "drawing board" and making significant as well as minor adjustments to the graphics and interactions. At this stage, it is essential to pay close attention to the input to prevent the need for major redesign requirements after a significant amount of preliminary effort has been put into the simulation. Further iterations of development and pilot testing are being conducted with the primary goal of ensuring that the simulation will assist the learner in meeting the learning goals that have been established.

Writing a script entails coming up with the dialogue that the different characters of a computer game or simulation will use. The virtual scenario will now include these scripts when it is complete. It is essential to run scripts for a variety of professions by subject matter experts to ascertain whether or not the scripts are accurate representations of usual statements, as well as whether or not the material is authentic.

When it comes to aiding the process from planning and scenario development all the way through execution, a project manager could be helpful. This individual will be responsible for developing a project plan, which will include both fundamental performance targets and important technical milestones. Above all else, it is crucial to keep the focus on the end goal, which is to enable the end user to achieve the specified learning objectives and intended educational results while being interested and challenged throughout the virtual simulation.

Virtual Simulation Debriefing and Feedback

Although real-time debriefing is challenging, virtual scenarios should have built-in automated feedback (Stathakarou, Kononowicz, Henningsohn, & McGrath, 2018). See Figure 4.

Figure 4. Built-in performance-based standardized feedback in mobile eHBB simulation

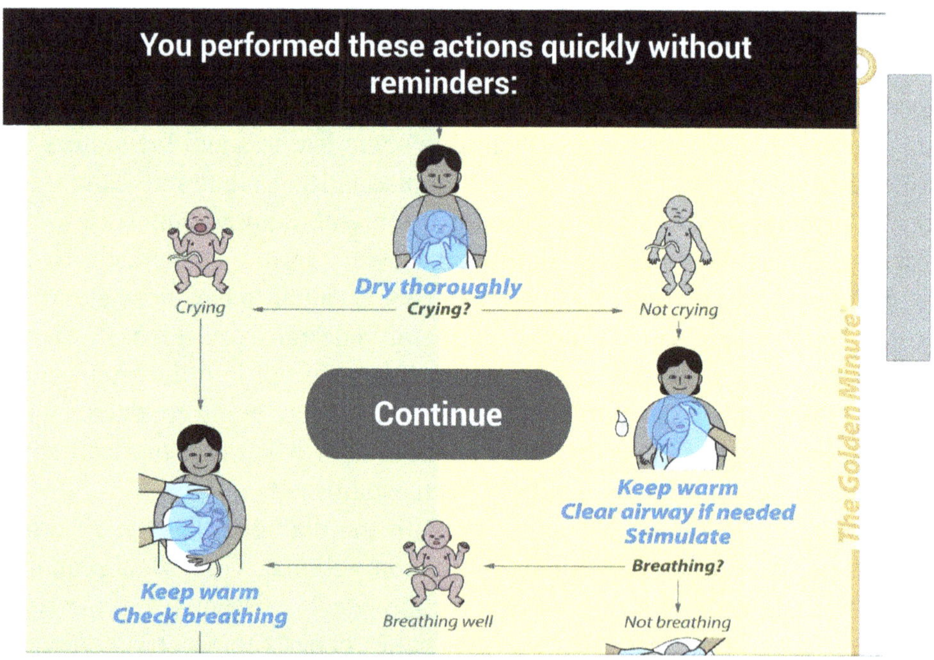

As an alternative, debriefing questions using a standardized format such as the following can be used as prompts such as:

What was the condition of the patient
What went well?
What didn't go well?
What will you do differently next time

Where possible, to demonstrate learning, have the learner indicate in the environment what they will do differently next time. This can be captured for evaluation of the activity. See Figure 5.

Figure 5. Debriefing question to promote learner reflection in mobile eHBB simulation

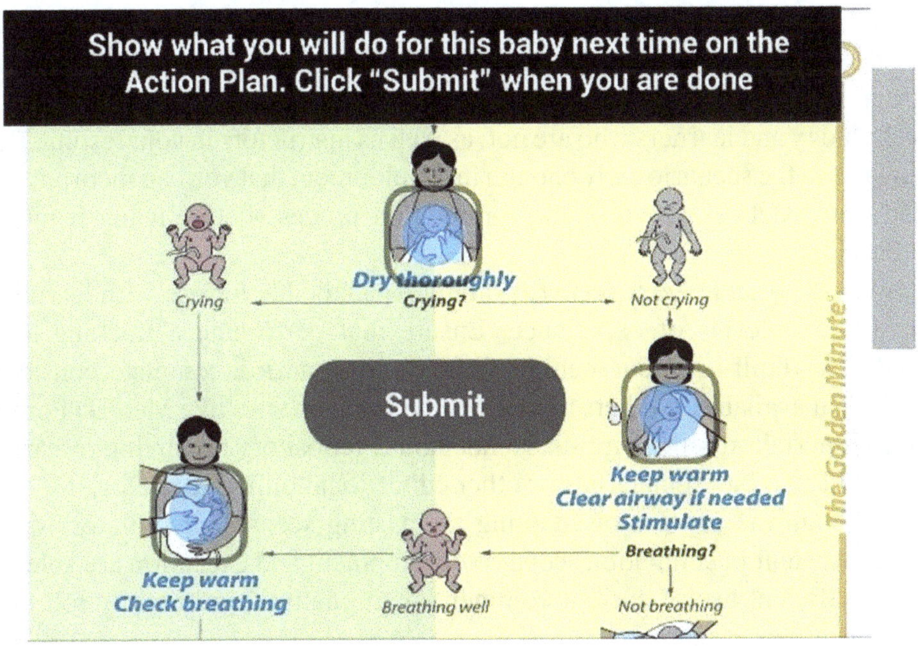

However, there are other ways to provide objective feedback through data collected through the scenario. We will discuss this in more detail in the Chapter 6. Evaluation of Simulation Performance. Learners can also respond to questions during debriefing done outside the scenario. In addition, learners can provide written responses to a standard set of questions to assess knowledge. For example, in the scenario on pericardial effusion, the scenario debriefer might ask:

What made you suspect a pericardial effusion? or
How would you diagnose a pericardial effusion?

SOLUTIONS AND RECOMMENDATIONS

Virtual simulations have been widely applied in health professional education and simulation educators should familiarize themselves with both virtual and augmented reality simulations. It is particularly important to identify suitable activities which can be readily accessed by learners and instructors and can be customized for various situations. When developing a new virtual scenario, utilize the expertise of content experts and software developers.

Test the new virtual scenario you have created with a small but representative group of learners. Consider including both learners who are familiar with technology and learners who are not; as well as instructors in your testing. Be sure to test the scenario early enough in development that you can incorporate end-user feedback and test your orientation process before using it more broadly.

Where possible, your scenario should be adaptable for use with learners of different levels of experience. Ensure that performance tracking and feedback is built-in to your scenario. When your scenario is complete, consider making it available to others through publication on sites like MedED Portal (mededportal.org), the Virginia Henderson E-repository of nursing research and evidence-based materials or other educational online repositories.

Through the process of adapting an existing scenario, facilitators who are competent in simulation scenario development and execution are able to make efficient use of current commercial simulations and rapidly roll out new scenarios to learners.

FUTURE RESEARCH DIRECTIONS

Areas for future research in virtual scenario development include incorporating adaptive learning elements and testing training effectiveness in various learner groups and settings. The goal of a simulation scenario is to provide medical professionals with the opportunity to improve their level of knowledge and comprehension to improve their ability to plan and prepare for potential actions that may be required of them in a clinical setting. However, to get the most out of the use of virtual scenarios, it is required for the learner as well as the teacher to have faith in the legitimacy, relevance, and worth of the process. This is the case to get the most of the use of virtual scenarios. The direct participation of stakeholders in the creation of scenarios as usability testers will ensure that they truly understand, own, and are consequently more likely to utilize or assist with the deployment of the scenarios. This can be accomplished by ensuring that they participate in the creation of the scenarios.

CONCLUSION

In conclusion, VR and AR simulation can be performed with a range of devices including mobile phones and head mounted displays or headsets. The choice of what type of device to use depends on the learning objectives, the learner characteristics, the availability of devices to learners, and the experience and comfort level of the facilitator. Virtual scenarios can be adapted or created to meet learning objectives. A good scenario is essentially a story, and a successful simulation facilitates learner engagement, attention and reflection. Text and graphics that will be represented along with the virtual environment for virtual reality simulations or the physical environment for augmented reality simulations can be planned using a "storyboard." This is a tool that can be used to plan the beginning, middle, and end stages of a simulation. Finally, new scenarios must be developed with expert input to ensure that learning objectives are met, and attention must be given to early end-user testing for newly created scenarios to ensure that they are easy to use and effective for the intended learner group.

REFERENCES

Agency for Healthcare Research and Quality TeamSTEPPS® 2.0. (2016). Retrieved from https://www.ahrq.gov/teamstepps/instructor/index.html

Akaike, M., Fukutomi, M., Nagamune, M., Fujimoto, A., Tsuji, A., Ishida, K., & Iwata, T. (2012). Simulation-based medical education in clinical skills laboratory. *The Journal of Medical Investigation*, *59*(1-2), 28–35. doi:10.2152/jmi.59.28 PMID:22449990

Ammanuel, S., Brown, I., Uribe, J., & Rehani, B. (2019). Creating 3D models from Radiologic Images for Virtual Reality Medical Education Modules. *Journal of Medical Systems*, *43*(6), 166–166. doi:10.100710916-019-1308-3 PMID:31053902

Andersen, D., Popescu, V., Cabrera, M. E., Shanghavi, A., Gomez, G., Marley, S., Mullis, B., & Wachs, J. P. (2016). Medical telementoring using an augmented reality transparent display. *Surgery*, *159*(6), 1646–1653. doi:10.1016/j.surg.2015.12.016 PMID:26804823

Andersen, D., Popescu, V., Cabrera, M. E., Shanghavi, A., Mullis, B., Marley, S., Gomez, G., & Wachs, J. P. (2017). An Augmented Reality-Based Approach for Surgical Telementoring in Austere Environments. *Military Medicine*, *182*(S1), 310–315. doi:10.7205/MILMED-D-16-00051 PMID:28291491

Andersen, S. A. W., Mikkelsen, P. T., Konge, L., Cayé-Thomasen, P., & Sørensen, M. S. (2016). Cognitive load in distributed and massed practice in virtual reality mastoidectomy simulation. *The Laryngoscope*, *126*(2), E74–E79. doi:10.1002/lary.25449 PMID:26153783

Andreatta, P. B., Klotz, J. J., Dooley-Hash, S. L., Hauptman, J. G., Biddinger, B., & House, J. B. (2015). Performance-based comparison of neonatal intubation training outcomes: simulator and live animal. *Advances in Neonatal Care: Official Journal of the National Association of Neonatal Nurses, 15*(1), 56-64. doi:10.1097/ANC.0000000000000130

Cao, C., & Cerfolio, R. J. (2019). Virtual or Augmented Reality to Enhance Surgical Education and Surgical Planning. *Thoracic Surgery Clinics*, *29*(3), 329–337. doi:10.1016/j.thorsurg.2019.03.010 PMID:31235302

Caylor, S., Aebersold, M., Lapham, J., & Carlson, E. (2015). The use of virtual simulation and a modified teamSTEPPS™ training for multiprofessional education. *Clinical Simulation in Nursing*, *11*(3), 163–171. doi:10.1016/j.ecns.2014.12.003

Ceccaldi, P.-F., Pirtea, P., Lemarteleur, V., Poulain, M., Ziegler, D. D., & Ayoubi, J.-M. (2019). Simulation and professional development: added value of 3D modelization in reproductive endocrinology and infertility and assisted reproductive technologies teamwork. *Gynecological Endocrinology: The Official Journal of the International Society of Gynecological Endocrinology, 35*(7), 559-563. doi:10.1080/09513590.2019.1588874

Chen, R., Grierson, L. E., & Norman, G. R. (2015). Evaluating the impact of high- and low-fidelity instruction in the development of auscultation skills. *Medical Education*, *49*(3), 276–285. doi:10.1111/medu.12653 PMID:25693987

Clements, M. B., Morrison, K. Y., & Schenkman, N. S. (2016). Evaluation of Laparoscopic Curricula in American Urology Residency Training: A 5-Year Update. *Journal of Endourology*, *30*(3), 347–353. doi:10.1089/end.2015.0561 PMID:26731240

Combs, C. D., & Combs, P. F. (2019). Emerging Roles of Virtual Patients in the Age of AI. *AMA Journal of Ethics*, *21*(2), E153–E159. doi:10.1001/amajethics.2019.153 PMID:30794125

De Oliveira, G. S. Jr, Glassenberg, R., Chang, R., Fitzgerald, P., & McCarthy, R. J. (2013). Virtual airway simulation to improve dexterity among novices performing fibreoptic intubation. *Anaesthesia*, *68*(10), 1053–1058. doi:10.1111/anae.12379 PMID:23952805

Evans, C. H., & Schenarts, K. D. (2016). Evolving Educational Techniques in Surgical Training. *The Surgical Clinics of North America*, *96*(1), 71–88. doi:10.1016/j.suc.2015.09.005 PMID:26612021

Farra, S., Hodgson, E., Miller, E. T., Timm, N., Brady, W., Gneuhs, M., Ying, J., Hausfeld, J., Cosgrove, E., Simon, A., & Bottomley, M. (2019). Effects of Virtual Reality Simulation on Worker Emergency Evacuation of Neonates. *Disaster Medicine and Public Health Preparedness*, *13*(2), 301–308. doi:10.1017/dmp.2018.58 PMID:30293544

Farra, S. L., Gneuhs, M., Hodgson, E., Kawosa, B., Miller, E. T., Simon, A., Timm, N., & Hausfeld, J. (2019). Comparative Cost of Virtual Reality Training and Live Exercises for Training Hospital Workers for Evacuation. *Computers, informatics, nursing. CIN*, *37*(9), 446–454. doi:10.1097/CIN.0000000000000540 PMID:31166203

Farra, S. L., Miller, E. T., & Hodgson, E. (2015). Virtual reality disaster training: Translation to practice. *Nurse Education in Practice*, *15*(1), 53–57. doi:10.1016/j.nepr.2013.08.017 PMID:24063793

Farra, S. L., Smith, S., Gillespie, G. L., Nicely, S., Ulrich, D. L., Hodgson, E., & French, D. (2015). Decontamination training: With and without virtual reality simulation. *Advanced Emergency Nursing Journal*, *37*(2), 125–133. doi:10.1097/TME.0000000000000059 PMID:25929223

Fraser, K., Ma, I., Teteris, E., Baxter, H., Wright, B., & McLaughlin, K. (2012). Emotion, cognitive load and learning outcomes during simulation training. *Medical Education*, *46*(11), 1055–1062. doi:10.1111/j.1365-2923.2012.04355.x PMID:23078682

Garner, S. L., Prater, L. S., Raj, L., Leena, G. V., & Anitha, A. J. J. (2018). Effectiveness of Peripheral Intravenous Skill Continuing Education Using Low-Fidelity Simulation Among Nurses in India. *Journal of Continuing Education in Nursing*, *49*(6), 255–261. doi:10.3928/00220124-20180517-05 PMID:29847683

Gerup, J., Soerensen, C. B., & Dieckmann, P. (2020). Augmented reality and mixed reality for healthcare education beyond surgery: An integrative review. *International Journal of Medical Education*, *11*, 1–18. doi:10.5116/ijme.5e01.eb1a PMID:31955150

Gray, M. M., Thomas, A. A., Burns, B., & Umoren, R. A. (2019). Identifying Crucial Equipment and Skills Needed to Evacuate Critically Ill Infants During Disasters: Using Nursing Expertise to Guide Training Targets. *Prehospital and Disaster Medicine*, *34*(4), 370–375. doi:10.1017/S1049023X19004473 PMID:31239004

Günay İsmailoğlu, E., & Zaybak, A. (2018). Comparison of the Effectiveness of a Virtual Simulator With a Plastic Arm Model in Teaching Intravenous Catheter Insertion Skills. *Computers, informatics, nursing. CIN*, *36*(2), 98–105. doi:10.1097/CIN.0000000000000405 PMID:29176359

Gutiérrez-Maldonado, J., Ferrer-García, M., Plasanjuanelo, J., Andrés-Pueyo, A., & Talarn-Caparrós, A. (2015). Virtual Reality to Train Diagnostic Skills in Eating Disorders. Comparison of two Low Cost Systems. *Studies in Health Technology and Informatics*, *219*, 75–81. https://pubmed.ncbi.nlm.nih.gov/26799883 PMID:26799883

Haerling, K. A. (2018). Cost-Utility Analysis of Virtual and Mannequin-Based Simulation. *Simulation in Healthcare: Journal of the Society for Simulation in Healthcare, 13*(1), 33-40. doi:10.1097/SIH.0000000000000280

Harvey, E. M., Wright, A., Taylor, D., Bath, J., & Collier, B. (2013). TeamSTEPPS(®) simulation-based training: An evidence-based strategy to improve trauma team performance. *Journal of Continuing Education in Nursing*, *44*(11), 484–485. doi:10.3928/00220124-20131025-92 PMID:24199639

Hunziker, S., Buhlmann, C., Tschan, F., Balestra, G., Legeret, C., Schumacher, C., Semmer, N. K., Hunziker, P., & Marsch, S. (2010). Brief leadership instructions improve cardiopulmonary resuscitation in a high-fidelity simulation: A randomized controlled trial. *Critical Care Medicine, 38*(4), 1086–1091. Advance online publication. doi:10.1097/CCM.0b013e3181cf7383 PMID:20124886

Isaza-Restrepo, A., Gómez, M. T., Cifuentes, G., & Argüello, A. (2018). The virtual patient as a learning tool: A mixed quantitative qualitative study. *BMC Medical Education, 18*(1), 297–297. doi:10.118612909-018-1395-8 PMID:30522478

Kaplan, A. D., Cruit, J., Endsley, M., Beers, S. M., Sawyer, B. D., & Hancock, P. (2020). The Effects of Virtual Reality, Augmented Reality, and Mixed Reality as Training Enhancement Methods: A Meta-Analysis. *Human Factors*. PMID:32091937

Keleekai, N. L., Schuster, C. A., Murray, C. L., King, M. A., Stahl, B. R., Labrozzi, L. J., . . . Glover, K. R. (2016). Improving Nurses' Peripheral Intravenous Catheter Insertion Knowledge, Confidence, and Skills Using a Simulation-Based Blended Learning Program: A Randomized Trial. *Simulation in Healthcare: Journal of the Society for Simulation in Healthcare, 11*(6), 376-384. doi:10.1097/SIH.0000000000000186

Kononowicz, A. A., Woodham, L. A., Edelbring, S., Stathakarou, N., Davies, D., Saxena, N., Tudor Car, L., Carlstedt-Duke, J., Car, J., & Zary, N. (2019). Virtual Patient Simulations in Health Professions Education: Systematic Review and Meta-Analysis by the Digital Health Education Collaboration. *Journal of Medical Internet Research, 21*(7), e14676. doi:10.2196/14676 PMID:31267981

Kuchenbecker, K. J., Parajon, R. C., & Maggio, M. P. (2017). Evaluation of a Vibrotactile Simulator for Dental Caries Detection. *Simulation in Healthcare: Journal of the Society for Simulation in Healthcare, 12*(3), 148-156. doi:10.1097/SIH.0000000000000201

Lin, D. W., Romanelli, J. R., Kuhn, J. N., Thompson, R. E., Bush, R. W., & Seymour, N. E. (2009). Computer-based laparoscopic and robotic surgical simulators: Performance characteristics and perceptions of new users. *Surgical Endoscopy, 23*(1), 209–214. doi:10.100700464-008-9805-3 PMID:18297349

Lopreiato, J. O., & Sawyer, T. (2015). Simulation-based medical education in pediatrics. *Academic Pediatrics, 15*(2), 134–142. doi:10.1016/j.acap.2014.10.010 PMID:25748973

Loukas, C., Nikiteas, N., Kanakis, M., & Georgiou, E. (2011). Evaluating the effectiveness of virtual reality simulation training in intravenous cannulation. *Simulation in Healthcare: Journal of the Society for Simulation in Healthcare, 6*(4), 213-217. doi:10.1097/SIH.0b013e31821d08a9

Loukas, C., Nikiteas, N., Kanakis, M., Moutsatsos, A., Leandros, E., & Georgiou, E. (2010). A virtual reality simulation curriculum for intravenous cannulation training. *Academic Emergency Medicine: Official Journal of the Society for Academic Emergency Medicine, 17*(10), 1142-1145. doi:10.1111/j.1553-2712.2010.00876.x

Mairami, A., Paton, C., Asangansi, I., Otuneye, A., Audu, L., Edgecombe, H., . . . Umoren, R. (2019). *eHBB: Preliminary testing and evaluation of a virtual reality simulation on neonatal resuscitation.* Paper presented at the 50th Annual General and Scientific Conference of the Paediatrics Association of Nigeria (PANCONF), Ibadan, Nigeria.

Marei, H. F., Donkers, J., Al-Eraky, M. M., & Van Merrienboer, J. J. G. (2019). Collaborative use of virtual patients after a lecture enhances learning with minimal investment of cognitive load. *Medical Teacher, 41*(3), 332–339. doi:10.1080/0142159X.2018.1472372 PMID:29798713

Motz, P., Gray, M., Sawyer, T., Kett, J., Danforth, D., Maicher, K., & Umoren, R. (2018). Virtual Antenatal Encounter and Standardized Simulation Assessment (VANESSA): Pilot Study. *JMIR Serious Games, 6*(2), e8. doi:10.2196/games.9611 PMID:29752249

Naur, T. M. H., Nilsson, P. M., Pietersen, P. I., Clementsen, P. F., & Konge, L. (2017). Simulation-Based Training in Flexible Bronchoscopy and Endobronchial Ultrasound-Guided Transbronchial Needle Aspiration (EBUS-TBNA): A Systematic Review. *Respiration: International Review of Thoracic Diseases, 93*(5), 355-362. doi:10.1159/000464331

Nifakos, S., & Zary, N. (2014). Virtual patients in a real clinical context using augmented reality: Impact on antibiotics prescription behaviors. *Studies in Health Technology and Informatics, 205*, 707–711. https://pubmed.ncbi.nlm.nih.gov/25160278 PMID:25160278

Nippita, S., Haviland, M. J., Voit, S. F., Perez-Peralta, J., Hacker, M. R., & Paul, M. E. (2018). Randomized trial of high- and low-fidelity simulation to teach intrauterine contraception placement. *American Journal of Obstetrics and Gynecology, 218*(2), 258.e251–258.e211. doi:10.1016/j.ajog.2017.11.553 PMID:29138033

Padilha, J. M., Machado, P. P., Ribeiro, A., Ramos, J., & Costa, P. (2019). Clinical Virtual Simulation in Nursing Education: Randomized Controlled Trial. *Journal of Medical Internet Research, 21*(3), e11529–e11529. doi:10.2196/11529 PMID:30882355

Patel, A., Koshy, N., Ortega-Barnett, J., Chan, H. C., Kuo, Y.-F., Luciano, C., Rizzi, S., Matulyauskas, M., Kania, P., Banerjee, P., & Gasco, J. (2014). Neurosurgical tactile discrimination training with haptic-based virtual reality simulation. *Neurological Research, 36*(12), 1035–1039. doi:10.1179/1743132814Y.0000000405 PMID:24984771

Peddle, M., McKenna, L., Bearman, M., & Nestel, D. (2019). Development of non-technical skills through virtual patients for undergraduate nursing students: An exploratory study. *Nurse Education Today, 73*, 94–101. doi:10.1016/j.nedt.2018.11.008 PMID:30610960

Riva, G., & Wiederhold, B. K. (2015). The New Dawn of Virtual Reality in Health Care: Medical Simulation and Experiential Interface. *Studies in Health Technology and Informatics, 219*, 3–6. https://pubmed.ncbi.nlm.nih.gov/26799868 PMID:26799868

Roussin, C. J., & Weinstock, P. (2017). SimZones: An Organizational Innovation for Simulation Programs and Centers. *Academic Medicine, 92*(8), 1114–1120. doi:10.1097/ACM.0000000000001746 PMID:28562455

Scholz, C., Mann, C., Kopp, V., Kost, B., Kainer, F., & Fischer, M. R. (2012). High-fidelity simulation increases obstetric self-assurance and skills in undergraduate medical students. *Journal of Perinatal Medicine, 40*(6), 607–613. doi:10.1515/jpm-2012-0052 PMID:23093253

See, K. W. M., Chui, K. H., Chan, W. H., Wong, K. C., & Chan, Y. C. (2016). Evidence for Endovascular Simulation Training: A Systematic Review. *European Journal of Vascular and Endovascular Surgery: The Official Journal of the European Society for Vascular Surgery, 51*(3), 441-451. doi:10.1016/j.ejvs.2015.10.011

Stathakarou, N., Kononowicz, A. A., Henningsohn, L., & McGrath, C. (2018). Modelling Feedback in Virtual Patients: An Iterative Approach. *Studies in Health Technology and Informatics*, *247*, 201–205. https://pubmed.ncbi.nlm.nih.gov/29677951 PMID:29677951

Stevens, R., Galloway, T., & Willemsen-Dunlap, A. (2019). Advancing Our Understandings of Healthcare Team Dynamics From the Simulation Room to the Operating Room: A Neurodynamic Perspective. *Frontiers in Psychology*, *10*, 1660. doi:10.3389/fpsyg.2019.01660 PMID:31456706

Stone, R. J. (2011). The (human) science of medical virtual learning environments. *Philosophical Transactions of the Royal Society of London. Series B, Biological Sciences*, *366*(1562), 276–285. doi:10.1098/rstb.2010.0209 PMID:21149363

Sweigart, L., & Hodson-Carlton, K. (2013). Improving student interview skills: The virtual avatar as client. *Nurse Educator*, *38*(1), 11–15. doi:10.1097/NNE.0b013e318276df2d PMID:23222623

Sweigart, L. U. R., Scott, P., Hodson-Carlton, K., Jones, J., Gossett, E., & McCabe, H. (2015). (Accepted). Virtual learning environment TeamSTEPPS simulations produce teamwork attitude changes among health professional students. *for Publication in the Journal of Nursing Education*.

Tolsgaard, M. G., Ringsted, C., Dreisler, E., Nørgaard, L. N., Petersen, J. H., Madsen, M. E., Freiesleben, N. L. C., Sørensen, J. L., & Tabor, A. (2015). Sustained effect of simulation-based ultrasound training on clinical performance: A randomized trial. *Ultrasound in Obstetrics & Gynecology*, *46*(3), 312–318. doi:10.1002/uog.14780 PMID:25580809

Umoren, R., Gray, M., Grace, D., Sawyer, T., Hou, S., Thompson, K., & Loren, D. (2018, June 20-22). *NICU TeamSTEPPS: Virtual Teamwork Training for NICU Professionals*. Paper presented at the AHA Team Training National Conference, San Diego, CA.

Umoren, R., Stadler, D. J., Gasior, S. L., Al-Sheikhly, D., Truman, B., & Lowe, C. (2014). Global collaboration and team-building through 3D virtual environments. *Innovations in Global Medical and Health Education*, 1.

Umoren, R. A., Poore, J. A., Sweigart, L., Rybas, N., Gossett, E., Johnson, M., Allen, M., Scott, P. J., Truman, B., & Das, R. (2017). TeamSTEPPS Virtual Teams: Interactive Virtual Team Training and Practice for Health Professional Learners. *Creative Nursing*, *23*(3), 184–191. doi:10.1891/1078-4535.23.3.184 PMID:28789739

Umoren, R. A., Scott, P. J., Sweigart, L., Gossett, E., Hodson-Carlton, K., Johnson, M., Jones, J. A., Poore, J. A., Rybas, N., Truman, B., & Das, R. (2018). A comparison of teamwork attitude changes with virtual TeamSTEPPS® simulations in health professional students. *Journal of Interprofessional Education & Practice*, *10*, 51–55. doi:10.1016/j.xjep.2017.12.001

Vaccaro, C. M., Crisp, C. C., Fellner, A. N., Jackson, C., Kleeman, S. D., & Pavelka, J. (2013). Robotic virtual reality simulation plus standard robotic orientation versus standard robotic orientation alone: A randomized controlled trial. *Female Pelvic Medicine & Reconstructive Surgery*, *19*(5), 266–270. doi:10.1097/SPV.0b013e3182a09101 PMID:23982574

Valdis, M., Chu, M. W. A., Schlachta, C., & Kiaii, B. (2016). Evaluation of robotic cardiac surgery simulation training: A randomized controlled trial. *The Journal of Thoracic and Cardiovascular Surgery*, *151*(6), 1498–1505. e1492. doi:10.1016/j.jtcvs.2016.02.016 PMID:26964911

Vishwanath, A., Kam, M., & Kumar, N. (2017). Examining Low-Cost Virtual Reality for Learning in Low-Resource Environments. *Proceedings of the 2017 Conference on Designing Interactive Systems*. 10.1145/3064663.3064696

Walker, R. B., Underwood, P. K., Bernhagen, M., Markin, N., & Boedeker, B. H. (2012). Virtual intubation training at a remote military site. *Studies in Health Technology and Informatics*, *173*, 540–542. https://pubmed.ncbi.nlm.nih.gov/22357054 PMID:22357054

Wang, E. E., Quinones, J., Fitch, M. T., Dooley-Hash, S., Griswold-Theodorson, S., Medzon, R., Korley, F., Laack, T., Robinett, A., & Clay, L. (2008). Developing technical expertise in emergency medicine—The role of simulation in procedural skill acquisition. *Academic Emergency Medicine*, *15*(11), 1046–1057. doi:10.1111/j.1553-2712.2008.00218.x PMID:18785939

Weinger, M. B., Banerjee, A., Burden, A. R., McIvor, W. R., Boulet, J., Cooper, J. B., Steadman, R., Shotwell, M. S., Slagle, J. M., DeMaria, S. Jr, Torsher, L., Sinz, E., Levine, A. I., Rask, J., Davis, F., Park, C., & Gaba, D. M. (2017). Simulation-based Assessment of the Management of Critical Events by Board-certified Anesthesiologists. *Anesthesiology*, *127*(3), 475–489. doi:10.1097/ALN.0000000000001739 PMID:28671903

Wetzel, E. A., Lang, T. R., Pendergrass, T. L., Taylor, R. G., & Geis, G. L. (2013). Identification of latent safety threats using high-fidelity simulation-based training with multidisciplinary neonatology teams. *Joint Commission Journal on Quality and Patient Safety*, *39*(6), 268–268. doi:10.1016/S1553-7250(13)39037-0 PMID:23789165

Wong, D. T., Mehta, A., Singh, K. P., Leong, S. M., Ooi, A., Niazi, A., You-Ten, E., Okrainec, A., Patel, R., Singh, M., & Wong, J. (2019). The effect of virtual reality bronchoscopy simulator training on performance of bronchoscopic-guided intubation in patients: A randomised controlled trial. *European Journal of Anaesthesiology*, *36*(3), 227–233. doi:10.1097/EJA.0000000000000890 PMID:30234669

Yousif, S., Machan, J. T., Alaska, Y., & Suner, S. (2017). Airway Management in Disaster Response: A Manikin Study Comparing Direct and Video Laryngoscopy for Endotracheal Intubation by Prehospital Providers in Level C Personal Protective Equipment. *Prehospital and Disaster Medicine*, *32*(4), 352–356. doi:10.1017/S1049023X17000188 PMID:28318455

Ziv, A., Erez, D., Munz, Y., Vardi, A., Barsuk, D., Levine, I., . . . Berkenstadt, H. (2006). The Israel Center for Medical Simulation: a paradigm for cultural change in medical education. Acad Med, 81(12), 1091-1097. 00001888-200612000-00014 doi:10.1097/01.ACM.0000246756.55626.1b

KEY TERMS AND DEFINITIONS

Augmented Reality: Computer generated holographic images can be viewed by the learner in the physical environment using a mobile device or specially designed headset.

High-Fidelity Manikin: This term refers to a technology-enabled manikin with features such as mechanical respiration and heart rate.

Low-Fidelity Manikin: This is typically a low cost, low technology manikin with minimal features.

Objective Structured Clinical Examination (OSCE): An: approach to assessment that involves defined objectives and anticipated actions, often with an accompanying checklist for assessment.

Simulation Debriefer: A simulation instructor who leads the learners through a reflective analysis of simulation events.

Simulation Facilitator: A simulation instructor who guides the learners through the scenario with the goal of meeting learning objectives.

Simulation Technician/Specialist: An individual who supports the practice of simulation through setting up and managing simulation manikins and supplies.

Teledebriefing: Teledebriefing describes a process in which learners who are participating in a simulation scenario undergo debriefing with a facilitator located at an off-site location.

Telefacilitation: The conduct of a telesimulation by a remote facilitator.

Telesimulation: Telesimulation is a process by which telecommunication and simulation resources are utilized to provide education, training, and/or assessment to learners at an off-site location.

Video-Assisted Debriefing: The practice of using video captured during simulation sessions for reflective discussions on learner and team performance.

Virtual Environment: 3D computer generated objects that can be viewed on a screen or in a head-mounted display.

Virtual Reality: Computer generated 3D images viewed by a learner in a virtual environment using a low-cost or high-end head mounted display.

Section 2

Process of Simulation Education and Evaluation

Chapter 5
Organizing Simulations for Interprofessional Learners

ABSTRACT

To successfully conduct simulation sessions, simulation facilitators must prepare the content and logistics including equipment and location. This chapter provides an overview of the methods and process of simulation instruction including preparation, facilitation, and debriefing simulation scenarios during simulation sessions. Simulation facilitation requires instructors to provide scenario details while simulation debriefers guide learners through a reflective session centered around the learning objectives. This chapter reviews the practical steps for organizing simulations and explores the basis for various approaches to simulation debriefing.

INTRODUCTION

The airline industry once suffered from the same dysfunction that undermines teamwork in healthcare today. In response to a series of human-error related crashes, the airline industry developed job training and information sharing processes known as Crew Resource Management (CRM) that enhance communication and teamwork (Littlepage et al., 2016). Healthcare professionals applying the lessons learned from aviation safety have found that lives can be saved, and patient care enhanced, by adapting the relevant lessons of aviation safety and teamwork (Boet et al., 2014; Fransen et al., 2017). Simulation can be used to promote safety culture through the

DOI: 10.4018/978-1-7998-4378-8.ch005

understanding that improving patient care and safety is not just a mission or value statement, but integral to daily practice (Cohen et al., 2004; Wong et al., 2016). The simulation facilitator is key in planning and implementing simulation education that supports behavior change. Organizing a successful simulation session begins with planning and preparation and culminates with a thorough debriefing session that supports learners in identifying lessons learned for implementation in future practice (Bowe et al., 2017; Griswold-Theodorson et al., 2015).

Facilitators of a simulation could either be faculty or peers. Because of concerns over learner stress as well as the effects the presence of an instructor has on the behavior of students, consideration has been given to the possible benefits of student-led simulation experiences that are led by their peers (Curtis et al., 2016; Kushnir, 1986). The facilitator and the learners will be in the same physical location in the vast majority of instances; nevertheless, remote facilitating has been documented (Ohta et al., 2017). This chapter focuses on fundamental concepts for the facilitation of simulations and the debriefing of such simulations. These principles are most applicable to in-person simulations, but remote facilitators can also make use of them. Chapter 7 "Telesimulation: Remote Learning, Facilitation, and Debriefing" goes into greater depth on the subject of remote learning and debriefing, as well as remote facilitation.

BACKGROUND

To successfully organize simulation education sessions for health professional learners, the facilitator must set aside time to adequately prepare for the session. If the opportunity presents itself, simulation educators should conduct a review of safety events to identify relevant learning points that can be emphasized throughout the simulation and the subsequent debrief. In cases when direct access to these records is not possible, it is helpful to elicit examples from learners of recent experiences that bring attention to the necessity of improving both systems and practices. Increasing the relevance of the training and facilitating its transfer to practice can be accomplished by the use of these instances into simulation training (Patterson et al., 2013). In many fields of study, the chances to learn about and gain experience with unusual occurrences are quite rare. Even while it is hoped that students would be exposed to a sufficient number of real-world scenarios to guarantee that they become competent, simulation can bridge this gap and help minimize accidents caused by a lack of knowledge or skills. Debriefing gives medical personnel the opportunity to practice the art of speaking up about medical errors and the consequences of those errors - not by pointing fingers, but by engaging in constructive discourse about how to make things better. The instructor of the simulation needs to explore more than just technical abilities to find possibilities to develop leadership and team communication.

It is essential for novice simulation educators to be familiar with the fundamental operational principles of delivering simulation activities and to build their simulation expertise by observing experienced simulation instructors, attending healthcare simulation conferences, and investing in available simulation references. It is also important for novice simulation educators to have access to simulation references. Even though a significant amount of effort will have been put into preparing and testing each scenario, facilitators of the simulation need to be willing to quickly adjust to unforeseen events that may take place. Unanticipated responses from students or co-facilitators, technological difficulties with the mannequin, or a lack of resources in the clinical or simulation environment could all be potential causes of these occurrences (for simulations that are conducted in situ). The facilitator of the simulation is responsible for reviewing and assessing any existing simulation scenarios, including those based on manikins and those conducted virtually, in order to find the most effective way to integrate and evaluate their utilization. This is especially true for applications of new and developing technologies to virtual simulation. This chapter provides an overview of the preparation that is required for running a simulation session, as well as standard approaches to the facilitation of the session and the debriefing that follows it. Please refer to Chapters 3 and 4 on "Scenario Development for Manikin-based Simulations" and "Scenario Development for Virtual Simulations" for additional information on scenario development for manikin-based and virtual simulation, respectively.

Adequate preparation for each simulation session is essential to the success of the event. The role of the simulation facilitator, once the students have arrived, is one of the most significant functions since it involves establishing the mood of the session as an opportunity for the students to exercise their abilities in a risk-free situation. The primary responsibility of the facilitator of a simulation is to ensure that participants continue to make progress toward the simulation's learning goals while also effectively managing the simulation's time and resources. During the debriefing session, the person in charge of the simulation looks for opportunities to highlight and stress certain learning objectives in order to consolidate students' new knowledge. Tracking the results of learning through the use of various teaching and assessment instruments is an important aspect that requires additional study. Please refer to Chapter 6 on "Evaluation of Simulation Performance" for an overview of the approaches used to analyze the performance of the learner during a simulation. This chapter focuses on the process of organizing simulations for interprofessional learners. Topics covered include critical considerations for preparation, facilitation, and debriefing of simulation sessions.

Preparation for the Simulation Session

The amount of preparation needed will vary depending on the learner type, scenario availability, available simulation equipment (manikins, hospital supplies) and location (clinical or classroom setting). Both clinical and classroom environments are particularly useful for simulation training and can be used to great success (Berkowitz, 2017; Haraldseid et al., 2015). On the other hand, in some instances, specialized simulation or clinical skills laboratories might need to be set up in advance in order to get ready for the session (Utz et al., 2015). Dedicated simulation centers can now be outfitted with high-fidelity manikins and clinical equipment, as well as 3D printing and visualization, virtual reality, and computerized simulation, thanks to advances in technology. These centers are used for training on procedures and developing visuospatial skills (Bernardo, 2017; Maxwell et al., 2016; Rinewalt et al., 2012; Sarwani et al., 2012). In addition, research simulation laboratories may also be equipped with hardware for tracking the subject's gaze, physiological stress monitors, and other forms of neurophysiological monitoring equipment in order to conduct research into human factors and the respective roles of workload and fatigue on performance (Bernardo, 2017).

If this is the first time that the session has been carried out, there may be a significant amount of time spent preparing. This is due to the fact that it is necessary to choose an appropriate location, collect the required equipment, and do practice runs of the situations that will be employed. Even if the location has been used in the past, it is essential for the facilitator of the simulation and the simulation technologist to arrive early, at least up to an hour before the learners are scheduled to arrive, in order to ensure that the simulation environment is set up, check the equipment, and display the appropriate signage indicating that a simulation event is taking place.

Learner Type

It is important during preparation to find out whether you will be working with novice or experienced learners when it comes to simulation education, learners from a single profession or multiple professions, learners who will be pulled from clinical service for the training (in situ simulations) or learners who will be attending the session without conflicting clinical responsibilities (Bullough et al., 2016), learners who are internal to the organization or external learners.

Novice learners who are attending a simulation education session for the first time will require additional time designated on the agenda for explanation of the role of simulation education in patient safety, time to discuss the opportunities provided by simulation training to make mistakes in a safe environment (Haraldseid et al., 2015; Lendahls & Oscarsson, 2017). An explanation of the rules of simulation which have been widely used to encourage learners to "suspend disbelief", engage fully in the role they occupy during the simulation, be supportive of other learners, and keep the scenario and participant actions during simulation confidential outside the session. In addition, an orientation to the simulator should be provided by the facilitator or simulation technologist (Lencioni et al., 2017). This orientation identifies unique features of the manikin or simulator and specifies features that may not function as expected. Experienced learners who have attended simulation sessions before may need a brief reminder of these rules, but not as much time will need to be spent in this regard.

Within the context of the clinical setting, it will be necessary to delegate responsibilities to learners belonging to a single profession that may differ from those that are often expected of them. Because of this, the facilitator might need to provide additional information about the scenario or additional orientation to the roles in order to support learners who might not be familiar with their position. It is possible to let members of the learner group adopt the clinical role that is typical for their profession if the learner group comprises persons from more than one profession. However, in order to aid with the facilitation and debriefing of role-specific actions, it is essential to have a session facilitator who is familiar with the fundamentals of each role and comes, ideally, from the same line of work as the other participants.

Learners who are able to attend the session without other duties that compete for their attention will be in a position to concentrate completely on the educational session. However, learners who are being pulled away from their clinical responsibilities in order to participate in the simulation session have extra time constraints, which need to be taken into consideration during the preparation stage of the session. The facilitator is responsible for being ready to start and conclude the session on time, adapting to changes in clinical acuity that may result in fewer people participating in the session or changing the location of the session owing to clinical care demands, and starting and ending the session on time.

Scenario Availability

The facilitator must consider whether a scenario exists to address the learning objectives of the session. An online search or search of institutional resources may reveal an existing scenario which matches the learning objectives or can be easily adapted to meet them. Modifications can often be made to existing scenarios designed by other facilitators (Hirsch et al., 2016; Khamis et al., 2016; Komorowski et al., 2017) or even created by learners (Gwin et al., 2017; Nguyen et al., 2016; Pheister et al., 2017; Tongdee et al., 2016). Additional information on adapting an existing scenario can be found in Chapter 3 on "Approach to scenario development for manikin-based simulation". If there is no existing scenario which can be adapted to meet the learning objectives, the facilitator may create a new scenario (Lee et al., 2015; Sannomiya et al., 2016). Additional guidance on creating a new simulation scenario can be found in Chapter 3: Approach to scenario development for manikin-based simulation. Each simulation scenario focuses on a defined clinical domain, critical knowledge and skills, and/or levels of competency. In some cases, scenarios present opportunities to reinforce evidenced-based practice guidelines and national patient safety goals. In other cases, scenarios highlight research - based design characteristics which enable the exploration and tracking of cognitive knowledge, cognitive load, emotion, adaptive responses and other human factors in patient safety and latent safety risks in the clinical environment (Deutsch et al., 2016; Fraser & McLaughlin, 2019; Hayden et al., 2018; Kobayashi et al., 2013; Schlairet et al., 2015; Uemura et al., 2014).

Simulation Equipment

Many established simulation or clinical skills laboratories maintain lists of equipment and supplies required for each simulation session. Scenarios may also contain a list of supplies needed for the scenario. The facilitator must identify and source the equipment needed to conduct the scenario. When the equipment is not listed as part of the scenario, the facilitator should systematically identify, and list required equipment and supplies. If a list must be developed, then start with identifying the most important items and build out the list to include less critical items. For example, a scenario with the learning objective to demonstrate intubation skills would require an manikin (low or high fidelity manikin may be acceptable), a laryngoscope, an appropriately sized endotracheal tube with or without a stylet, a bag and mask device to provide positive pressure ventilation; a stethoscope and end-tidal CO2 detector to assess for correct position of the endotracheal tube tip, and medical tape or other device to secure the endotracheal tube. Other equipment such as a pulse oximeter, suction, supplemental oxygen, or a mechanical ventilator would add to the realism of the scenario. However, this equipment may be considered optional as the focus is on the intubation procedure itself, and not ventilator management. Additional equipment or supplies may vary with the patient age and clinical condition. For example, a newborn manikin would require a blanket and may be placed on a radiant warmer.

Session Location

The location of the simulation session deserves special consideration. Simulations can be held "in situ" i.e., in the clinical environment where patient care occurs, in a simulated clinical care setting or simulation center or in a classroom setting which is converted for simulation purposes. There are some advantages to using in-situ simulation, one of which is that the tools and materials that trainees employ are an exact match for the setting in which they engage in practice (Bradley et al., 2018; Theilen et al., 2017; Wetzel et al., 2013; Zimmermann et al., 2015). In-situ simulation is very useful for the process of putting into practice new therapeutic protocols (Marzano et al., 2016). The knowledge gained from participating in in-situ simulations may be applicable in clinical practice (Surcouf et al., 2013; Theilen et al., 2017). In addition, the simulation may discover certain safety hazards that were previously unknown, known as "latent safety risks," such as the breakdown of equipment, the location of equipment that is inaccessible, or delays in acquiring supplies using the workflow or processes that are now in place (Kerner et al., 2016; Wetzel et al., 2013). The early detection of these dangers by means of simulation paves the way for the creation of an opportunity to enhance both the security and the quality of medical care. See Table 1 for a comparison of the typical settings that are used for simulation sessions, which include in-situ hospital or clinic rooms, simulation or clinical skills centers, and classrooms. These settings can be found all around the world.

Table 1. Comparison of typical locations used for simulation sessions

	In-situ (clinical)	Simulation center	Classroom
Convenience for facilitators	+	+++	++
Convenience for health practitioners	+++	++	+
Convenience for health professional students	+	++	+++
Potential for interference with clinical care	++	-	-
Availability of clinical supplies/ equipment	+++	++	-
Identification of latent safety threats	+++	+	-

Session Logistics

Other logistics for setting up simulation training include:

- **Reserving a Venue**: For sessions that will occur outside the clinical environment, reserve the simulation center and for in-situ simulations, work with clinical leaders to secure a clinical space
- **Advertise:** Create and post flyers or other advertisements for the simulation session
- **Register Participants:** Create a sign-up method for registering and relaying session information to participants
- **Refreshments:** Order refreshments which may include breakfast and lunch for an all-day session
- **Equipment Reservations**: Reserving manikins and other equipment
- **Identifying Assistants:** Identifying co-facilitators and simulation technologists to assist with set up, facilitating and/or debriefing the scenario

Facilitating the Simulation Session

Introductions

The simulation facilitator role begins long before the learners enter the simulation session. The facilitator of the simulation needs to have knowledge of the fundamentals of education based on simulations, the ability to keep the session interactive without intimidating new learners, the desire to encourage learners to share their knowledge and skills with others in the session, and the ability to support a safe learning environment through their words and actions. It is not unheard of to have students in a single classroom who come from a variety of professional backgrounds and who possess a broad spectrum of skill levels and variable degrees of prior experience with simulation-based education. When trying to understand your learner group, it can be helpful to establish the background of your learners early on in the session through introductions and a brief explanation of what they hope to gain from the session. This can be a key step in the process. Be sure to keep these learner goals in mind since you will likely want to refer back to them both throughout the session and after it's over to make sure they're being met.

Role of Simulation

After introductions, the agenda should include an explanation of the role of simulation education in patient safety if learners are not already familiar with this information. Then briefly go over the expectations for the session. This typically includes elements that encourage learners to "suspend disbelief" or engage fully in the scenario "as though the manikin was an actual patient". It is also important to make a statement to the effect that the session is a safe and respectful environment where mistakes can be made without endangering the patient. You must state by words and actions that you consider your learners to be intelligent, hard-working, and doing their best. Only the facilitator can begin or terminate the scenario. Learner performance will be kept confidential.

Beginning the Scenario

When you are ready to begin, meet briefly (huddle) with your co-facilitators and/or simulation technologists to clarify which scenario you will be starting with (if not already done prior to the session). You may have the participants identify a team leader if appropriate to the scenario and assign roles while you are doing this. When ready, the facilitator begins the scenario by reading the introductory information to the participant in the role designated to engage with the patient first. This participant will evaluate the patient and relay the information they elicit, along with the details of the case to their team. It is typical that additional healthcare team members will be called to assist and that the healthcare team involvement will expand to meet the demands posed by the deterioration in the patient's clinical condition as the scenario moves from the Beginning Stage to the Middle Stage. See Chapter 3: Approach to scenario development for manikin-based simulation for details on the Beginning, Middle and End Stages of scenarios. See Figure 1 for an illustration of facilitator and learners during bedside simulation facilitation.

Figure 1. Schematic illustration of facilitator and learners during bedside facilitation

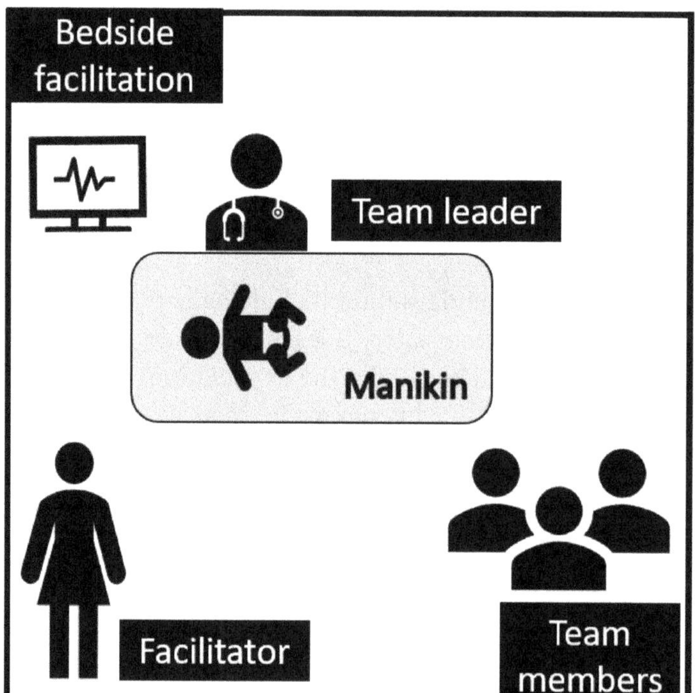

Facilitating the Scenario

During the course of the scenario, participants may seek assistance from the facilitator in order to accomplish the learning objectives. Facilitators should only present information that is provided by the facilitator notes on the scenario. This will ensure that learning objectives are satisfied. In most cases, the scope of this information is limited to recent updates on the patient's clinical status, investigations, or x-rays that have been requested, and it should be pertinent to the stage at which the scenario is currently at.

If it is the goal of the scenario for the participants to find the diagnosis or show a diagnostic or therapeutic action, then the scenario facilitators should refrain from providing this information to the participants while they are engaged in the scenario. When the learning objective is centered on a diagnostic or therapeutic intervention, it is possible that the diagnosis will be presented right away at the beginning of the scenario.

Whenever a participant appears to be having significant difficulty or is working toward a goal that is not congruent with the learning objectives of the session, the facilitator should intervene. When this occurs, it is probable that the facilitator had miscalculated the amount of difficulty of the scenario, and it is possible that the facilitator will need to assist in order to achieve the learning objectives.

Working with Problem Learners

Working with problem learners to enable everyone to get the greatest benefit from the session is a high-level facilitation skill. Some learners may not engage with simulation-based sessions due to lack of preparation and fear of being judged by the instructor or their peers (Haraldseid et al., 2015).

Lack of Preparation

If learners are unprepared, the facilitator may opt to present pertinent information relevant to the scenario as part of the introduction. For example, a scenario focused on team performance during pediatric sepsis may include a brief lecture on the management of pediatric sepsis before the scenario starts. This allays learner anxiety by revealing not on the diagnosis but also the recommended management of pediatric sepsis, so that the focus can be on the scenario learning objectives of team communication and performance (Wong et al., 2016).

Performance Anxiety

It is important to prepare learners who may be anxious about their performance during simulation education. Emotion and cognitive load may have an impact on performance (Schlairet et al., 2015). Learners who have performance anxiety around being observed or assessed by the facilitator or their peers should be reminded that mistakes are expected, even welcome. In fact, everyone makes mistakes, and the goal of the simulation is to provide an opportunity to make mistakes when patient safety is not at risk. We all learn from mistakes, both the ones we make and those of others. Both facilitators and learners must adhere to the principles of confidentiality during simulation: "What occurs in simulation, stays in simulation". As such, it is not appropriate for facilitators to bring up examples of earlier failures in subsequent training sessions. As one of the objectives of simulation is to learn, and learning occurs best in a safe environment, confidentiality about mistakes occurring during simulation is expected and required.

Failure to Align Scenario Objectives with Learner Needs

Poor alignment of scenario objectives with learner needs and interests may pose a significant barrier to learner engagement. When experienced learners are given a scenario that is too easy, they arrive at the diagnosis or carry out the intervention quickly and find that there is little to no challenge or opportunity to learn. Some learners in this situation will disengage while others will take over the narrative and delay or disrupt the session unless the facilitator can introduce additional challenges such as systems issues or complications to increase the learning opportunities in the scenario. Novice learners who find the scenario too challenging and are unable to perform the desired actions or tasks to move from the Middle Stage to the End Stage of the scenario may also disengage unless the facilitator can provide information to one or all of the participants that guides the team to the diagnosis. In some cases, inserting a co-facilitator into the scenario as a "helpful" consultant, or calling a "time out" to debrief the progress in the scenario may give the team an opportunity to regroup and get on the right track. In some cases, learner self-efficacy scores decline following the simulation because initial perceptions of proficiency were inaccurate (Karabacak et al., 2019).

Failure to "Suspend Disbelief"

Learners who are unfamiliar with simulation education may experience difficulty with the concept of "suspending disbelief". However, the unwillingness to suspend disbelief is often a symptom of lack of preparation or fear as discussed in the preceding sections. There are certain signs that identify a learner who has not suspended disbelief. Such learners may not perform actions such as wearing provided gloves, may omit steps such as sterilizing skin before central line placement or may not verbalize to the "patient" that they are about to perform a painful procedure. When a learner does not carry out actions as though the manikin were an actual patient, it interferes with the ability of other participants to engage with the scenario. It is necessary for the facilitator to address potential underlying issues such as a gap in knowledge or fear of judgment and remind all learners at the start of the session to perform tasks as they would on an actual patient.

Table 2. Strategies for working with "problem learners"

Challenge	Strategy
Lack of preparation	• Include pertinent information as an introductory lecture or pre-brief
Performance anxiety	• Emphasize principles of confidentiality • Discuss how mistakes are expected, even welcome during simulation
Scenario mismatch with learner needs	Scenario too easy: • Introduce additional challenges such as systems issues or complications Scenario too difficult: • Provide additional hints • Introduce a co-facilitator into the scenario as a "helpful" consultant • Call a "time out" to give the participants a chance to regroup
Failure to "suspend disbelief"	• Set expectations that tasks are performed as they would be on an actual patient • Address underlying knowledge gaps or anxiety

Debriefing the Simulation Session

In healthcare, where errors lead to loss of life, it is critical to identify ways to improve practice and provide better care. Debriefing, also referred to as "after action review" is the process by which the learners are guided through a discussion of the events that occurred during the scenario (Sawyer et al., 2016; Sawyer & Deering, 2013). The primary objective for debriefing is to promote learning by self-reflection at an individual and a team level (Dufrene & Young, 2014; Severson et al., 2014). Debriefing takes place immediately after the scenario ends. The facilitator may conduct the debriefing session or may delegate the role to another facilitator whose role during the scenario was to observe the participant's actions and conduct the debriefing session.

Debriefing may occur at or away from the simulated patient's bedside. See Figure 2 for a schematic illustration of classroom debriefing.

Figure 2. Schematic illustration of facilitators and learners with video-assisted classroom debriefing

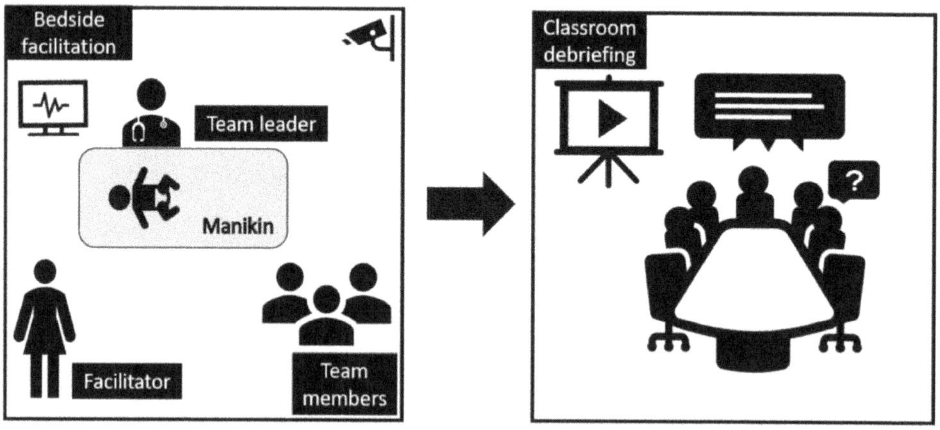

There are many described approaches to debriefing (Dufrene & Young, 2014; Levett-Jones & Lapkin, 2014; Lyons et al., 2015; Maestre & Rudolph, 2015). In general, for a debriefing to be successful, the debriefer should try to ask as many open-ended questions as possible, avoid directly criticizing performance, but be willing to validate incorrect actions identified by participants (Husebø et al., 2013; Rudolph et al., 2007). The debriefer should ensure that learning objectives are discussed during the debriefing while keeping most of the discussion between the participants. Data collected by the facilitator during the simulation using a structured checklist, video or eye-tracking may be used to support debriefing sessions (Henneman et al., 2014; Sawyer et al., 2012; Syed et al., 2014; Szulewski et al., 2018). A recent review of 23 studies on video-assisted debriefing showed that while this approach improved learners' experience, attitude and performance, it did not have an advantage over verbal debriefing on knowledge acquisition (Zhang et al., 2019). Learner-centered debriefing may help facilitators identify and address learner needs while building learner engagement. This approach differs from instructor-centered approaches where instructors maintain control over the debriefing with limited input from learners (Cheng et al., 2016). Students can also be encouraged to engage in self-debriefing which may be through discussion or written (Reed, 2015). In some studies, performance improved regardless of whether the debriefing was self- or instructor led (Boet et al., 2011). Debriefing is an important skill, but one that can be challenging to for many instructors to master (McKechnie, 2016; Ulmer et al., 2018). Structured tools have been described to aid instructors and provide coaching and peer-assessment to improve faculty effectiveness in conducing debriefing sessions (Cheng et al., 2017; Saylor et al., 2016).

Debriefing can occur during or after the simulation session. In some cases, it is necessary for the facilitator to pause the simulation to highlight specific learning objectives or because the learners are clearly going "off-track" and there is a risk of the learning objectives not being met. This use of a "pause button" can trigger in-simulation debriefing or "debriefing-on-demand" (Gaylle, 2019; McMullen et al., 2016). See Figure 2 for a schematic illustration of bedside debriefing during or after the simulation session.

Figure 3. Schematic illustration of facilitator and learners with bedside debriefing during or after the simulation

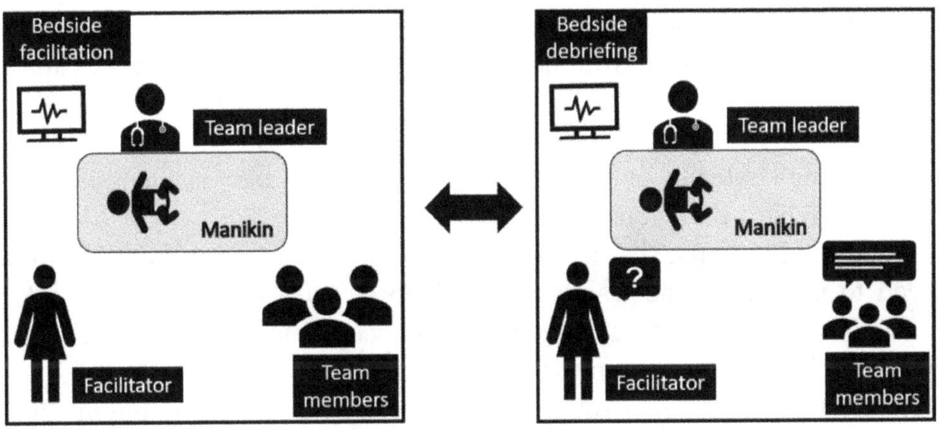

Facilitators should be aware that the learners' cognitive load, perceptions of their performance during the simulation or prior clinical experiences may trigger an emotional response (Fraser et al., 2012; Fraser & McLaughlin, 2019; Schlairet et al., 2015). After a simulation concludes, many instructors will allow for a few minutes of decompression where learners may talk freely about the events of the simulation or how it made them feel (Lilot et al., 2018). In a randomized controlled trial of 149 residents, this five minute "relaxation break" before debriefing was found to enhance recall of critical messages three months after the session (Lilot et al., 2018).

At the start of post-simulation debriefing, some debriefers will allow further exploration of how the simulation made the learners' feel while others prefer to stick to the facts of the session by asking the team leader to relay what they thought were the primary issues encountered in the case. After the team leader concludes their summary of events. The debriefer may ask other team members if they agree and provide an opportunity for them to add additional facts or expand on their own perceptions of the events. Then it is typical for the debriefer to ask the team what, in their opinion, went well during the scenario and after exploring these items, what could have gone better. If after the team has exhausted their account of correctly or incorrectly performed actions or behaviors, there are additional actions to discuss, the debriefer should prompt the mention of these by asking questions around these actions.

The level of the team's knowledge of the subject matter in relation to the learning objectives can be inferred from the responses that they provided. A team that has done sufficient preparation will have the tendency to express their knowledge of the content and where they went wrong very quickly. For instance, "When was the level of oxygen increased to 100% during the scenario?" A team that is well-prepared may answer by saying something along the lines of "We should have done that at the beginning of chest compressions, but we forgot." This makes it possible for the debriefer to offer follow-up questions to investigate the causes behind the error and guide the team in establishing strategies on how to avoid it in the future by asking questions such as "What would you do differently the next time?"

While this occurs, the debriefer may come to the conclusion that they need to investigate the team's knowledgebase by asking more particular questions, such as "What level of oxygen concentration should be delivered when beginning chest compressions?" If the team says "100% oxygen," the facilitator will ask, "Was 100% oxygen delivered at the beginning of chest compressions?" If the team says "Yes," the facilitator will move on to the next question. On the other hand, the group can respond "No" or indicate that it was launched later.

There are cultural considerations that impact the quality and type of debriefing sessions. These affect the interaction time, participant initiative for interactions, debriefing content and discussion of non-technical skills. Using a power distance index (PDI), a value reflecting social hierarchy, Ulmer et al., 2018 found a clear correlation between PDI and debriefer-participant behavior patterns with the higher the PDI, the more the debriefer determines the course of the debriefing and the more difficult it becomes to address non-technical skills (Ulmer et al., 2018).

SOLUTIONS AND RECOMMENDATIONS

Adequate preparation and attention to creating a safe learning environment contribute to a successful simulation training session. For facilitators, focusing on structured, learner-centered debriefing strategies and soliciting peer feedback following debriefing sessions can enhance debriefing skills. Consideration of cultural prototypes and their impact on simulation facilitation and debriefing will help facilitators adapt to the prevailing educational expectations in their setting. Additional information on simulation facilitation and debriefing can be acquired through attending simulation facilitator courses which provide opportunities for instructors to hone their skills. Simulation facilitator courses are available through institutions of higher learning, particularly those with a long history of simulation education.

Establishing the background of your learners early on in the session through introductions and a brief explanation of what they hope to gain from the session can be helpful when trying to gain an understanding of your learner group. In the event that the learners have not adequately prepared for the scenario, the facilitator may decide to provide the important background information or brief the group on what to expect as part of the introduction. When a student does not act as though the manikin were an actual patient, it interferes with the ability of other participants to interact with the scenario. It is necessary for the facilitator to address potential underlying issues such as a gap in knowledge or fear of judgment and to remind all learners to perform tasks as they would on an actual patient.

FUTURE RESEARCH DIRECTIONS

Areas of future research revolve around refining approaches to scenario facilitation and debriefing to successfully achieve scenario learning objectives. Recognizing the role of cognitive load and emotions during simulation and debriefing will lead to more learner-focused sessions. A new frontier in simulation and debriefing will be the expanded use of physiological tracking during simulation and debriefing along with its application to performance. In general, for a debriefing to be successful, the debriefer should strive to ask as many open-ended questions as they possibly can, avoid outright criticizing participants' performances, but be willing to confirm erroneous behaviors that are identified by participants. In general, for a debriefing to be successful, the debriefer should strive to ask as many open-ended questions as they possibly can, avoid outright criticizing participants' performances, but be willing to confirm erroneous behaviors that are identified by participants. Defining approaches to prebriefing and debriefing continue to evolve and remain a subject of investigation by simulation researchers.

CONCLUSION

In conclusion, the preparation of a simulation session is essential to the success of the session. Facilitators must be knowledgeable and organized. Simulation scenarios should be conducted professionally, with clear learning objectives and assurances of a safe learning environment. Debriefing sessions should learner driven and focus on objective facts to reinforce correct actions and identify ways to improve future performance.

REFERENCES

Berkowitz, S. S. (2017). Teaching Transnasal Endoscopy to Graduate Students Without a Hospital or Simulation Laboratory: Pool Noodles and Cadavers. *American Journal of Speech-Language Pathology*, *26*(3), 709–715. doi:10.1044/2017_AJSLP-15-0119 PMID:28637051

Bernardo, A. (2017). Establishment of Next-Generation Neurosurgery Research and Training Laboratory with Integrated Human Performance Monitoring. *World Neurosurgery*, *106*, 991–1000. doi:10.1016/j.wneu.2017.06.160 PMID:28985669

Boet, S., Bould, M. D., Bruppacher, H. R., Desjardins, F., Chandra, D. B., & Naik, V. N. (2011). Looking in the mirror: Self-debriefing versus instructor debriefing for simulated crises. *Critical Care Medicine*, *39*(6), 1377–1381. doi:10.1097/CCM.0b013e31820eb8be PMID:21317645

Boet, S., Bould, M. D., Fung, L., Qosa, H., Perrier, L., Tavares, W., Reeves, S., & Tricco, A. C. (2014). Transfer of learning and patient outcome in simulated crisis resource management: a systematic review. *Canadian journal of anaesthesia = Journal canadien d'anesthesie, 61*(6), 571-582. doi:10.1007/s12630-014-0143-8

Bowe, S. N., Johnson, K., & Puscas, L. (2017). Facilitation and Debriefing in Simulation Education. *Otolaryngologic Clinics of North America, 50*(5), 989–1001. doi:10.1016/j.otc.2017.05.009 PMID:28822579

Bradley, N. L., Innes, K., Dakin, C., Sawka, A., Lakha, N., & Hameed, S. M. (2018). Multidisciplinary in-situ simulation to evaluate a rare but high-risk process at a level 1 trauma centre: the "Mega-Sim" approach. *Canadian journal of surgery. Journal canadien de chirurgie, 61*(5), 357-360. doi:10.1503/cjs.005417

Bullough, A. S., Wagner, S., Boland, T., Waters, T. P., Kim, K., & Adams, W. (2016). Obstetric team simulation program challenges. *Journal of Clinical Anesthesia, 35*, 564–570. doi:10.1016/j.jclinane.2016.08.019 PMID:27871594

Cheng, A., Grant, V., Huffman, J., Burgess, G., Szyld, D., Robinson, T., & Eppich, W. (2017). Coaching the Debriefer: Peer Coaching to Improve Debriefing Quality in Simulation Programs. *Simulation in Healthcare: Journal of the Society for Simulation in Healthcare, 12*(5), 319-325. doi:10.1097/SIH.0000000000000232

Cheng, A., Morse, K. J., Rudolph, J., Arab, A. A., Runnacles, J., & Eppich, W. (2016). Learner-Centered Debriefing for Health Care Simulation Education: Lessons for Faculty Development. *Simulation in Healthcare: Journal of the Society for Simulation in Healthcare, 11*(1), 32-40. doi:10.1097/SIH.0000000000000136

Cohen, M. M., Kimmel, N. L., Benage, M. K., Hoang, C., Burroughs, T. E., & Roth, C. A. (2004). Implementing a hospitalwide patient safety program for cultural change. *Joint Commission Journal on Quality and Safety, 30*(8), 424–431. doi:10.1016/S1549-3741(04)30048-1 PMID:15357132

Curtis, E., Ryan, C., Roy, S., Simes, T., Lapkin, S., O'Neill, B., & Faithfull-Byrne, A. (2016). Incorporating peer-to-peer facilitation with a mid-level fidelity student led simulation experience for undergraduate nurses. *Nurse Education in Practice, 20*, 80–84. doi:10.1016/j.nepr.2016.07.003 PMID:27509080

Deutsch, E. S., Dong, Y., Halamek, L. P., Rosen, M. A., Taekman, J. M., & Rice, J. (2016). Leveraging Health Care Simulation Technology for Human Factors Research: Closing the Gap Between Lab and Bedside. *Human Factors, 58*(7), 1082–1095. doi:10.1177/0018720816650781 PMID:27268996

Dufrene, C., & Young, A. (2014). Successful debriefing - best methods to achieve positive learning outcomes: A literature review. *Nurse Education Today*, *34*(3), 372–376. doi:10.1016/j.nedt.2013.06.026 PMID:23890542

Fransen, A. F., van de Ven, J., Schuit, E., van Tetering, A., Mol, B. W., & Oei, S. G. (2017). Simulation-based team training for multi-professional obstetric care teams to improve patient outcome: A multicentre, cluster randomised controlled trial. *BJOG*, *124*(4), 641–650. doi:10.1111/1471-0528.14369 PMID:27726304

Fraser, K., Ma, I., Teteris, E., Baxter, H., Wright, B., & McLaughlin, K. (2012). Emotion, cognitive load and learning outcomes during simulation training. *Medical Education*, *46*(11), 1055–1062. doi:10.1111/j.1365-2923.2012.04355.x PMID:23078682

Fraser, K., & McLaughlin, K. (2019). Temporal pattern of emotions and cognitive load during simulation training and debriefing. *Medical Teacher*, *41*(2), 184–189. doi:10.1080/0142159X.2018.1459531 PMID:29687734

Gaylle, D. (2019). In-simulation Debriefing Increases Therapeutic Communication Skills. *Nurse Educator*, *44*(6), 295–299. doi:10.1097/NNE.0000000000000643 PMID:30640799

Griswold-Theodorson, S., Ponnuru, S., Dong, C., Szyld, D., Reed, T., & McGaghie, W. C. (2015). Beyond the simulation laboratory: A realist synthesis review of clinical outcomes of simulation-based mastery learning. *Academic Medicine*, *90*(11), 1553–1560. doi:10.1097/ACM.0000000000000938 PMID:26375271

Gwin, T., Villanueva, C., & Wong, J. (2017). Student Developed and Led Simulation Scenarios. *Nursing Education Perspectives*, *38*(1), 49–50. doi:10.1097/01.NEP.0000000000000080 PMID:29194248

Haraldseid, C., Friberg, F., & Aase, K. (2015). Nursing students' perceptions of factors influencing their learning environment in a clinical skills laboratory: A qualitative study. *Nurse Education Today*, *35*(9), e1–e6. doi:10.1016/j.nedt.2015.03.015 PMID:25873478

Hayden, E. M., Wong, A. H., Ackerman, J., Sande, M. K., Lei, C., Kobayashi, L., Cassara, M., Cooper, D. D., Perry, K., Lewandowski, W. E., & Scerbo, M. W. (2018). Human Factors and Simulation in Emergency Medicine. *Academic Emergency Medicine: Official Journal of the Society for Academic Emergency Medicine, 25*(2), 221-229. doi:10.1111/acem.13315

Henneman, E. A., Cunningham, H., Fisher, D. L., Plotkin, K., Nathanson, B. H., Roche, J. P., Marquard, J. L., Reilly, C. A., & Henneman, P. L. (2014). Eye tracking as a debriefing mechanism in the simulated setting improves patient safety practices. *Dimensions of critical care nursing. Dimensions of Critical Care Nursing, 33*(3), 129–135. doi:10.1097/DCC.0000000000000041 PMID:24704737

Hirsch, J., Generoso, J. R., Latoures, R., Acar, Y., & Fidler, R. L. (2016). Simulation Manikin Modifications for High-Fidelity Training of Advanced Airway Procedures. *A & A Case Reports, 6*(9), 268–271. doi:10.1213/XAA.0000000000000278 PMID:26752178

Husebø, S. E., Dieckmann, P., Rystedt, H., Søreide, E., & Friberg, F. (2013). The relationship between facilitators' questions and the level of reflection in postsimulation debriefing. *Simulation in Healthcare: Journal of the Society for Simulation in Healthcare, 8*(3), 135-142. doi:10.1097/SIH.0b013e31827cbb5c

Karabacak, U., Unver, V., Ugur, E., Kocatepe, V., Ocaktan, N., Ates, E., & Uslu, Y. (2019). Examining the effect of simulation based learning on self-efficacy and performance of first-year nursing students. *Nurse Education in Practice, 36*, 139–143. doi:10.1016/j.nepr.2019.03.012 PMID:30978577

Kerner, R. L., Jr., Gallo, K., Cassara, M., D'Angelo, J., Egan, A., & Simmons, J. G. (2016). Simulation for Operational Readiness in a New Freestanding Emergency Department: Strategy and Tactics. *Simulation in Healthcare: Journal of the Society for Simulation in Healthcare, 11*(5), 345-356. doi:10.1097/SIH.0000000000000180

Khamis, N. N., Satava, R. M., Alnassar, S. A., & Kern, D. E. (2016). A stepwise model for simulation-based curriculum development for clinical skills, a modification of the six-step approach. *Surgical Endoscopy, 30*(1), 279–287. doi:10.100700464-015-4206-x PMID:25899812

Kobayashi, L., Parchuri, R., Gardiner, F. G., Paolucci, G. A., Tomaselli, N. M., Al-Rasheed, R. S., Bertsch, K. S., Devine, J., Boss, R. M., Gibbs, F. J., Goldlust, E., Monti, J. E., O'Hearn, B., Portelli, D. C., Siegel, N. A., Hemendinger, D., & Jay, G. D. (2013). Use of in situ simulation and human factors engineering to assess and improve emergency department clinical systems for timely telemetry-based detection of life-threatening arrhythmias. *BMJ Quality & Safety, 22*(1), 72–83. doi:10.1136/bmjqs-2012-001134 PMID:23060389

Komorowski, J., Andrighetti, T., & Benton, M. (2017). Modification of Obstetric Emergency Simulation Scenarios for Realism in a Home-Birth Setting. *Journal of Midwifery & Women's Health*, *62*(1), 93–100. doi:10.1111/jmwh.12527 PMID:28002642

Kushnir, T. (1986). Stress and social facilitation: The effects of the presence of an instructor on student nurses' behaviour. *Journal of Advanced Nursing*, *11*(1), 13–19. doi:10.1111/j.1365-2648.1986.tb01215.x PMID:3632980

Lee, J. J., Jeong, H.-C., Kang, K.-A., Kim, Y.-J., & Lee, M.-N. (2015). Development of a Simulation Scenario and Evaluation Checklist for Patients With Asthma in Emergency Care. *Computers, informatics, nursing. CIN*, *33*(12), 546–554. doi:10.1097/CIN.0000000000000193 PMID:26509408

Lencioni, R. D., Ragle, C. A., Kinser, M. L., Coffey, T., & Fransson, B. A. (2017). Effect of simulator orientation during skills training on performance of basic laparoscopic tasks by veterinary students. *Journal of the American Veterinary Medical Association*, *251*(10), 1196–1201. doi:10.2460/javma.251.10.1196 PMID:29099249

Lendahls, L., & Oscarsson, M. G. (2017). Midwifery students' experiences of simulation- and skills training. *Nurse Education Today*, *50*, 12–16. doi:10.1016/j.nedt.2016.12.005 PMID:28006699

Levett-Jones, T., & Lapkin, S. (2014). A systematic review of the effectiveness of simulation debriefing in health professional education. *Nurse Education Today*, *34*(6), e58–e63. doi:10.1016/j.nedt.2013.09.020 PMID:24169444

Lilot, M., Evain, J.-N., Bauer, C., Cejka, J.-C., Faure, A., Balança, B., Vassal, O., Payet, C., Bui Xuan, B., Duclos, A., Lehot, J.-J., & Rimmelé, T. (2018). Relaxation before Debriefing during High-fidelity Simulation Improves Memory Retention of Residents at Three Months: A Prospective Randomized Controlled Study. *Anesthesiology*, *128*(3), 638–649. doi:10.1097/ALN.0000000000002045 PMID:29303790

Littlepage, G. E., Hein, M. B., Moffett, R. G. III, Craig, P. A., & Georgiou, A. M. (2016). Team Training for Dynamic Cross-Functional Teams in Aviation: Behavioral, Cognitive, and Performance Outcomes. *Human Factors*, *58*(8), 1275–1288. doi:10.1177/0018720816665200 PMID:27549389

Lyons, R., Lazzara, E. H., Benishek, L. E., Zajac, S., Gregory, M., Sonesh, S. C., & Salas, E. (2015). Enhancing the effectiveness of team debriefings in medical simulation: More best practices. *Joint Commission Journal on Quality and Patient Safety*, *41*(3), 115–125. doi:10.1016/S1553-7250(15)41016-5 PMID:25977127

Maestre, J. M., & Rudolph, J. W. (2015). Theories and styles of debriefing: The good judgment method as a tool for formative assessment in healthcare. *Revista Española de Cardiología (English Ed.)*, *68*(4), 282–285. doi:10.1016/j.rec.2014.05.018 PMID:25239179

Marzano, D., Smith, R., Mhyre, J. M., Seagull, F. J., Curran, D., Behrmann, S., Priessnitz, K., & Hammoud, M. (2016). Evaluation of a simulation-based curriculum for implementing a new clinical protocol. *International Journal of Gynaecology and Obstetrics: the Official Organ of the International Federation of Gynaecology and Obstetrics*, *135*(3), 333–337. doi:10.1016/j.ijgo.2016.06.022 PMID:27614788

Maxwell, W. D., Mohorn, P. L., Haney, J. S., Phillips, C. M., Lu, Z. K., Clark, K., Corboy, A., & Ragucci, K. R. (2016). Impact of an Advanced Cardiac Life Support Simulation Laboratory Experience on Pharmacy Student Confidence and Knowledge. *American Journal of Pharmaceutical Education*, *80*(8), 140–140. doi:10.5688/ajpe808140 PMID:27899836

McKechnie, A. (2016). The importance and practice of debrief in medical simulation. *British Journal of Hospital Medicine*, *77*(3), 184-187. doi:10.12968/hmed.2016.77.3.184

McMullen, M., Wilson, R., Fleming, M., Mark, D., Sydor, D., Wang, L., Zamora, J., Phelan, R., & Burjorjee, J. E. (2016). "Debriefing-on-Demand": A Pilot Assessment of Using a "Pause Button" in Medical Simulation. *Simulation in Healthcare: Journal of the Society for Simulation in Healthcare*, *11*(3), 157-163. doi:10.1097/SIH.0000000000000140

Nguyen, N., Watson, W. D., & Dominguez, E. (2016). An Event-Based Approach to Design a Teamwork Training Scenario and Assessment Tool in Surgery. *Journal of Surgical Education*, *73*(2), 197–207. doi:10.1016/j.jsurg.2015.10.005 PMID:26774937

Ohta, K., Kurosawa, H., Shiima, Y., Ikeyama, T., Scott, J., Hayes, S., Gould, M., Buchanan, N., Nadkarni, V., & Nishisaki, A. (2017). The Effectiveness of Remote Facilitation in Simulation-Based Pediatric Resuscitation Training for Medical Students. *Pediatric Emergency Care*, *33*(8), 564–569. doi:10.1097/PEC.0000000000000752 PMID:27261952

Patterson, M. D., Geis, G. L., LeMaster, T., & Wears, R. L. (2013). Impact of multidisciplinary simulation-based training on patient safety in a paediatric emergency department. *BMJ Quality & Safety*, *22*(5), 383–393. doi:10.1136/bmjqs-2012-000951 PMID:23258388

Pheister, M., Stagno, S., Cotes, R., Prabhakar, D., Mahr, F., Crowell, A., & Schwartz, A. (2017). Simulated Patients and Scenarios to Assess and Teach Psychiatry Residents. *Academic Psychiatry: The Journal of the American Association of Directors of Psychiatric Residency Training and the Association for Academic Psychiatry, 41*(1), 114-117. doi:10.1007/s40596-015-0477-8

Reed, S. J. (2015). Written debriefing: Evaluating the impact of the addition of a written component when debriefing simulations. *Nurse Education in Practice*, *15*(6), 543–548. doi:10.1016/j.nepr.2015.07.011 PMID:26299701

Rinewalt, D., Du, H., & Velasco, J. M. (2012). Evaluation of a novel laparoscopic simulation laboratory curriculum. *Surgery*, *152*(4), 550–556. doi:10.1016/j.surg.2012.08.009 PMID:23021133

Rudolph, J. W., Simon, R., Rivard, P., Dufresne, R. L., & Raemer, D. B. (2007). Debriefing with good judgment: Combining rigorous feedback with genuine inquiry. *Anesthesiology Clinics*, *25*(2), 361–376. doi:10.1016/j.anclin.2007.03.007 PMID:17574196

Sannomiya, Y., Muranaka, Y., Teraoka, M., Suzuki, S., Saito, Y., Yamato, H., & Ishii, M. (2016). Proposal of Comprehensive Model of Teaching Basic Nursing Skills Under Goal-Based Scenario Theory. *Studies in Health Technology and Informatics*, *225*, 1055–1056. https://pubmed.ncbi.nlm.nih.gov/27332480 PMID:27332480

Sarwani, N., Tappouni, R., & Flemming, D. (2012). Use of a simulation laboratory to train radiology residents in the management of acute radiologic emergencies. *AJR. American Journal of Roentgenology*, *199*(2), 244–251. doi:10.2214/AJR.11.7892 PMID:22826384

Sawyer, T., Eppich, W., Brett-Fleegler, M., Grant, V., & Cheng, A. (2016). More Than One Way to Debrief: A Critical Review of Healthcare Simulation Debriefing Methods. *Simulation in Healthcare: Journal of the Society for Simulation in Healthcare, 11*(3), 209-217. doi:10.1097/SIH.0000000000000148

Sawyer, T., Sierocka-Castaneda, A., Chan, D., Berg, B., Lustik, M., & Thompson, M. (2012). The effectiveness of video-assisted debriefing versus oral debriefing alone at improving neonatal resuscitation performance: a randomized trial. *Simulation in Healthcare: Journal of the Society for Simulation in Healthcare, 7*(4), 213-221. doi:10.1097/SIH.0b013e3182578eae

Sawyer, T. L., & Deering, S. (2013). Adaptation of the US Army's after-action review for simulation debriefing in healthcare. *Simulation in Healthcare, 8*(6), 388–397. doi:10.1097/SIH.0b013e31829ac85c PMID:24096913

Saylor, J. L., Wainwright, S. F., Herge, E. A., & Pohlig, R. T. (2016). Peer-Assessment Debriefing Instrument (PADI): Assessing Faculty Effectiveness in Simulation Education. *Journal of Allied Health, 45*(3), e27–e30. PMID:27585622

Schlairet, M. C., Schlairet, T. J., Sauls, D. H., & Bellflowers, L. (2015). Cognitive load, emotion, and performance in high-fidelity simulation among beginning nursing students: A pilot study. *The Journal of Nursing Education, 54*(3, Suppl), S5–S11. doi:10.3928/01484834-20150218-10 PMID:25692940

Severson, M. A., Maxson, P. M., Wrobleski, D. S., & Dozois, E. J. (2014). Simulation-based team training and debriefing to enhance nursing and physician collaboration. *Journal of Continuing Education in Nursing, 45*(7), 297–305. doi:10.3928/00220124-20140620-03 PMID:24972099

Surcouf, J. W., Chauvin, S. W., Ferry, J., Yang, T., & Barkemeyer, B. (2013). Enhancing residents' neonatal resuscitation competency through unannounced simulation-based training. *Medical Education Online, 18*(1), 1–7. doi:10.3402/meo.v18i0.18726 PMID:23522399

Syed, S. A., Nukala, S., Marcano, J. L., Bedwell, W. L., Haubner, L., & Raij, A. (2014). Sensing and visualization tools for objective assessment and debriefing of high-risk neonatal resuscitation training scenarios. *Studies in Health Technology and Informatics, 196*, 416–422. https://pubmed.ncbi.nlm.nih.gov/24732547 PMID:24732547

Szulewski, A., Braund, H., Egan, R., Hall, A. K., Dagnone, J. D., Gegenfurtner, A., & van Merrienboer, J. J. G. (2018). Through the Learner's Lens: Eye-Tracking Augmented Debriefing in Medical Simulation. *Journal of Graduate Medical Education, 10*(3), 340–341. doi:10.4300/JGME-D-17-00827.1 PMID:29946395

Theilen, U., Fraser, L., Jones, P., Leonard, P., & Simpson, D. (2017). Regular in-situ simulation training of paediatric Medical Emergency Team leads to sustained improvements in hospital response to deteriorating patients, improved outcomes in intensive care and financial savings. *Resuscitation, 115*, 61–67. doi:10.1016/j.resuscitation.2017.03.031 PMID:28359769

Tongdee, P., Tiansri, K., Srisawat, S., Ngamnoun, A., Pinwanna, K., & Nimkuntod, P. (2016). Mobile Content and Scenario-Based Manikin for Improving Learning Outcomes in Obstetrics of Preclinical Medical Students. *Journal of the Medical Association of Thailand = Chotmaihet thangphaet, 99*(7), S49-S53. https://pubmed.ncbi.nlm.nih.gov/29901908

Uemura, M., Tomikawa, M., Nagao, Y., Yamashita, N., Kumashiro, R., Tsutsumi, N., Ohuchida, K., Ieiri, S., Ohdaira, T., & Hashizume, M. (2014). Significance of metacognitive skills in laparoscopic surgery assessed by essential task simulation. *Minimally Invasive Therapy & Allied Technologies, 23*(3), 165-172. doi:10.3109/13645706.2013.867273

Ulmer, F. F., Sharara-Chami, R., Lakissian, Z., Stocker, M., Scott, E., & Dieckmann, P. (2018). Cultural Prototypes and Differences in Simulation Debriefing. *Simulation in Healthcare: Journal of the Society for Simulation in Healthcare, 13*(4), 239-246. doi:10.1097/SIH.0000000000000320

Utz, B., Kana, T., & van den Broek, N. (2015). Practical aspects of setting up obstetric skills laboratories—A literature review and proposed model. *Midwifery, 31*(4), 400–408. doi:10.1016/j.midw.2014.11.010 PMID:25535017

Wetzel, E. A., Lang, T. R., Pendergrass, T. L., Taylor, R. G., & Geis, G. L. (2013). Identification of latent safety threats using high-fidelity simulation-based training with multidisciplinary neonatology teams. *Joint Commission Journal on Quality and Patient Safety, 39*(6), 268–273. doi:10.1016/S1553-7250(13)39037-0 PMID:23789165

Wong, A. H.-W., Gang, M., Szyld, D., & Mahoney, H. (2016). Making an "Attitude Adjustment": Using a Simulation-Enhanced Interprofessional Education Strategy to Improve Attitudes Toward Teamwork and Communication. *Simulation in Healthcare: Journal of the Society for Simulation in Healthcare, 11*(2), 117-125. doi:10.1097/SIH.0000000000000133

Zhang, H., Mörelius, E., Goh, S. H. L., & Wang, W. (2019). Effectiveness of Video-Assisted Debriefing in Simulation-Based Health Professions Education: A Systematic Review of Quantitative Evidence. *Nurse Educator, 44*(3), E1–E6. doi:10.1097/NNE.0000000000000562 PMID:30015683

Zimmermann, K., Holzinger, I. B., Ganassi, L., Esslinger, P., Pilgrim, S., Allen, M., Burmester, M., & Stocker, M. (2015). Inter-professional in-situ simulated team and resuscitation training for patient safety: Description and impact of a programmatic approach. *BMC Medical Education, 15*(1), 189–189. doi:10.118612909-015-0472-5 PMID:26511721

KEY TERMS AND DEFINITIONS

Augmented Reality: Computer generated holographic images can be viewed by the learner in the physical environment using a mobile device or specially designed headset.

High-Fidelity Manikin: This term refers to a technology-enabled manikin with features such as mechanical respiration and heart rate.

Low-Fidelity Manikin: This is typically a low cost, low technology manikin with minimal features.

Objective Structured Clinical Examination (OSCE): An approach to assessment that involves defined objectives and anticipated actions, often with an accompanying checklist for assessment.

Simulation Debriefer: A simulation instructor who leads the learners through a reflective analysis of simulation events.

Simulation Facilitator: A simulation instructor who guides the learners through the scenario with the goal of meeting learning objectives.

Simulation Technician/Specialist: An individual who supports the practice of simulation through setting up and managing simulation manikins and supplies.

Teledebriefing: Teledebriefing describes a process in which learners who are participating in a simulation scenario undergo debriefing with a facilitator located at an off-site location.

Telefacilitation: The conduct of a telesimulation by a remote facilitator.

Telesimulation: Telesimulation is a process by which telecommunication and simulation resources are utilized to provide education, training, and/or assessment to learners at an off-site location.

Video-Assisted Debriefing: The practice of using video captured during simulation sessions for reflective discussions on learner and team performance.

Virtual Environment: 3D computer generated objects that can be viewed on a screen or in a head-mounted display.

Virtual Reality: Computer generated 3D images viewed by a learner in a virtual environment using a low-cost or high-end head mounted display.

Chapter 6
Evaluation of Simulation Performance

ABSTRACT

Simulation can be used for formative and summative evaluation of learner performance. This chapter describes tools and approaches for evaluation of simulation performance through direct and indirect observation, video review, and other metrics of data capture for manikin-based and virtual simulation. Simulation instructors are guided through an approach to evaluating team performance using validated tools. Special considerations for evaluating individual and team performance are discussed, including the impact of stress on performance, minimizing bias, and evaluating large groups of learners.

INTRODUCTION

Simulation-based performance evaluations are undertaken by instructors using specific performance metrics based on the learning goals and objectives and type of simulation activity. The wide range of simulation types from procedural manikin-based simulation to virtual simulation means that the approach to evaluation must be tailored to the activity and purpose of the evaluation. Evaluations may be formative, intended to guide the learner or summative, intended for assessment of performance (Aeder et al., 2007; Mangold et al., 2015; Solheim et al., 2017). Regardless of the simulation type, establishing learning objectives during simulation development is key to the proper evaluation of simulation performance. For more information,

DOI: 10.4018/978-1-7998-4378-8.ch006

see Chapter 3 on "Scenario Development for Manikin-based Simulation". The evaluation needs to be adjusted based on the level of the learner, the nature of the scenario, and the amount of time that is available. The evaluation may concentrate on the individual or the team, and it may be carried out in person or virtually by instructors, external assessors, or even simulated patients. It may also focus on either the individual or the team. Determining the method by which data will be collected on the performance of learners is the first step in getting started with an evaluation. Video and audio recordings are two methods of data collection that have seen widespread use in simulation training. These recordings, along with validated, standardized checklists and manikin-based data, have been used for evaluation purposes. It is possible to configure virtual simulations so that they record information about the timing and frequency of a learner's actions. In recent times, strategies that have been used to reduce the burden of direct observation or video review include crowdsourcing manual video review, the outsourcing of manual video review, and the automation of video review through the use of artificial intelligence.

APPROACH TO EVALUATION OF SIMULATION PERFORMANCE

Formative Evaluation

Examination scores do not provide a comprehensive measurement of performance, and it is widely acknowledged that training programs need to incorporate a variety of methods for evaluating their trainees. Formative assessment can be provided by simulation, which can help students improve their learning and performance, as well as provide feedback to both individual students and the team. The necessity of engaging in repeated practice up until one's desired level of competence necessitated the development of the concept of mastery learning. The theory of deliberative practice developed by Ericsson provides support for the use of simulation education due to the fact that it is interactive and gives students the opportunity to practice their abilities repeatedly while receiving immediate feedback (Ericsson, 2004). The majority of the assessments carried out during simulations are formative. This indicates that the information gained from the assessment is used to improve performance and address deficiencies prior to a summative performance evaluation being carried out. Formative evaluations may employ straightforward checklists or more complex formats such as objective structured clinical examinations (OSCE) in order to investigate knowledge gaps and encourage practice (Mangold et al., 2015). This method is suitable for assessing a wide variety of performance metrics, including clinical decision-making, procedural skills, as well as communication with patients and other team members.

Summative Evaluation

Summative performance evaluations are high-stakes assessments in which learner competence is evaluated for the purposes of advancement or certification (Ghoman et al., 2020; Szasz et al., 2016). The reason for the evaluation is what makes it formative or summative. The approaches used for summative evaluations are similar to those used with formative evaluations. For instance, the Objective Structured Clinical Examinations (OSCE) A and OSCE B found in the Helping Babies Breathe curriculum are examples of summative evaluations of neonatal resuscitation performance. The users of these checklists are the observers, and they contain the actions that are expected to be carried out. Nevertheless, there are a few obstacles to consider when conducting summative simulation assessments. The simulations need to be designed appropriately and in a way that is consistent with the goals of the program. Validity and dependability are required of the evaluation tools. The degree to which an assessment measures the intended metric and accurately reflects the actual practices of a healthcare provider is what's meant to be measured by the validity of the assessment. It is essential to take measures to ensure the ratings can be trusted. The same scores would be reproduced in a highly reliable test by different evaluators as well as by the same evaluator at a later time. Evaluators shouldn't have any prior knowledge of the students whose work they're assessing, and ratings should be carried out without any outside assistance whenever it's possible. Training programs for evaluators are required if accurate and consistent performance ratings are to be achieved (Oermann et al., 2016). To guarantee that students receive objective evaluations, it is necessary to proceed in this manner. It's possible that many times, teachers will find it more useful to make use of the data that was gathered directly through manikin-based or virtual simulation software programs. It's possible that these data are significantly more objective than those obtained using human raters, given that even experienced raters can have different opinions.

Figure 1. Direct observation

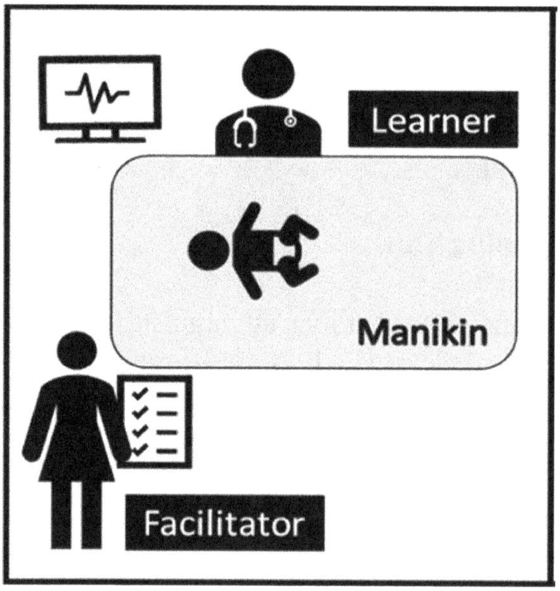

TYPES OF DATA COLLECTION

Standardized Checklists

Standardized checklists are used for assessing learner performance. For the purpose of learner assessment, there is a substantial quantity of checkpoints that have been validated in a variety of fields (Solheim et al., 2017). Both technical and non-technical skills should be taken into consideration because they cover the most ground. It is essential that you ascertain whether or not the checklist you choose has been validated in the learner population with which you are currently collaborating. The checklist can be modified to fit the characteristics of your population if that proves necessary; however, changing the wording of any of the items on the checklist could render it useless. Validation can be a time-consuming process, but if there are no checklists currently available in the area of interest, it may be necessary to conduct validation of your own checklist in order to encourage other researchers to use it. Validation can be done in a number of different ways. For the purposes of education as well as formative evaluations, a checklist that has not been validated can be used and shared. Nevertheless, when conducting research, it is recommended that only validated checklists be used. Refer to Chapter 9, "Research and Data

Collection Strategies for Simulation Educators" for additional information on the process of developing and validating standardized checklists.

Technical Skills Checklists

Technical skills can be assessed using performance checklists for specific tasks such as central venous line placement, endotracheal intubation and chest compressions. Skills-based checklist have been used to evaluate skill efficiency and often focus on time to task completion of checklist items. This may be done in a single assessment or over time in the context of a training rotation where didactics, simulation and clinical experiences may impact skills. For example, Nwachukwu et al., described a checklist to assess orthopedic surgery resident diagnostic knee and shoulder arthroscopic efficiency (Geeraerts & Le Guen, 2018; Nwachukwu et al., 2017). Examples of crisis checklists or cognitive aids include the cognitive aids in Anesthesia and Critical care from the French Society of Anesthesia and Intensive Care Medicine (SFAR) (http://www.sfar.org/espace-professionel/). The use of the SFAR checklist improved non-technical performance in critical actions such the correct and complete administration of medications during simulation training (Hardy et al., 2018). The Neonatal Resuscitation Performance Evaluation (NRPE) Tool is used to evaluate neonatal resuscitation performance (Sawyer et al., 2012a). Similarly, the Society for Pediatric Anesthesia has developed a set of critical-event checklists and cognitive aids. In general these, aids are designed to serve as evidence-based information to guide responses and management of critical events and as a method to facilitate shared understanding of required actions among team members during a critical event (Clebone et al., 2017).

Non-Technical Skills Checklists

Non-technical skills include leadership, communication and teamwork. Effective communication is essential for improving healthcare outcomes. Good physician-patient communication ensures that patients adequately understand their diagnoses, treatment options, medications, plans for referral and prognosis (Setyonugroho et al., 2015). Examples of verbal communication behaviors that have been positively associated with health outcomes include empathy, reassurance and support, explanations, positive reinforcement, humor, psychosocial talk, information sharing, friendliness, courtesy, summarization and clarification (Beck et al., 2002). Verbal behaviors have been classified into: 1) data gathering to understand the patient (gathering information); 2) development of rapport and responding to the patient's emotions (developing a therapeutic relationship); and 3) patient education and behavioral management (decision-making and management) (Beck et al., 2002). See Figure 2 for a schematic representation derived from the Bird and Cohen-Cole model. Similar categorization schemes have been described by Roter and Hall, Ong et al., and Beisecker and Beisecker (Beck et al., 2002).

Figure 2. Relationship between the domains of provider-patient communication
Legend: Adapted from Domains of communication in the provider-patient relationship in Beck RS, Daughtridge R, Sloane PD. Physician-patient communication in the primary care office: a systematic review. The Journal of the American Board of Family Practice. 2002 Jan 1;15(1):25-38.(Beck et al., 2002)

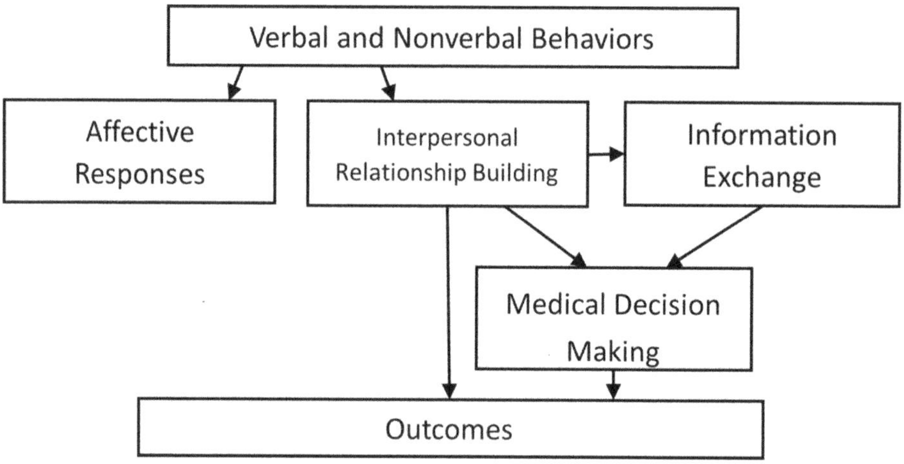

Nonverbal behaviors positively associated with outcomes included head nodding, forward lean, direct body orientation, uncrossed legs and arms, arm symmetry, and less mutual gaze (Beck et al., 2002). Harrigan and Rosenthal grouped nonverbal behavior by anatomic position into the categories of trunk, arms, legs, head, and proximity or touch. Behaviors associated with unfavorable outcomes included more patient gaze, body orientation 45 to 90 degrees away from the patient, indirect body orientation, backward lean, crossed arms, task touch and frequent touch (Beck et al., 2002).

Checklists designed for crisis situations such as cardiac arrest or post-partum hemorrhage feature not just technical skills, but also nontechnical skills including critical elements of leadership and communication (Geeraerts & Le Guen, 2018). General and specific checklists designed to rate provider-patient interactions have been described. An example of a generic checklist is the common ground (CG) instrument. Specific communication checklists that focus on history-taking, physician-patient communication, interviewing, negotiating treatment, information giving, empathy and other domains. Instruments such as the Anaesthestists' Non-technical Skills Scale (ANTS) (Fletcher et al., 2003) have been used to evaluate teamwork skills.

Manikin-Based Data

The use of manikin-based data has increased with the availability of high-fidelity electronic manikins and accessories such as the Zoll defibrillator pads. These manikins contain pressure and flow sensors that can be used to return data on adequate performance of procedures. Due to the presence of these sensors, the high-fidelity manikin is able to identify certain procedures as being accomplished successfully such as the placement of the endotracheal tube during endotracheal intubation and to be able to detect complications such as right-main stem intubation where the endotracheal tube is malpositioned in the right bronchus.

The volume of air delivered during positive pressure ventilation can be determined using flow sensor calculations. Pressure sensors can detect the amount of pressure delivered with each breath and the rate of positive pressure ventilation can be delivered and reported. The depth and rate of chest compression can also be detected and feedback provided in real time using specialized defibrillator pads and on certain high-fidelity manikins. In obstetric care, sensors can determine the degree of torque or pulling of the head relative to the neck and shoulder of the newborn during a delivery complicated by shoulder dystocia that could result in Erb's palsy or other neurologic complications can be detected on certain birthing manikins. Using these types of visualized data and reports generated by manikin-based sensors, the instructor is able to assess performance in real-time and the learner receives formative feedback to improve their performance and reduce the risk of complications in patient care.

Even though the method of providing feedback through the use of manikins is still being developed, in most cases the instructor is present and provides the feedback. There are now new possibilities available that could make it possible for students to practice on their own and get feedback in predetermined areas within their clinical setting. However, due to the high cost of high-fidelity manikins as well as their relative scarcity, it can be challenging for simulation centers to make these readily available for asynchronous learning.

Audiovisual Data

Simple camera setup: It has been extensively described how audiovisual methods can be used to collect data while simulations are being run. The use of dedicated video-recording cameras, wearable devices, cell phone cameras, or webcams are all viable options for capturing a straightforward video recording. It is important that the devices be positioned in such a way that they can record the actions that are being carried out on the manikin. In certain circumstances, it is essential to record the interactions between the members of the healthcare team. In the majority of situations in which a straightforward video capture is desired, a single camera, typically a phone or webcam, is mounted to a stationary holder or stand and then trained on a manikin. Figure 3. A live video feed can be accessed through the webcam, which is connected to a laptop. Software that is capable of video recording as well as screen capture makes it possible to save the video recording and retrieve it at a later time. Because of recent advancements in video conferencing platforms, it is now possible to configure these platforms so that they stream live video to remote facilitators. It is also possible to record videos while simultaneously archiving the files for later retrieval.

Figure 3. Remote observation via camera

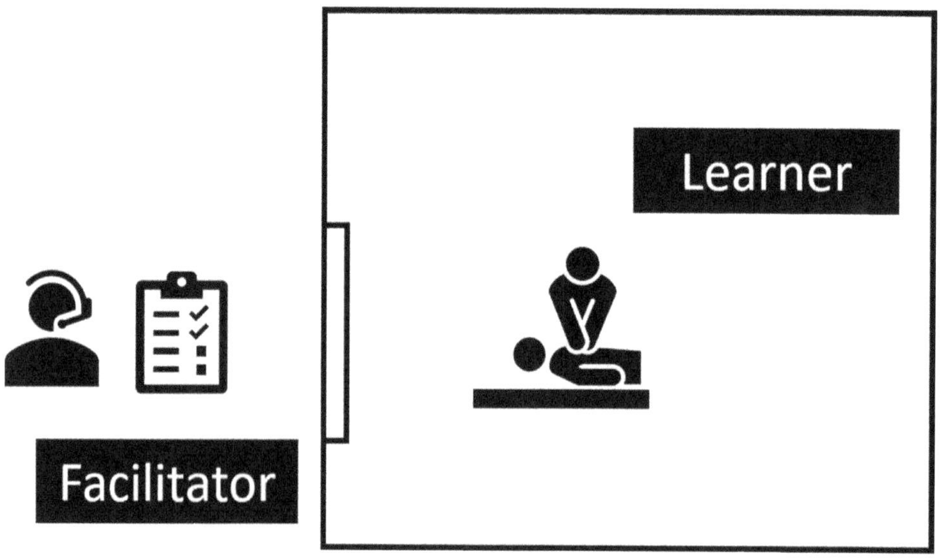

Wearable Devices

For the purpose of video capture, some facilitators have used a camera that was mounted on one of the team members, such as the team leader, in order to record both the perspective of the team leader as well as the actions taken by the participants while they were participating in the simulation. Wearable devices such as Google Glass or the augmented reality glasses made by Microsoft HoloLens are examples of one option that have been used to capture video for livestreaming or for recording. It might be helpful to simulate the patient's experience from their point of view if the simulation is focused on the patient's journey through the healthcare system. In situations like these, the camera is mounted on the manikin so that it can capture a view of the surrounding area as well as the healthcare team.

Multi-Camera Systems

In some cases, two or more cameras, capturing the view of the team leader, team members and the manikin may be used. Commercially available software programs are used to capture and synchronize video feeds from more than one camera. This allows for audio and video recordings to be stored, retrieved and analyzed for educational and research purposes. The use of these software programs also allows facilitators to annotate areas of interest for video debriefing following the simulation. Audio and video recordings can be used to evaluate learners and provide formative and summative feedback on learner performance. In research projects, they can be used by trained raters to describe learner performance during events such as codes, delivery resuscitations and teamwork simulations.

Simulated Patient Evaluations

Standardized Patients

Standardized patient (SP) clinical examinations are used in undergraduate and postgraduate health sciences education to present the care of patients presenting with episodic illnesses and to evaluate students' skill in performing history taking or physical examination as well as assessments and medical decision making as it is applied to the delivery of health care. With SPs, the level of difficulty and the amount of information presented by the patient can be correlated with the skill level of the student with adaptation of cases with higher levels of difficulty for more advanced students.

SPs can be a means of indirect observation during simulated assessments. SPs are trained in interview, communication, physical assessment, and feedback strategies. They are often provided with an assessment form to document learner actions. In addition, these forms may contain a field for open-ended comments that have been found to be revealing of concerns in areas such as communication and interpersonal skills, as well as in history taking, and the physical exam. SPs evaluations may be used primarily for formative feedback rather than assessment, but in some cases, their perspectives have been invaluable for highlighting positive attributes or deficiencies that were not identified by scores on the traditional assessment forms (Boulet, 2012). For example, positive communication behaviors like good listening skills or difficulties with communication such as lack of empathy or lack of connection to the patient. They can also identify deficiencies in history taking and physical examination (Blatt et al., 2016).

Virtual Standardized Patients

Virtual Standardized Patients (VSPs) have been used to support learning experiences, developing knowledge, skill and practice of NTS categories including communication, situation awareness, teamwork, decision-making skills and duty, advocacy and empathy (Foster et al., 2016; Peddle et al., 2019; Stevens et al., 2006). However, they may be better received by students in professions where patient interactions are limited. A qualitative study of learners in pharmacy and medicine found that pharmacy students perceived increased value in using VSPs due to their limited access to patients during their education while medical students challenged the role of VPs in their clinical development. The primary concerns expressed were that VSPs lack the flexibility required by doctors to use their judgement and work with uncertainty (Timmis et al., 2018). Studies in clinical psychiatry showed that students who were taught using a computer-based software method were better able to answer a standard series of questions designed to evaluate their understanding of dementia than those who were taught in a conventional manner (Matsumura et al., 2018). The advantage of well-designed VSPs over SPs may be in more objective evaluation of performance using standardized metrics (Georg et al., 2018; Huwendiek et al., 2009; Urresti-Gundlach et al., 2017).

Longitudinal Standardized Patient Experiences

Another approach to using SPs is through Longitudinal standardized patient (LSP) experiences. Students are given the opportunity to interact with standardized patients over the course of this experience, much like they would in a clinic. Learners are able to develop an appreciation for the continuum of care as a result of the use of LSP cases, which allow for the practice, evaluation, and feedback in clinical skills that might otherwise be lacking (Block et al., 2018). It is recommended that students, faculty, and SPs be purposefully paired with one another in order to improve relationship-building and feedback (Block et al., 2018).

Virtual Simulation Data

During virtual simulations, it is possible for data to be captured automatically using metrics identified during simulation design, processed using algorithmic or artificial intelligence (AI) approaches, and feedback to be delivered without the input of the instructor. The automation of the feedback enables the learner to engage in deliberate practice, which consists of the learner repeating actions or tasks until they have achieved mastery. The incorporation of gamification into virtual simulations can assist in ensuring that, even though certain actions must be performed repeatedly, there are built-in rewards and incentives to keep the process interesting. There are a number of important advantages to adopting this methodology, most notably for students who possibly do not have convenient access to simulation facilities.

Detailed data can also be collected more quickly and accurately through the use of virtual simulations as opposed to human observations. For instance, specific information on the amount of time required for certain actions can be reported as timestamped actions, information on the sequence of actions, and information on the relationship between the chosen actions and certain outcomes. Even though the time it takes to complete actions in virtual simulations might not have a strong correlation with the time it takes to complete these actions in a clinical setting, the trends can still be investigated. The performance of an individual learner or an entire group of students can be compared across multiple attempts using these metrics for measuring performance.

Table 1. Data sources and types for simulation evaluations

Data sources	Data types	Simulation evaluation
Standardized checklists	Technical skills checklists	Procedural skills
	Non-technical skills checklists	Leadership Teamwork Communication (verbal and non-verbal)
Manikin-based data	Flow sensors Pressure sensors	Procedural skills e.g., chest compressions, endotracheal intubation
Audiovisual data	Single cameras (video recording camera, cell phone camera, webcams)	Procedural skills Leadership Teamwork Communication (verbal and non-verbal)
	Multi-camera systems	
	Wearable devices	
Simulated patient evaluations	Standardized Patients (SP)	Communication Cognitive skills Physical Examination skills
	Virtual standardized patients	
Virtual simulation data	Action timing Action sequence	Cognitive skills Teamwork skills Procedural skills

EVALUATING TEAM PERFORMANCE

When health professionals coordinate care, communicate effectively, and support one another in crisis situations, they deliver high quality patient care. Non-technical skills have been demonstrated to be critical for patient safety and there have been several training curricula such designed for crew-resource management, including the Team Strategies and Tools for Performance and Patient Safety (TeamSTEPPS) (King et al., 2008). Teamwork training is essential to support the growth of teamwork knowledge, attitudes, and behaviors, and it has been described how manikin-based and virtual simulation can be used for teamwork training and assessment. Teamwork training is important to support the development of teamwork knowledge, attitudes, and behaviors (Sawyer et al., 2013; Sweigart et al., 2016; Umoren et al., 2017; Umoren et al., 2018). Evaluation of team performance is made possible by the utilization of objective ratings that may be performed either during or after the simulation to evaluate the level of teamwork.

Teamwork Assessment Tools

The assessment of team performance and feedback on areas for improvement requires validated tools and measures. There are two types of scales typically used to evaluate communication skills: 1) behavioral checklists and 2) global rating scales. Global rating scales have been demonstrated to have higher internal consistency when compared to checklists. Using both global rating scales and checklists in combination can improve content validity and internal consistency (Setyonugroho et al., 2015). For example, the Assessment of Obstetrical Team Performance (AOTP) and Global Assessment of Obstetrical Team Performance (GAOTP) (Morgan et al., 2012) have an internal consistency for AOTP of 0.96 and GAOTP of 0.91. Collectively, as a 22-point scale, the internal consistency was very high at 0.97. Systematic literature reviews have been conducted to identify validated teamwork assessment tools in specialty specific training such as in Obstetric emergencies (Onwochei et al., 2017) and in Internal Medicine (Havyer et al., 2014). A recent review conducted by Wooding et al., (Wooding et al., 2020) focused on assessing the validity of teamwork tools used in simulation-based interprofessional teamwork training for health professionals and students, building on a prior systematic literature review of teamwork assessment tools in undergraduate education (Havyer et al., 2016). Common contexts for teamwork training during simulation are pediatric and neonatal emergencies, particularly resuscitation, emergency room trauma, anesthetic or surgical complications mid-operation and obstetric emergencies (Wooding et al., 2020).

Many validated tools have been developed for the assessment of team performance. See Table 1. Some of the earliest teamwork scales included the Anaesthetists' Non-Technical Skills Scale (ANTS) (Fletcher et al., 2003), the Mayo High Performance Teamwork Scale (Malec et al., 2007), the Clinical Teamwork Scale (CTS) (Guise et al., 2008), and the Team Emergency Assessment Measure (TEAM) (Cooper et al., 2010). The KidSIM Team Performance Scale (KidSIM) (Sigalet et al., 2013) was developed in 2013 from the Mayo Scale (Malec et al., 2007) and Clinical Teamwork Scale (Guise et al., 2008). Other teamwork scales include Communication and Teamwork Skills (CATS) (Frankel et al., 2007), Observational Skill-based Clinical Assessment tool for Resuscitation (OSCAR) (Walker et al., 2011), Objective Teamwork Assessment System (OTAS) (Passauer-Baierl et al., 2014; Phitayakorn et al., 2015), Operating Room Team Assessment Scale (ORTAS) (Hull et al., 2011; Paige et al., 2014), Team Average Performance

Assessment Scale (TAPAS) (Oriot et al., 2016), Team Performance Observation Tool (TPOT) (Zhang et al., 2015), and the Assessment of Obstetrical Team Performance (AOTP) (Morgan et al., 2012). Some teamwork scales such as Checklist of Expected Actions (Daniels et al., 2008), Neonatal Resuscitation Program (NRP) Performance Checklist (Sawyer et al., 2012b) and the Trauma Simulation Evaluation Tool (Auerbach et al., 2014) have been described for use in retrospective video review and direct observation of simulated encounters but have not undergone psychometric validation.

Table 2. Validated team performance scales

Tool	Acronym	Early studies	Other studies	Study population	Evaluation context
Anaesthetists' Non-Technical Skills Scale	ANTS	Fletcher et al., 2003	Jankouskas et al., 2007 Patterson et al., 2013	Pediatricians, anesthetists, nurses, paramedics, respiratory therapists, patient care assistants, others	Retrospective video review
Assessment of Obstetrical Team Performance	AOTP	Tregunno, et al., 2009	Morgan et al., 2012	Anesthetists, nurses, obstetricians, family doctors	Retrospective video review
Clinical Teamwork Scale	CTS	Guise et al., 2008		Obstetricians, nurses	Retrospective video review
KidSIM Team Performance Scale	KidSIM		Sigalet et al., 2013	Nursing, medical and respiratory therapy students	Retrospective video review
Mayo High Performance Teamwork Scale	MHPTS	Malec et al., 2007 Hobgood et al., 2010 (adapted Mayo scale)	Burton et al., 2011 Weller et al., 2011	Doctors, nurses and respiratory therapists	Retrospective video review
Objective Teamwork Assessment System	OTAS	Passauer-Baierl et al., 2014	Phitayakorn et al., 2015	Nurses, scrub technicians, anesthetic residents, surgical residents	Retrospective video review
Observational Skill-based Clinical Assessment tool for Resuscitation	OSCAR	Walker et al., 2011		Anesthetists, nurses, physicians	Retrospective video review
Operating Room Team Assessment Scale	ORTAS	Hull et al., 2011	Paige et al., 2014	Medical students, nursing anesthesia students, nursing students	Direct observation
Team Average Performance Assessment Scale	TAPAS	Oriot et al., 2016	Ghazali et al., 2016	Physicians, nurses, ambulance drivers	Direct observation
Team Emergency Assessment Measure	TEAM	Cooper et al., 2010	Rovamo et al., 2015	Medical students, nursing students, pediatricians, anesthetists, obstetricians, midwives, neonatal nurses	Direct observation
Team Performance Observation Tool	TPOT	Zhang et al., 2015		Physical therapy and nursing students	Retrospective video review

Selecting a Teamwork Assessment Tool

When selecting a teamwork assessment tool, it is important to first determine whether it is a validated tool. This can be done by reviewing publications in which the tool appears to determine whether psychometric assessments such as internal consistency or reliability (Cronbach's alpha) and inter-rater reliability using the intraclass correlation coefficient (ICC) or Pearson's correlation coefficient. However, the validity and reliability of some communication skills checklists has been brought into question due to studies showing that the agreement between reviewers can be as low as 0.45 (Setyonugroho et al., 2015). While this may be attributed to the differences in the rubrics used for assessment of communication skills, in many cases, additional reviewer training to improve agreement is needed. Where checklists are not optimally used, it may be difficult to reliably assess learner performance. Always consider the context i.e., direct observation of simulations or retrospective video review and learner type (profession and level) in which the tool was validated to determine if these match the context and learner e.g., undergraduate medical and nursing students, in which it will be used. Poor internal consistency or interrater reliability may make the tool difficult to use or the results difficult to interpret.

Rater Training

Prior to using checklists for learner assessment, instructors must first participate in rater training to ensure that they are familiar with their structure and how to use them. The profession of the assessor ought to be comparable to that of the students, and it ought to be a factor in determining the aims and purposes of the simulation. Every assessor needs to be given training on how to use the assessment tool, and if at all possible, there should be two or more raters involved in each assessment. This is of utmost significance in the event that the assessor does not have a profession or skill level that is equivalent to or higher than that of the learners, such as a teaching assistant. When there is a lot at stake in an evaluation, it is especially important to use multiple people to evaluate it. In order to make the evaluation more consistent, it is essential to make sure that all of the evaluators receive the appropriate training regarding the evaluation tool and that they participate in the inter-rater reliability assessments.

OTHER CONSIDERATIONS

Decreasing the Impact of Stress on Performance

Factors that affect learner performance during simulations should be considered as having potential impact on performance evaluations. Elevated stress levels can impair performance on tasks that require working memory, divided attention, and critical decision-making and is a predictor for dose calculation and documentation errors (Harvey et al., 2012; LeBlanc et al., 2005). Stress can also impair team performance during simulated critical events such as codes (Bjørshol et al., 2011; Harvey et al., 2012; Hunziker et al., 2011; Hunziker et al., 2012; LeBlanc et al., 2005; LeBlanc et al., 2012). It is possible that stress levels may impact both individual and team performance during simulations. This is because it has been reported that simulations cause anxiety in some of the learners who participate in them. When Boostel et al. compared the perception of stressors by nursing students before and after a high-fidelity clinical simulation or a conventional laboratory practice class, they discovered that the simulation group was significantly more worried about six factors related to a lack of competence and to interpersonal relationships (Boostel et al., 2018). It is essential for the person who is facilitating the simulation to make a concerted effort early on in the session to alleviate the anxiety felt by the participants by outlining what they can expect. The participants should be informed by the facilitators that the primary purpose of the session is to identify opportunities for learning, that "mistakes are ok," and that the information regarding their performance will be kept confidential. If the learner is remotely observed by the instructor from outside the simulation area, either through the use of a camera (Figure 3) or a one-way mirror, this may be an additional method that can be utilized to alleviate the stress that is caused by being directly observed (Figure 4).

Figure 4. Remote observation via a one-way mirror.

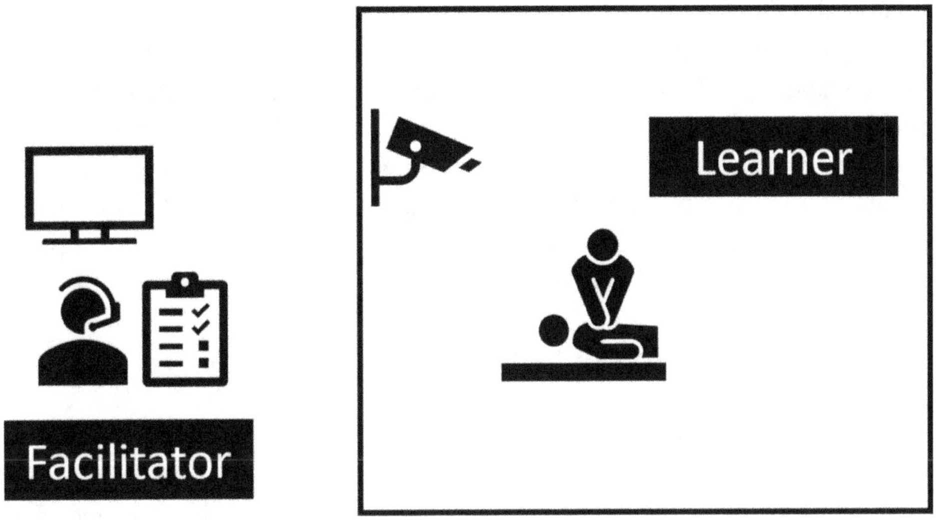

Minimizing Bias

When conducting performance evaluations, it is important to ensure that the evaluation focuses on performance and not the preferences or biases of the assessor. While an indepth discussion of minimizing evaluator bias is beyond the scope of this chapter, strategies such as blinding of assessors is an important way to minimize bias. Blinding of assessors means that they do not have knowledge of the student, include past performance and other factors which may bias the assessment. External assessors can also help to meet this criterion for fair assessments. When assessors are not blinded, well-defined assessment objectives, attention to rater training, utilizing two or more raters, recording the session for video review, and employing validated tools may help to minimize bias. Longitudinal or repeated assessments can also be used to track individual and team performance over time.

Evaluating Large Groups of Learners

Simulations are typically small-group activities with a high instructor to learner ratio of approximately 1:6. Large scale simulations may be indicated because the event reflected in the simulation is large e.g. mass casualty event, disaster evacuation or because there are many learners who require the simulation experience e.g. certification training. The approach to evaluating simulation experiences with a large volume of learners is similar to that utilized for smaller simulation groups. In many cases, conducting large scale simulations in a virtual environment increases feasibility and reduces cost. Similar to smaller scale simulations, observers are provided with a checklist of actions or behaviors to document in real-time or video recordings are captured using a camera system linked to a central location where the facilitator can monitor events as they occur. The video recordings can also facilitate debriefing. Utilizing a screen capture software for virtual simulations can also support information capture and debriefing.

Dealing with Equipment Failure

Failure of equipment during a simulation can be distracting; however, experienced simulation facilitators are able to quickly address issues or pivot to ensure that the experience of the participants is not harmed. The failure of the primary manikin, an issue with the controller, problems with the monitor, or an issue with the video recording systems are all potential causes of equipment failure. In high-stakes situations, where a malfunction in the equipment affects the assessment of primary simulation objectives, it is possible that the simulation will need to be paused and then restarted. In other situations, where the evaluation is formative, either allowing the case to continue developing despite the manikin's failure to do so in order to obtain additional teaching points or terminating the case early and discussing additional teaching points during the debriefing process are both viable options.

SOLUTIONS AND RECOMMENDATIONS

In health professional schools, students complete standardized tests that measure their readiness to progress in their program. Simulation-based assessments complement these standardized tests and enable instructors to identify gaps and provide feedback. These assessments must be carefully implemented in order to validly measure the knowledge and skills they are intended to assess. While simulation has been more commonly used for formative than summative assessments, there is increasing interest and emerging use of simulation, particularly virtual simulations for summative assessments. In these cases, rather than the performance metrics being assessed directly by the instructor which might be prone to bias, the metrics are collected directly by the virtual simulation software. Whether in-person or virtual simulation-based assessments should utilize validated assessment rubrics or tools. These tools should focus on individual or team performance and should be used in the appropriate contexts and learner groups.

Because high-fidelity electronic manikins and attachments collect data, there are opportunities for utilization of data obtained by pressure and flow sensors built into them to determine whether or not procedures were performed correctly. Reporting functions on the correct placement of the endotracheal tube during endotracheal intubation, and detection of complications, such as right-main stem intubation, in which the endotracheal tube is malpositioned in the right bronchus can be determined based on calculations made with a flow sensor that determines the amount of air that is provided during positive pressure ventilation.

In some contexts, conducting large-scale simulations in a virtual environment improves accessibility and feasibility while also lowering the associated costs. Large-scale simulations may be required either because the event that is modeled in the simulation is significant (such as a mass casualty event or a catastrophe evacuation), or because there are a large number of students who need to get expertise with the simulation.

FUTURE RESEARCH DIRECTIONS

Areas for future research include more sophisticated approaches for data collection during the simulation such as motion and gaze tracking to facilitate learner assessment and minimize bias. When carrying out performance evaluations, it is essential to make certain that the evaluation focuses on performance and not the preferences or prejudices of the individual carrying out the evaluation. With the increasing availability of virtual simulations and virtual simulated patients, instructors now have an array of tools to implement and evaluate simulations in both small and large groups of learners. With a wide array of validated tools designed for communication and teamwork training, facilitators are able to select tools that apply to their context and learners. The emergence of innovative approaches to analyzing and providing objective, performance-based feedback to learners may utilize artificial intelligence or crowd-sourced review of audio and video data to decrease the burden on instructors. The primary purpose of an SP's evaluations may be to provide formative feedback rather than assessment, but in certain circumstances, their points of view have been helpful in uncovering favorable characteristics or weaknesses that were not identified by standard assessment scores. More research is needed on how to utilize SP input and contributions to learner assessment.

CONCLUSION

In conclusion, learner assessment using simulation is highly feasible, but summative assessments require careful attention to data collection using validated tools by trained observers. Instructors evaluate simulation-based performance based on learning goals, objectives, and simulation type. As simulations differ from procedural manikin-based to virtual, the evaluation approach must be matched to the activity and learning objectives. Formative evaluations instruct the student while summative evaluations assess performance. Evaluations should be based on learner level, scenario type, and time. Instructors, external assessors, or simulated patients can evaluate individuals or teams in-person or electronically. There are several options for collecting learner performance data and digital recordings, validated, standardized checklists, and manikin-based data are commonly employed in simulation training. Virtual simulations can be set up to record learner action sequences and frequency and support objective evaluation of learner performance. Recent solutions to lessen the strain of direct observation or video review include employing artificial intelligence to automate video review and crowdsourcing manual video review.

REFERENCES

Aeder, L., Altshuler, L., Kachur, E., Barrett, S., Hilfer, A., Koepfer, S., Schaeffer, H., & Shelov, S. P. (2007). The "Culture OSCE"—introducing a formative assessment into a postgraduate program. *Education for health (Abingdon, England)*, *20*(1), 11. PMID:17647178

Auerbach, M., Roney, L., Aysseh, A., Gawel, M., Koziel, J., Barre, K., Caty, M. G., & Santucci, K. (2014). In situ pediatric trauma simulation: Assessing the impact and feasibility of an interdisciplinary pediatric in situ trauma care quality improvement simulation program. *Pediatric Emergency Care*, *30*(12), 884–891. doi:10.1097/PEC.0000000000000297 PMID:25407035

Beck, R. S., Daughtridge, R., & Sloane, P. D. (2002). Physician-patient communication in the primary care office: A systematic review. *The Journal of the American Board of Family Practice*, *15*(1), 25–38. PMID:11841136

Bjørshol, C. A., Myklebust, H., Nilsen, K. L., Hoff, T., Bjørkli, C., Illguth, E., Søreide, E., & Sunde, K. (2011). Effect of socioemotional stress on the quality of cardiopulmonary resuscitation during advanced life support in a randomized manikin study. *Critical Care Medicine*, *39*(2), 300–304. doi:10.1097/CCM.0b013e3181ffe100 PMID:21076285

Blatt, B., Plack, M., Simmens, S., Lopreiato, J., Berg, K., Klevan, J., & Lewis, K. (2016). Do Standardized Patients Have Concerns About Students Not Captured by Traditional Assessment Forms? *Teaching and Learning in Medicine*, *28*(4), 395–405. doi:10.1080/10401334.2016.1176573 PMID:27152446

Block, L., Brenner, J., Conigliaro, J., Pekmezaris, R., DeVoe, B., & Kozikowski, A. (2018). Perceptions of a longitudinal standardized patient experience by standardized patients, medical students, and faculty. *Medical Education Online*, *23*(1), 1548244–1548244. doi:10.1080/10872981.2018.1548244 PMID:30560720

Boostel, R., Felix, J. V. C., Bortolato-Major, C., Pedrolo, E., Vayego, S. A., & Mantovani, M. F. (2018). Stress of nursing students in clinical simulation: A randomized clinical trial. *Revista Brasileira de Enfermagem*, *71*(3), 967–974. doi:10.1590/0034-7167-2017-0187 PMID:29924167

Boulet, J. R. (2012). Using SP-based assessments to make valid inferences concerning student abilities: Pitfalls and challenges. *Medical Teacher*, *34*(9), 681–682. doi:10.3109/0142159X.2012.708465 PMID:22905654

Burton, K. S., Pendergrass, T. L., Byczkowski, T. L., Taylor, R. G., Moyer, M. R., Falcone, R. A., & Geis, G. L. (2011). Impact of simulation-based extracorporeal membrane oxygenation training in the simulation laboratory and clinical environment. *Simulation in Healthcare*, *6*(5), 284–291. doi:10.1097/SIH.0b013e31821dfcea PMID:21642905

Clebone, A., Burian, B. K., Watkins, S. C., Gálvez, J. A., Lockman, J. L., & Heitmiller, E. S. (2017). The Development and Implementation of Cognitive Aids for Critical Events in Pediatric Anesthesia: The Society for Pediatric Anesthesia Critical Events Checklists. *Anesthesia and Analgesia*, *124*(3), 900–907. doi:10.1213/ANE.0000000000001746 PMID:28079584

Cooper, S., Cant, R., Porter, J., Sellick, K., Somers, G., Kinsman, L., & Nestel, D. (2010). Rating medical emergency teamwork performance: Development of the Team Emergency Assessment Measure (TEAM). *Resuscitation*, *81*(4), 446–452. doi:10.1016/j.resuscitation.2009.11.027 PMID:20117874

Daniels, K., Lipman, S., Harney, K., Arafeh, J., & Druzin, M. (2008). Use of simulation based team training for obstetric crises in resident education. *Simulation in Healthcare*, *3*(3), 154–160. doi:10.1097/SIH.0b013e31818187d9 PMID:19088659

Ericsson, K. A. (2004). Deliberate practice and the acquisition and maintenance of expert performance in medicine and related domains. *Academic Medicine*, *79*(10, Suppl), S70–S81. doi:10.1097/00001888-200410001-00022 PMID:15383395

Fletcher, G., Flin, R., McGeorge, P., Glavin, R., Maran, N., & Patey, R. (2003). Anaesthetists' Non-Technical Skills (ANTS): Evaluation of a behavioural marker system. *British Journal of Anaesthesia*, *90*(5), 580–588. doi:10.1093/bja/aeg112 PMID:12697584

Foster, A., Chaudhary, N., Kim, T., Waller, J. L., Wong, J., Borish, M., Cordar, A., Lok, B., & Buckley, P. F. (2016). Using Virtual Patients to Teach Empathy: A Randomized Controlled Study to Enhance Medical Students' Empathic Communication. *Simulation in Healthcare: Journal of the Society for Simulation in Healthcare*, *11*(3), 181-189. doi:10.1097/SIH.0000000000000142

Frankel, A., Gardner, R., Maynard, L., & Kelly, A. (2007). Using the communication and teamwork skills (CATS) assessment to measure health care team performance. *Joint Commission Journal on Quality and Patient Safety*, *33*(9), 549–558. doi:10.1016/S1553-7250(07)33059-6 PMID:17915529

Geeraerts, T., & Le Guen, M. (2018). Checklists and cognitive aids in simulation training and daily critical care practice: Simple tools to improve medical performance and patient outcome. *Anaesthesia Critical Care & Pain Medicine*, *37*(1), 3–4. doi:10.1016/j.accpm.2017.12.004 PMID:29362161

Georg, C., Karlgren, K., Ulfvarson, J., Jirwe, M., & Welin, E. (2018). A Rubric to Assess Students' Clinical Reasoning When Encountering Virtual Patients. *The Journal of Nursing Education*, *57*(7), 408–415. doi:10.3928/01484834-20180618-05 PMID:29958310

Ghoman, S. K., Cutumisu, M., & Schmölzer, G. M. (2020). Simulation-Based Summative Assessment of Neonatal Resuscitation Providers Using the RETAIN Serious Board Game—A Pilot Study. *Frontiers in Pediatrics*, *8*, 14. https://www.ncbi.nlm.nih.gov/pmc/articles/PMC7006050/pdf/fped-08-00014.pdf. doi:10.3389/fped.2020.00014 PMID:32083041

Guise, J.-M., Deering, S. H., Kanki, B. G., Osterweil, P., Li, H., Mori, M., & Lowe, N. K. (2008). Validation of a tool to measure and promote clinical teamwork. *Simulation in Healthcare*, *3*(4), 217–223. doi:10.1097/SIH.0b013e31816fdd0a PMID:19088666

Hardy, J.-B., Gouin, A., Damm, C., Compère, V., Veber, B., & Dureuil, B. (2018). The use of a checklist improves anaesthesiologists' technical and non-technical performance for simulated malignant hyperthermia management. *Anaesthesia Critical Care & Pain Medicine*, *37*(1), 17–23. doi:10.1016/j.accpm.2017.07.009 PMID:28939466

Harvey, A., Bandiera, G., Nathens, A. B., & Leblanc, V. R. (2012). Impact of stress on resident performance in simulated trauma scenarios. *The Journal of Trauma and Acute Care Surgery*, *72*(2), 497–503. doi:10.1097/TA.0b013e31821f84be PMID:22439221

Havyer, R. D., Nelson, D. R., Wingo, M. T., Comfere, N. I., Halvorsen, A. J., McDonald, F. S., & Reed, D. A. (2016). Addressing the Interprofessional Collaboration Competencies of the Association of American Medical Colleges: A systematic review of assessment instruments in undergraduate medical education. *Academic Medicine*, *91*(6), 865–888. doi:10.1097/ACM.0000000000001053 PMID:26703415

Havyer, R. D., Wingo, M. T., Comfere, N. I., Nelson, D. R., Halvorsen, A. J., McDonald, F. S., & Reed, D. A. (2014). Teamwork assessment in internal medicine: A systematic review of validity evidence and outcomes. *Journal of General Internal Medicine*, *29*(6), 894–910. doi:10.100711606-013-2686-8 PMID:24327309

Hobgood, C., Sherwood, G., Frush, K., Hollar, D., Maynard, L., Foster, B., Sawning, S., Woodyard, D., Durham, C., & Wright, M. (2010). Teamwork training with nursing and medical students: Does the method matter? Results of an interinstitutional, interdisciplinary collaboration. *Quality & Safety in Health Care*, *19*(6), e25–e25. PMID:20427311

Hull, L., Arora, S., Kassab, E., Kneebone, R., & Sevdalis, N. (2011). Observational teamwork assessment for surgery: content validation and tool refinement. *Journal of the American College of Surgeons, 212*(2), 234-243. e235.

Hunziker, S., Laschinger, L., Portmann-Schwarz, S., Semmer, N. K., Tschan, F., & Marsch, S. (2011). Perceived stress and team performance during a simulated resuscitation. *Intensive Care Medicine*, *37*(9), 1473–1479. doi:10.100700134-011-2277-2 PMID:21695475

Hunziker, S., Semmer, N. K., Tschan, F., Schuetz, P., Mueller, B., & Marsch, S. (2012). Dynamics and association of different acute stress markers with performance during a simulated resuscitation. *Resuscitation*, *83*(5), 572–578. doi:10.1016/j.resuscitation.2011.11.013 PMID:22115935

Huwendiek, S., Reichert, F., Bosse, H. M., de Leng, B. A., van der Vleuten, C. P., Haag, M., Hoffmann, G. F., & Tönshoff, B. (2009). Design principles for virtual patients: A focus group study among students. *Medical Education*, *43*(6), 580–588. doi:10.1111/j.1365-2923.2009.03369.x PMID:19493183

Jankouskas, T., Bush, M. C., Murray, B., Rudy, S., Henry, J., Dyer, A. M., Liu, W., & Sinz, E. (2007). Crisis resource management: Evaluating outcomes of a multidisciplinary team. *Simulation in Healthcare*, *2*(2), 96–101. doi:10.1097/SIH.0b013e31805d8b0d PMID:19088613

King, H. B., Battles, J., Baker, D. P., Alonso, A., Salas, E., Webster, J., Toomey, L., & Salisbury, M. (2008). TeamSTEPPS™: team strategies and tools to enhance performance and patient safety. *Advances in Patient Safety: new directions and alternative approaches (Vol. 3: performance and tools).*

LeBlanc, V. R., MacDonald, R. D., McArthur, B., King, K., & Lepine, T. (2005). Paramedic performance in calculating drug dosages following stressful scenarios in a human patient simulator. *Prehospital Emergency Care*, *9*(4), 439–444. doi:10.1080/10903120500255255 PMID:16263679

LeBlanc, V. R., Regehr, C., Tavares, W., Scott, A. K., MacDonald, R., & King, K. (2012). The impact of stress on paramedic performance during simulated critical events. *Prehospital and Disaster Medicine*, *27*(4), 369–374. doi:10.1017/S1049023X12001021 PMID:22831965

Malec, J. F., Torsher, L. C., Dunn, W. F., Wiegmann, D. A., Arnold, J. J., Brown, D. A., & Phatak, V. (2007). The mayo high performance teamwork scale: Reliability and validity for evaluating key crew resource management skills. *Simulation in Healthcare*, *2*(1), 4–10. doi:10.1097/SIH.0b013e31802b68ee PMID:19088602

Mangold, K. A., Jeffers, J. M., Burns, R. A., Trainor, J. L., Unti, S. M., Eppich, W., & Adler, M. D. (2015). An Objective Structured Clinical Examination to Improve Formative Assessment for Senior Pediatrics Residents. *Journal of Graduate Medical Education*, *7*(3), 470–474. doi:10.4300/JGME-D-14-00777.1 PMID:26457159

Matsumura, Y., Shinno, H., Mori, T., & Nakamura, Y. (2018). Simulating Clinical Psychiatry for Medical Students: a Comprehensive Clinic Simulator with Virtual Patients and an Electronic Medical Record System. *Academic Psychiatry: The Journal of the American Association of Directors of Psychiatric Residency Training and the Association for Academic Psychiatry, 42*(5), 613-621. doi:10.1007/s40596-017-0860-8

Morgan, P. J., Tregunno, D., Pittini, R., Tarshis, J., Regehr, G., Desousa, S., Kurrek, M., & Milne, K. (2012). Determination of the psychometric properties of a behavioural marking system for obstetrical team training using high-fidelity simulation. *BMJ Quality & Safety*, *21*(1), 78–82. doi:10.1136/bmjqs-2011-000296 PMID:21994358

Nwachukwu, B., Gaudiani, M., Hammann-Scala, J., & Ranawat, A. (2017). A Checklist Intervention to Assess Resident Diagnostic Knee and Shoulder Arthroscopic Efficiency. *Journal of Surgical Education*, *74*(1), 9–15. doi:10.1016/j.jsurg.2016.07.007 PMID:27561628

Oermann, M. H., Kardong-Edgren, S., & Rizzolo, M. A. (2016). Summative Simulated-Based Assessment in Nursing Programs. *The Journal of Nursing Education*, *55*(6), 323–328. doi:10.3928/01484834-20160516-04 PMID:27224460

Onwochei, D. N., Halpern, S., & Balki, M. (2017). Teamwork assessment tools in obstetric emergencies: A systematic review. *Simulation in Healthcare*, *12*(3), 165–176. doi:10.1097/SIH.0000000000000210 PMID:28009653

Oriot, D., Bridier, A., & Ghazali, D. (2016). Development and assessment of an evaluation tool for team clinical performance: The Team Average Performance Assessment Scale (TAPAS). *Health Care. Current Reviews*, *4*(164), 2. doi:10.4172/2375-4273.1000164

Paige, J. T., Garbee, D. D., Kozmenko, V., Yu, Q., Kozmenko, L., Yang, T., Bonanno, L., & Swartz, W. (2014). Getting a head start: High-fidelity, simulation-based operating room team training of interprofessional students. *Journal of the American College of Surgeons*, *218*(1), 140–149. doi:10.1016/j.jamcollsurg.2013.09.006 PMID:24183570

Passauer-Baierl, S., Hull, L., Miskovic, D., Russ, S., Sevdalis, N., & Weigl, M. (2014). Re-validating the Observational Teamwork Assessment for Surgery tool (OTAS-D): Cultural adaptation, refinement, and psychometric evaluation. *World Journal of Surgery*, *38*(2), 305–313. doi:10.100700268-013-2299-8 PMID:24154575

Patterson, M. D., Geis, G. L., Falcone, R. A., LeMaster, T., & Wears, R. L. (2013). In situ simulation: Detection of safety threats and teamwork training in a high risk emergency department. *BMJ Quality & Safety*, *22*(6), 468–477. doi:10.1136/bmjqs-2012-000942 PMID:23258390

Peddle, M., McKenna, L., Bearman, M., & Nestel, D. (2019). Development of non-technical skills through virtual patients for undergraduate nursing students: An exploratory study. *Nurse Education Today*, *73*, 94–101. doi:10.1016/j.nedt.2018.11.008 PMID:30610960

Phitayakorn, R., Minehart, R. D., Hemingway, M. W., Pian-Smith, M. C., & Petrusa, E. (2015). The relationship between intraoperative teamwork and management skills in patient care. *Surgery*, *158*(5), 1434–1440. doi:10.1016/j.surg.2015.03.031 PMID:25999257

Rovamo, L., Nurmi, E., Mattila, M.-M., Suominen, P., & Silvennoinen, M. (2015). Effect of a simulation-based workshop on multidisplinary teamwork of newborn emergencies: An intervention study. *BMC Research Notes*, *8*(1), 671. doi:10.118613104-015-1654-2 PMID:26563963

Sawyer, T., Laubach, V. A., Hudak, J., Yamamura, K., & Pocrnich, A. (2013). Improvements in teamwork during neonatal resuscitation after interprofessional TeamSTEPPS training. *Neonatal Network*, *32*(1), 26–33. doi:10.1891/0730-0832.32.1.26 PMID:23318204

Sawyer, T., Sierocka-Castaneda, A., Chan, D., Berg, B., Lustik, M., & Thompson, M. (2012a). The effectiveness of video-assisted debriefing versus oral debriefing alone at improving neonatal resuscitation performance: a randomized trial. *Simulation in Healthcare: Journal of the Society for Simulation in Healthcare, 7*(4), 213-221. doi:10.1097/SIH.0b013e3182578eae

Sawyer, T., Sierocka-Castaneda, A., Chan, D., Berg, B., Lustik, M., & Thompson, M. (2012b). The effectiveness of video-assisted debriefing versus oral debriefing alone at improving neonatal resuscitation performance: A randomized trial. *Simulation in Healthcare, 7*(4), 213–221. doi:10.1097/SIH.0b013e3182578eae PMID:22673159

Setyonugroho, W., Kennedy, K. M., & Kropmans, T. J. (2015). Reliability and validity of OSCE checklists used to assess the communication skills of undergraduate medical students: A systematic review. *Patient Education and Counseling, 98*(12), 1482–1491. doi:10.1016/j.pec.2015.06.004 PMID:26149966

Sigalet, E., Donnon, T., Cheng, A., Cooke, S., Robinson, T., Bissett, W., & Grant, V. (2013). Development of a team performance scale to assess undergraduate health professionals. *Academic Medicine, 88*(7), 989–996. doi:10.1097/ACM.0b013e318294fd45 PMID:23702524

Solheim, E., Plathe, H. S., & Eide, H. (2017). Nursing students' evaluation of a new feedback and reflection tool for use in high-fidelity simulation - Formative assessment of clinical skills. A descriptive quantitative research design. *Nurse Education in Practice, 27*, 114–120. doi:10.1016/j.nepr.2017.08.021 PMID:28888157

Stevens, A., Hernandez, J., Johnsen, K., Dickerson, R., Raij, A., Harrison, C., DiPietro, M., Allen, B., Ferdig, R., Foti, S., Jackson, J., Shin, M., Cendan, J., Watson, R., Duerson, M., Lok, B., Cohen, M., Wagner, P., & Lind, D. S. (2006). The use of virtual patients to teach medical students history taking and communication skills. *American Journal of Surgery, 191*(6), 806–811. doi:10.1016/j.amjsurg.2006.03.002 PMID:16720154

Sweigart, L. I., Umoren, R. A., Scott, P. J., Carlton, K. H., Jones, J. A., Truman, B., & Gossett, E. J. (2016). Virtual TeamSTEPPS(®) Simulations Produce Teamwork Attitude Changes Among Health Professions Students. *The Journal of Nursing Education, 55*(1), 31–35. doi:10.3928/01484834-20151214-08 PMID:26812380

Szasz, P., Grantcharov, T. P., Sweet, R. M., Korndorffer, J. R. Jr, Pedowitz, R. A., Roberts, P. L., & Sachdeva, A. K. (2016). Simulation-based summative assessments in surgery. *Surgery*, *160*(3), 528–535. doi:10.1016/j.surg.2016.03.030 PMID:27206332

Timmis, J., Orlu, M., & Park, S. (2018). Educational potential of using virtual patients for promoting interprofessional learning between medical and pharmacy students: A qualitative study. *Journal of Interprofessional Care*, *32*(6), 794–796. doi:10.1080/13561820.2018.1513461 PMID:30142278

Tregunno, D., Pittini, R., Haley, M., & Morgan, P. (2009). Development and usability of a behavioural marking system for performance assessment of obstetrical teams. *BMJ Quality & Safety*, *18*(5), 393–396. doi:10.1136/qshc.2007.026146 PMID:19812103

Umoren, R. A., Poore, J. A., Sweigart, L., Rybas, N., Gossett, E., Johnson, M., Allen, M., Scott, P. J., Truman, B., & Das, R. (2017). TeamSTEPPS Virtual Teams: Interactive Virtual Team Training and Practice for Health Professional Learners. *Creative Nursing*, *23*(3), 184–191. doi:10.1891/1078-4535.23.3.184 PMID:28789739

Umoren, R. A., Scott, P. J., Sweigart, L., Gossett, E., Hodson-Carlton, K., Johnson, M., Jones, J. A., Poore, J. A., Rybas, N., Truman, B., & Das, R. (2018). A comparison of teamwork attitude changes with virtual TeamSTEPPS® simulations in health professional students. *Journal of Interprofessional Education & Practice*, *10*, 51–55. doi:10.1016/j.xjep.2017.12.001

Urresti-Gundlach, M., Tolks, D., Kiessling, C., Wagner-Menghin, M., Härtl, A., & Hege, I. (2017). Do virtual patients prepare medical students for the real world? Development and application of a framework to compare a virtual patient collection with population data. *BMC Medical Education*, *17*(1), 174–174. doi:10.118612909-017-1013-1 PMID:28938884

Walker, S., Brett, S., McKay, A., Lambden, S., Vincent, C., & Sevdalis, N. (2011). Observational Skill-based Clinical Assessment tool for Resuscitation (OSCAR): Development and validation. *Resuscitation*, *82*(7), 835–844. doi:10.1016/j.resuscitation.2011.03.009 PMID:21481519

Weller, J., Frengley, R., Torrie, J., Shulruf, B., Jolly, B., Hopley, L., Hendersdon, K., Dzendrowskyj, P., Yee, B., & Paul, A. (2011). Evaluation of an instrument to measure teamwork in multidisciplinary critical care teams. *BMJ Quality & Safety*, *20*(3), 216–222. doi:10.1136/bmjqs.2010.041913 PMID:21209142

Wooding, E. L., Gale, T., & Maynard, V. (2020). Evaluation of teamwork assessment tools for interprofessional simulation: A systematic literature review. *Journal of Interprofessional Care*, *34*(2), 162–172. doi:10.1080/13561820.2019.1650730 PMID:31552752

Zhang, C., Miller, C., Volkman, K., Meza, J., & Jones, K. (2015). Evaluation of the team performance observation tool with targeted behavioral markers in simulation-based interprofessional education. *Journal of Interprofessional Care*, *29*(3), 202–208. doi:10.3109/13561820.2014.982789 PMID:25421454

KEY TERMS AND DEFINITIONS

Augmented Reality: Computer generated holographic images can be viewed by the learner in the physical environment using a mobile device or specially designed headset.

High-Fidelity Manikin: This term refers to a technology-enabled manikin with features such as mechanical respiration and heart rate.

Low-Fidelity Manikin: This is typically a low cost, low technology manikin with minimal features.

Objective Structured Clinical Examination (OSCE): An approach to assessment that involves defined objectives and anticipated actions, often with an accompanying checklist for assessment.

Simulation Debriefer: A simulation instructor who leads the learners through a reflective analysis of simulation events.

Simulation Facilitator: A simulation instructor who guides the learners through the scenario with the goal of meeting learning objectives.

Simulation Technician/Specialist: An individual who supports the practice of simulation through setting up and managing simulation manikins and supplies.

Teledebriefing: Teledebriefing describes a process in which learners who are participating in a simulation scenario undergo debriefing with a facilitator located at an off-site location.

Telefacilitation: The conduct of a telesimulation by a remote facilitator.

Telesimulation: Telesimulation is a process by which telecommunication and simulation resources are utilized to provide education, training, and/or assessment to learners at an off-site location.

Video-Assisted Debriefing: The practice of using video captured during simulation sessions for reflective discussions on learner and team performance.

Virtual Environment: 3D computer generated objects that can be viewed on a screen or in a head-mounted display.

Virtual Reality: Computer generated 3D images viewed by a learner in a virtual environment using a low-cost or high-end head mounted display.

Chapter 7
Telesimulation:
Remote Learning, Facilitation, and Debriefing

ABSTRACT

Telesimulation involves conducting simulation-based education remotely using generic or specially developed video platforms. The learners and the facilitator or debriefer are in geographically separated locations. The content of telesimulation training varies from clinical scenarios to technical training on how to use telemedicine platforms and best practices of telemedicine. This chapter provides an overview of the key elements and types of video conferencing platforms and their use for telesimulation facilitation and debriefing, assessment of remote learners, and telementoring. Technical considerations are reviewed regarding devices, software, internet access, and technical support.

INTRODUCTION

Telesimulation is a process by which telecommunication and simulation resources are utilized to provide education, training and/or assessment to learners at an off-site location (Christopher Eric McCoy et al., 2017). Telemedicine using video enabled conferencing systems is an increasingly important tool for healthcare delivery (Fang et al., 2016; Gross et al., 2020; Umoren et al., 2018). The rise of telemedicine as an option for inpatient

DOI: 10.4018/978-1-7998-4378-8.ch007

and outpatient care has been fueled by global events such as the COVID-19 pandemic. This has enabled patients to receive care while socially distancing themselves and conserving personal protective equipment (Keilman et al., 2020; Shur et al., 2021). By the year 2020, it is anticipated that 76% of hospitals in the United States will have implemented telemedicine programs in order to connect with patients remotely through the use of video, audio, chat, email, and other technologies (Intelligence, 2020). Telesimulation, which refers to the process of performing simulation through the use of telecommunication, has also become more common in the training and education of healthcare teams in a variety of fields, including surgery, anesthesia, nursing, emergency medicine, and pediatrics, to name a few. (Rami A. Ahmed et al., 2016; Fang et al., 2014; Christopher Eric McCoy et al., 2017; Umoren et al., 2018; Wang et al., 2017).

The ability to train learners at a remote location is one of the many advantages offered by telesimulation. Other advantages include the reduction of geographical and temporal barriers to the delivery of content, the facilitation of institutional partnerships and collaboration, and cost reduction. Telesimulation research has been used to demonstrate that the use of video telemedicine in clinical assessments and resuscitation support that were previously conducted by phone call can decrease the amount of time required to appropriately stabilize and support decision-making during the triage and care of pediatric patients while they are being transported (Fang et al., 2014; Umoren et al., 2018). There is a trend toward more conservative approaches in some situations, such as the use of non-invasive respiratory support rather than endotracheal intubation, with the addition of video to support the decision-making process in these cases (Umoren et al., 2018). This finding was supported by a clinical study on the use of telemedicine in transportation settings (Curfman et al., 2020).

However, the delivery of telesimulation training sessions can be technically challenging, and it is necessary to have knowledge of the video platform as well as potential means to be able to deliver the experience and provide access to learners who may not already have this knowledge or access to the platform. This is because telesimulation training sessions are designed to replicate real-world conditions as closely as possible (Brei et al., 2020). There are two different kinds of platforms that can be used for telesimulation: ones that are designed for video conferencing that can be used for any purpose, and others that are designed for video-based use that can be used for telemedicine. The first part of this chapter provides an overview of the technological characteristics of platforms that are frequently used for video conferencing.

The platforms are then investigated with regard to their potential educational applications, specifically teleeducation and telesimulation.

BACKGROUND

At the beginning of the 1990s, asynchronous communication between individuals was made possible through the use of e-mail and increased computer connectivity through a variety of networks. On the other hand, new avenues for synchronous communication via text and multimedia were being investigated at the same time. Text, graphics, and images are examples of standard data types, and multimedia is the combination of these standard data types with time-sensitive data (Pearl, 1992). Sun Microsystems provided a description of a prototype for a digital, integrated video conference application in the year 1992. The application was called "videoconf" (Pearl, 1992).

Types of Video Platforms

On-Premises Platforms

In the beginning, video conferencing could only be used for training purposes by large companies. These companies had the financial resources to purchase the necessary equipment, set up the necessary infrastructure, and hire the necessary personnel in order to implement an on-premises solution that was accessible to employees who were physically present at the location. These endpoints were installed in conference rooms and were connected to local networks that were protected by firewalls (Erickson et al., 2010). However, video conferencing systems are now widely available on a variety of endpoint devices including personal computers, smartphones, tablets, and even augmented reality headsets such as the Microsoft HoloLens [Microsoft]. The requirements for bandwidth and the complexity of the network and infrastructure also increase as the number and variety of endpoints grow, which leads to an increase in the amount of money that an organization must spend.

Cloud Platforms

The need to address these organizational costs while providing services to an expanding number of on-site and off-site participants led to the rise of cloud solutions such as Zoom [Zoom Technologies], Webex [Cisco Technologies], Join.me [LogMeIn], TeamViewer Meeting [TeamViewer], and MS Teams [Microsoft] that provide all of the essential video infrastructure as a fully supported hosted service charged on an annual basis. These solutions include Zoom [Zoom Technologies], Webex [Cisco Technologies], Join.me [LogMeIn]. The majority of these options provide free services that enable video conferences to take place between two or more participants for a predetermined amount of time, such as forty-five minutes. The participants are responsible for providing their own endpoints and covering the costs of their own internet data, but the Cloud provider is the one who is in charge of the interconnectivity and must ensure that it supports multipoint capability.

Features of Video Conferencing Platforms

Networking

Finding participants and their video cameras (webcams), providing access control and security, sharing resources, and sharing network bandwidth are the fundamental requirements for a video conferencing application. The process of initiating a video conference by entering a number into a software application such as FaceTime [Apple], Zoom [Zoom Technologies], or Webex [Cisco] is something that a lot of people who work in the healthcare industry are familiar with. Smartphones, tablets, and computers with media-playing capabilities can all be used to host video conferences that can accommodate two or more callers at once. It is necessary for mobile data networks (3G/4G/5G) to integrate with pre-existing wireless (wifi) networks. This is made easier by the international telecommunications standards that have been established by the International Telecommunications Union (ITU), which is an agency of the United Nations, and the Internet Engineering Task Force (IETF). Users of products that adhere to these standards have the ability to take part in a conference using any device they choose (Solutions). The advancements in communications that have helped faster connections by increasing available bandwidth and reducing network loading have improved the quality as well as the capacity of video conferences. These conferences can now support thousands of networked callers and are utilized for multi-site meetings and conferences all over the world. There is scant evidence to suggest that faster connections have any bearing on the efficacy of telehealth care. In a study conducted by Winter et al. (2019), the researchers compared the technical parameters of 4G and 3G connections within the context of simulated stroke evaluations performed by neurologists. There were no significant differences in assessment duration or treatment decisions, indicating that other factors likely contribute to these aspects of telehealth practice once an appropriate audiovisual connection is made. Remote examiners graded audio and video quality higher with 4G connections. However, there were no significant differences (Winter et al., 2019).

Security

The presence of security mechanisms prevents unauthorized individuals from remotely accessing connected cameras and microphones in order to eavesdrop. These mechanisms are of the utmost significance in the healthcare system in the United States as well as in other contexts that call for adherence to privacy regulations such as the Health Insurance Portability and Accountability Act, which was passed as a federal law in 1996 and restricts access to the private medical information of individuals (Act, 1996). Internet service providers may offer virtual private networks (VPN), which generate a secure tunnel over the provider network by applying encryption between sites. This results in a connection that is both more secure and faster than traditional methods. However, higher encryption levels can cause delays in the transmission of audio and video, which is especially problematic in environments with low bandwidth.

Video, Audio and Data Control Standards

The image quality as well as the effectiveness of video transmission are both determined by the video standards or codecs. Adaptive technologies allow for the transmission of video of a high quality over networks that have varying amounts of bandwidth. While some codecs send one video data stream for each resolution, frame rate, and quality, others send just one stream that contains multiple layers of all the resolutions, frame rates, and quality. This is determined by what the devices and network that serve as the endpoints are able to support. Some codecs send one video data stream for every resolution, frame rate, and quality. Because of this scalability, calls can be made all over the world. At each endpoint, users can select which layers of video to view without any additional encoding or decoding being required. When the network is busy, the video quality of the call automatically degrades for the caller, but the call itself is not interrupted in any way (Solutions). There is a need for audio standards in order to support high-quality audio with low delay, silence suppression, and the generation of comfort noise (Solutions). The Data and Control standards define the procedures and protocol for establishing communications between multiple audio-visual terminals, storing and retrieving video and audio, and controlling the far end camera. This function is typically included in video-based telemedicine platforms. However, investments in the delivery of telemedicine have outpaced those required to build capacity among healthcare workers for the utilization of telemedicine.

TELESIMULATION

It has been demonstrated that simulation is an effective method for the training of people who work in the healthcare industry (Fincher et al., 2010; Zigmont et al., 2011). As a direct consequence of this, simulation is being utilized more frequently in the healthcare industry to cultivate both technical and non-technical skills in healthcare teams (Kononowicz et al., 2019; McGaghie et al., 2016; Umoren et al., 2017). By putting the fundamental principles of learning theory into practice through simulation, it is possible to improve one's abilities through direct practice in a setting that is accurate to life. This is made possible because simulation makes it possible to put those fundamental principles into practice (Jain et al., 2010; Zigmont et al., 2011). The application of recently gained knowledge and skills, which is made possible by the simulation learning method, is further aided by the processes of reflection and debriefing (Poore et al., 2019; Salik & Paige, 2020). Because it ensures that the process of providing care via telemedicine is represented as accurately as possible, telesimulation is an essential component of telemedicine education. However, the applications of telesimulation go beyond telemedicine and can be applied to clinical settings as well as best practices for providing medical care. Telemedicine is just one of these settings where telesimulation can be utilized. In their recent study, Bond et al. (2019) outlined a straightforward and cost-effective approach to the integration of telehealth interprofessional team members while in-situ simulating clinical scenarios (Bond et al., 2019).

The method required for developing manikin-based simulation, which is outlined in Chapter 3 as the scenario development process for manikin-based simulation, is analogous to the method required for developing telesimulation scenarios. As was mentioned earlier, those who facilitate simulations are responsible for defining the learning objectives for each simulation, as well as identifying the learner, the clinical setting, and the characteristics of the patient. When conducting a telesimulation, it is of the utmost importance to take into consideration the hardware and software that will be necessary in order to carry out the simulation. Existing scenarios that were designed to be carried out in-person on manikins are very easily adaptable to be carried out via telesimulation. When developing new scenarios, it is important to keep in mind both the locations of the facilitators and the learners, as well as the devices that will be utilized in the scenario. Both the facilitators and the learners can be located anywhere in the world where it is possible to access the internet using end-point devices that are connected to mobile data networks or wireless networks (Hayden et al., 2018). For instance, a number of studies describe experiences with transcontinental high-fidelity manikin based telesimulation (Beissel et al., 2017; Bruns et al., 2016; McCoy et al., 2019; Mikrogianakis et al., 2011). Research that compared how students felt about telesimulation and traditional simulation came to the conclusion that there was no discernible difference between the two (Dang et al., 2020; C Eric McCoy et al., 2017).

Telefacilitation

The method of telefacilitation is very similar to the method of organizing simulations for learners who are physically present. Please refer to Chapter 5 on "Organizing Simulations for Interprofessional Learners" for more information on how to organize simulations for health professional learners. However, when working with remote learners, time zone differences, especially when they are significant, need to be taken into consideration during the scheduling process. This is done to ensure that the session takes place at a time that is convenient for both the facilitators and the learners. Learners ought to be informed of the session times as well as the materials at least one week before the session itself in order to provide sufficient time for preparation. It's possible that novice students who are taking part in a telesimulation for the very first time will need some additional assistance. For the session to be successful, it is essential to pay attention to the logistics of the session as well as the technical considerations, as there may be a need to coordinate with other simulation specialists and faculty either on-site or off-site. In telesimulation, you have the option of using either low- or high-fidelity manikins. For further information regarding simulation using manikins, please refer to Chapter 3 on "Approach to scenario development for manikin-based simulation". Learners might have easier access to manikins with a lower level of realism. On the other hand, high-fidelity manikins are accompanied by specialized software platforms. These software platforms give facilitators or simulation specialists the ability to control the manikins by using the software to interact with the manikins. However, the process for facilitating the telesimulation session follows the same approach as the process for facilitating in-person sessions.

When simulation specialists are available to support the simulation session by setting up and managing the manikin or monitoring equipment as the simulation progresses, it is possible that they will not be co-located with the manikin. However, it is possible that they will be. Whether or not it is necessary for the learners to be in the same physical location as the manikin is dependent on the learning objectives. Co-location is frequently required for the demonstration of procedural skills within simulations whose primary focus is on procedures. See Figure 1.

Figure 1. Telesimulation with remote facilitator and simulation specialist

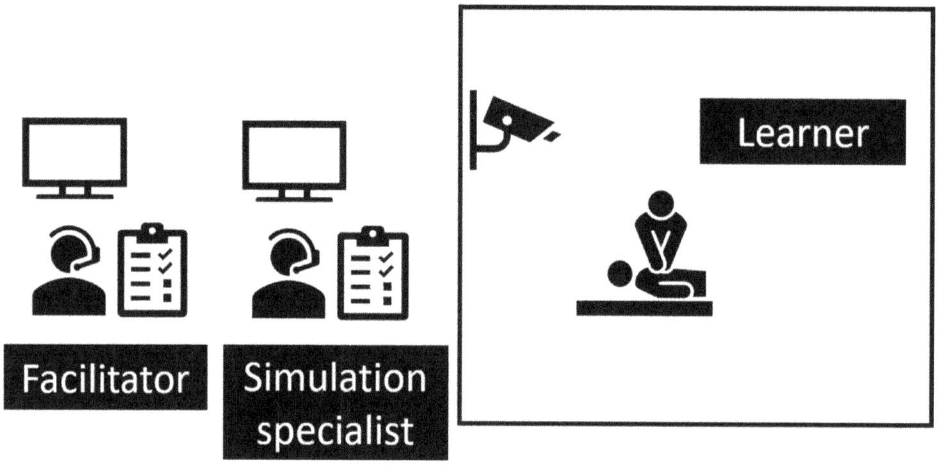

However, in simulations that focus on medical decision-making, communication and teamwork, learners may be distributed, and the simulation specialist may take on the role of a bedside provider directed by the team to perform certain procedures. Where the facilitator is located remotely, with advances in video conferencing platforms, it is feasible to make remote adjustments to the high-fidelity manikin's responses through remotely controlling the computer that is running the manikin software. Figure 2.

Figure 2. Telesimulation with remote facilitator and learner

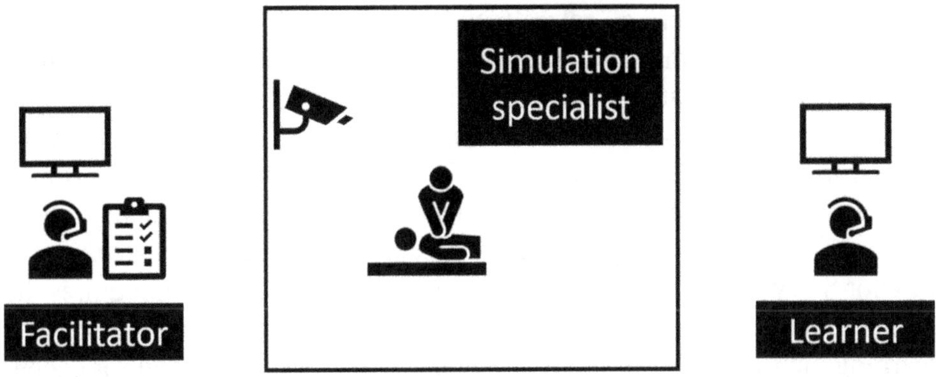

In other cases, a learner or group of learners may observe remotely while another learner participates in in-person simulations. The facilitator may be either on-site or off-site. The facilitator then debriefs learners on the simulation either in-person or remotely depending on the learner location. Figure 3.

Figure 3. Telesimulation with off-site facilitator and both on-site and off-site learners

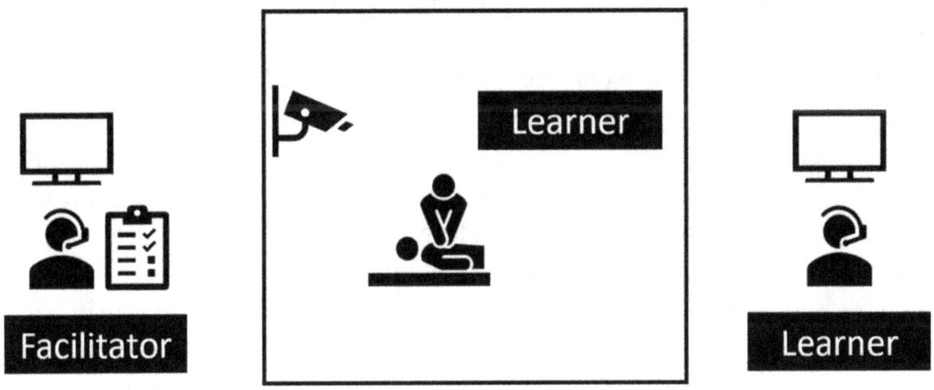

When a manikin is unavailable, telesimulations may be conducted entirely over the video conferencing platform using pre-recorded videos of simulated patients and monitors showing changes in vital signs as the simulation progresses. This approach has been adopted by the American College of Emergency Physicians TeleSIM Box program (Thomas et al., 2021).

Teledebriefing

The term "teledebriefing" refers to a process in which students who are taking part in a simulation scenario have a debriefing session with a facilitator who is located in an off-site location (Christopher Eric McCoy et al., 2017). The post-scenario debriefing that takes place after a simulation is widely regarded as the most crucial aspect of educational simulations; however, many educational establishments do not have a sufficient number of qualified teachers or subject-matter specialists who can facilitate this step (Taylor Sawyer et al., 2016; T. Sawyer et al., 2016). Debriefing requires the facilitation of reflective self-discovery of the learners' performance in a safe learning environment. The ultimate goal of debriefing is to gain a deeper understanding of the learning objectives, which will ultimately lead to the retention and application of newly acquired skills (Kolbe et al., 2015; Salik & Paige, 2020). In tandem with the advantages of telesimulation, which include a reduction in the burden of travel, cost, and time away from other obligations, the practice of teledebriefing has emerged in response to a growing demand for qualified subject matter expertise.

Learners do not object to participating in teledebriefing, which is consistent with the findings of previous research on telesimulation. According to the findings of a study that compared the efficacy of on-site and teledebriefing debriefing, learner ratings were high for both types of debriefing (on a scale from 1 to 7), with on-site receiving a rating of 6.6 and teledebriefing receiving a rating of 6.1. Even though students regularly rated teledebriefing and on-site debriefing as "consistently effective/very good," a small but statistically significant gap favored on-site debriefing (Rami A Ahmed et al., 2016). This could be an indication that teledebriefing instructors require more support and preparation than they are currently receiving.

It is essential to pay attention to cues and nonverbal communication in order to conduct teledebriefings that are successful. It's possible that in order to connect with the students and get past the effect that distance has on you, you'll need to be more expressive or empathic. Debriefers who are demonstrating appropriate maneuvers or procedures that might be done physically by on-site debriefers might need to show pictures or video instead and rely on learners to perform the actions themselves while providing feedback. This is because on-site debriefers may be limited in their mobility. In addition, it is essential to be able to acknowledge the possibility that, just like during the facilitation and debriefing that took place on-site, some actions may have been overlooked while participating in a teledebriefing. At the beginning of the scenario, designating a separate person to act as both the facilitator and the debriefer is one strategy that could be utilized to reduce the cognitive load. As a result, the simulation instructor who is tasked with debriefing can steer clear of the distractions brought on by the simulation's facilitation in order to pay close attention to the actions taken by the students.

Assessment of Remote Learners

Evaluations of student performance based on simulations are carried out by teachers in the same manner as evaluations of student performance based on on-site simulations. Please refer to Chapter 6 on "Evaluation of Simulation Performance". Although telesimulations have been described for use in formative assessments in a wide variety of fields, relatively little has been written about their application in summative assessments. An illustration of this can be seen in the program Helping Babies Breathe, which includes a summative examination consisting of two Objective Structured Clinical Examination (OSCE) simulation scenarios, which comes after a course that lasts for an entire day (Jones-Bamman et al., 2019).

The use of audiovisual data is utilized to a greater extent in telesimulations in comparison to on-site simulations, with the exception of those in which the instructor is located outside of the room. Because of this, capturing and playing back video for video-assisted debriefing is highly feasible with telesimulations, as is archiving video recordings for later use in research and analysis.

The use of data and reports derived from manikins, which can be accessed remotely by both teachers and students, is yet another method for evaluating the progress of individual students. Real-time data transfer is feasible and can be communicated to the remote facilitator thanks to the sensors that are embedded in high-fidelity manikins. This data transfer can take place via Bluetooth or wired connections. This makes it possible to conduct a remote assessment and makes teledebriefing easier.

TELEMENTORING

Telementoring is one of the other primary use cases for video conferencing platforms in the educational setting. The growing availability and ease of access to video platforms has led to an increase in the use of these mediums in general education sessions, which includes meetings and conferences. This training might be in the form of telementoring, which is essentially providing direction on how to handle actual clinical cases (Bond et al., 2019; Brei et al., 2020; Honda & McCoy, 2020; Jones-Bamman et al., 2019; McCoy et al., 2019; Sartori et al., 2019). The term "telementoring" refers to a relationship that is made possible by modern forms of communication technology and in which an experienced professional (the Mentor) guides a less knowledgeable student (the Mentee) from a remote location (Schlachta et al., 2016). The Project Extension for Community Healthcare Outcomes, also known as Project ECHO, is responsible for the development of some of the most prominent use cases of telementoring. This project utilized tele-education in order to close the knowledge gap that existed between primary care providers working in remote areas and specialists working in academic health centers (Zhou et al., 2016).

The Project ECHO model increased access to telementoring by establishing a virtual knowledge network on a wide variety of subject areas, including care for patients. In the first ECHO project, university specialists were linked with rural and prison-based clinicians in order to improve the quality of care for people in New Mexico who suffered from chronic hepatitis (Arora et al., 2007). Later projects that utilized these same methods concentrated on the treatment of chronic pain, rheumatology, geriatrics, hypertension, diabetes, behavioral health, and palliative care (Ball et al., 2018; Katzman et al., 2016; Zhou et al., 2016). Zhou et al. (2016) conducted a comprehensive review that included 39 studies that focused on 17 different medical conditions. Even though evaluation was frequently lacking, there were instances in which this approach was successful in changing provider behaviors, improving patient outcomes, and reducing costs (Arora et al., 2007). The ideas behind telementoring have also been applied to procedural training in surgical care (Erridge et al., 2019; Ponsky et al., 2014; Rosser et al., 2017) and neonatal resuscitation (Erridge et al., 2019; Ponsky et al., 2014; Rosser et al., 2017). (Jain et al., 2010; Jones-Bamman et al., 2019). The authors of a recent review on surgical telementoring, Erridge et al., described the use of video, audio, and telestration (drawing on a screen viewed by the learner) in 66 studies.

This review focused on surgical telementoring (Erridge et al., 2019). Seven out of the 12 studies that compared on-site mentoring to telementoring found no difference in outcomes, and none of the studies found that telementoring resulted in worse outcomes post-operatively. On-site mentoring was found to be more effective overall (Erridge et al., 2019). The success of these programs demonstrates that telementoring can be used for training healthcare workers in situations where attendance at in-person training sessions is limited due to cost, scheduling challenges, or geographic restrictions.

TECHNICAL CONSIDERATIONS

To avoid disruptions to the training session, it is important to recognize the key role played by choices of devices, software and internet connectivity to the instructor and learner experience.

Devices

Telesimulation can be carried out on any electronic device that is capable of running software for video conferencing. However, it is the responsibility of the facilitators to determine whether or not the participants in the session have access to suitable devices and the internet. Smartphones, tablets, and telehealth carts (Brei et al., 2020) are just some of the devices that are utilized. Augmented reality headsets like Google Glass are also utilized (McCoy et al., 2019). Because not all locations may have charging outlets, it may not be convenient to keep them plugged in throughout the session, or the connecting cables may create a hazard, it is important to choose devices that are dependable and able to maintain a charge for the entirety of the session. The software needed for video conferencing or telemedicine should be pre-downloaded onto any and all devices that will be used during the session so that they are ready to go when the session begins.

Software

When it comes to telemedicine training, it is essential to make use of software and hardware that are comparable to what is used in clinical settings, despite the fact that it is possible to use any device. For instance, telesimulation training with the Teladoc [Teladoc Health] or Amwell [Amwell] telemedicine carts use software that has additional features such as the ability to control a remote camera and a Bluetooth stethoscope. Using these specialized telemedicine features and troubleshooting issues with specialized carts requires additional learner exposure when compared to the straightforward video interface and devices used for generic video conferencing software such as Zoom [Zoom Technologies], Webex [Cisco Technologies], or MS Teams [Microsoft]. Examples of such software include Zoom [Zoom Technologies], Webex [Cisco Technologies], and MS Teams [Microsoft] (Brei et al., 2020; Rudolph et al., 2017; Sampsel et al., 2014). Before the telesimulation can begin, both the learner and the facilitator will need to complete additional preparations, which include downloading specialized software onto devices that are compatible with the experience.

Internet Access

The use of technology is extremely important for telesimulation and debriefing. The location where the simulation will take place at the site needs to be able to connect to a mobile network or wifi (wifi is preferred) and have a strong network signal, or it needs to have the ability to connect using an ethernet cable. Learners should also connect from locations that have a strong signal for either their mobile networks or their wifi networks. Learners need to be informed of the length of the session as well as the required amount of data when using internet connections that require prepayment.

Technical Support

It is essential to make certain that an on-site technical support person who possesses the necessary education and experience is always available for initial set up, troubleshooting, and take down after the session has concluded. When conducting sessions that involve an on-site component, such as manikin-based telesimulation, it is essential to have on-site support in order to prevent the loss of or damage to sensitive high-fidelity manikins and audiovisual equipment. In-person support makes it possible to troubleshoot problems and provides support for the session by reengaging participants in the event that technical issues arise while the session is being facilitated or debriefed. It is possible that during the actual simulations, subtle or inaudible communication may be missed due to a lack of direction of the camera or technical issues with the audiovisual connections during the simulation. This may be the case if there are any issues. The presence of in-person simulation experts or facilitators could be of assistance in mitigating these issues.

SOLUTIONS AND RECOMMENDATIONS

Telesimulation and teledebriefing are two innovative ways to address the difficulties associated with learner location and scheduling, as well as the scarcity of widely available expertise in simulation facilitation, debriefing, and particular subject matter areas. in the same way that recent advances in telemedicine have made it easier for more people to receive medical care. It is anticipated that not only will the use of telesimulation for the training of telemedicine professionals increase, but that it will also serve as a substitute for on-site simulation in order to reach a greater number of students. The development of video conferencing platforms, the widespread availability of internet connectivity, and the rise in the use of video conferencing as a result of the COVID-19 pandemic have created the conditions necessary for the global expansion of teleeducation, telementoring, and telesimulation programs. The fields of telemedicine, virtual reality, augmented reality, and artificial intelligence are all intertwined in the practice of telesimulation. It is anticipated that as these technologies and the devices that support them continue to advance, new possibilities will emerge in the future for facilitating and debriefing remote simulations. These possibilities are anticipated to arise as a result of advancements in these technologies.

FUTURE RESEARCH DIRECTIONS

To determine the extent to which telesimulation supports learning and how this compares with on-site simulation, areas for future exploration in telesimulation include more comparative evaluations of telesimulation and teledebriefing with on-site simulation. Telesimulation and teledebriefing are two types of remote simulation. In addition to this, it is essential to evaluate the degree to which the knowledge gained through participation in telesimulation sessions can be applied in other simulated or clinical environments. Transferring what is learned in a simulation into actual practice is an extremely important step, particularly in the field of healthcare, where the primary focus is on ensuring the safety of patients as a result of the knowledge gained from simulated scenarios. It will be necessary to adapt both new and existing tools and assessments in order to validate them across all learner groups. These tools and assessments support and facilitate assessments while taking place during telesimulation. The use of telesimulation across healthcare settings and teams has the potential to provide new insights into team performance and communication. This is especially true when simulations are carried out across a wide range of different environments and settings.

CONCLUSION

In conclusion, telesimulation is a developing subfield of simulation-based education. It has the potential to open doors for students who previously lacked access to simulation-based education, allowing them to receive supplementary assistance in the form of remote facilitation and/or teledebriefing. Telesimulation is an area of simulation-based education. Learners have shown an openness to this method, despite the fact that basic technical knowledge, advanced preparation, and on-site support considerations are essential for successful telesimulation. It is necessary to conduct additional research in order to determine the ways in which the knowledge gained through telesimulation can be applied in practice. On the other hand, developments in technology and the increasing prevalence of telemedicine will facilitate expansion in this particular subfield of simulation education.

REFERENCES

Act, A. (1996). Health insurance portability and accountability act of 1996. *Public Law, 104*, 191.

Ahmed, R. A., Atkinson, S. S., Gable, B., Yee, J., & Gardner, A. K. (2016). Coaching From the Sidelines: Examining the Impact of Teledebriefing in Simulation-Based Training. *Simulation in healthcare: journal of the Society for Simulation in Healthcare, 11*(5), 334-339. doi:10.1097/SIH.0000000000000177

Ahmed, R. A., Atkinson, S. S., Gable, B., Yee, J., & Gardner, A. K. (2016). Coaching from the sidelines: Examining the impact of teledebriefing in simulation-based training. *Simulation in Healthcare*, *11*(5), 334–339. doi:10.1097/SIH.0000000000000177 PMID:27388866

Arora, S., Geppert, C. M., Summers Kalishman, D., Dion, D., Pullara, F., Bjeletich, M. B., Simpson, G., Alverson, D. C., Moore, L. B., & Kuhl, D. (2007). Academic health center management of chronic diseases through knowledge networks: Project ECHO. *Academic Medicine*, *82*(2), 154–160. doi:10.1097/ACM.0b013e31802d8f68 PMID:17264693

Ball, S., Wilson, B., Ober, S., & Mchaourab, A. (2018). SCAN-ECHO for pain management: Implementing a regional telementoring training for primary care providers. *Pain Medicine*, *19*(2), 262–268. doi:10.1093/pm/pnx122 PMID:28525633

Beissel, A., Lilot, M., Bauer, C., Beaulieu, K., Hanacek, C., Desebbe, O., Cannesson, M., Lehot, J.-J., & Ricks, C. (2017). A trans-atlantic high-fidelity mannequin based telesimulation experience. *Anaesthesia Critical Care & Pain Medicine*, *36*(4), 239–241. doi:10.1016/j.accpm.2016.09.006 PMID:27720982

Bond, W. F., Barker, L. T., Cooley, K. L., Svendsen, J. D., Tillis, W. P., Vincent, A. L., Vozenilek, J. A., & Powell, E. S. (2019). A Simple Low-Cost Method to Integrate Telehealth Interprofessional Team Members During In Situ Simulation. *Simulation in Healthcare: Journal of the Society for Simulation in Healthcare, 14*(2), 129-136. doi:10.1097/SIH.0000000000000357

Brei, B. K., Neches, S., Gray, M. M., Handley, S., Castera, M., Hedstrom, A., D'Cruz, R., Kolnik, S., Strandjord, T., Mietzsch, U., Cooper, C., Moore, J. M., Billimoria, Z., Sawyer, T., & Umoren, R. (2020). Telehealth Training During the COVID-19 Pandemic: A Feasibility Study of Large Group Multiplatform Telesimulation Training. *Telemedicine Journal and E-Health: The Official Journal of the American Telemedicine Association*. doi:10.1089/tmj.2020.0357

Bruns, N. E., Irtan, S., Rothenberg, S. S., Bogen, E. M., Kotobi, H., & Ponsky, T. A. (2016). Trans-Atlantic Telementoring with Pediatric Surgeons: Technical Considerations and Lessons Learned. *Journal of Laparoendoscopic & Advanced Surgical Techniques. Part A.*, *26*(1), 75–78. doi:10.1089/lap.2015.0131 PMID:26698191

Curfman, A., Groenendyk, J., Markham, C., Quayle, K., Turmelle, M., Tieken, B., Brancato, C., & Saunders, S. (2020). Implementation of Telemedicine in Pediatric and Neonatal Transport. *Air Medical Journal*, *39*(4), 271–275. doi:10.1016/j.amj.2020.04.008 PMID:32690303

Dang, B. K., O'Leary-Kelley, C., Palicte, J. S., Badheka, S., & Vuppalapati, C. (2020). Comparing Virtual Reality Telepresence and Traditional Simulation Methods: A Pilot Study. *Nursing Education Perspectives*, *41*(2), 119–121. doi:10.1097/01.NEP.0000000000000496 PMID:31107394

Erickson, D., Greer, L., Belard, A., Tinnel, B., & O'Connell, J. (2010). A hybrid integrated services digital network-internet protocol solution for resident education. *Telemedicine Journal and E-Health: The Official Journal of the American Telemedicine Association, 16*(4), 454-460. doi:10.1089/tmj.2009.0132

Erridge, S., Yeung, D. K., Patel, H. R., & Purkayastha, S. (2019). Telementoring of surgeons: A systematic review. *Surgical Innovation*, *26*(1), 95–111. doi:10.1177/1553350618813250 PMID:30465477

Fang, J. L., Carey, W. A., Lang, T. R., Lohse, C. M., & Colby, C. E. (2014). Real-time video communication improves provider performance in a simulated neonatal resuscitation. *Resuscitation*, *85*(11), 1518–1522. doi:10.1016/j.resuscitation.2014.07.019 PMID:25132477

Fang, J. L., Collura, C. A., Johnson, R. V., Asay, G. F., Carey, W. A., Derleth, D. P., Lang, T. R., Kreofsky, B. L., & Colby, C. E. (2016). Emergency Video Telemedicine Consultation for Newborn Resuscitations: The Mayo Clinic Experience: The Mayo Clinic Experience. *Mayo Clinic Proceedings*, *91*(12), 1735–1743. doi:10.1016/j.mayocp.2016.08.006 PMID:27887680

Fincher, R.-M. E., White, C. B., Huang, G., & Schwartzstein, R. (2010). Toward hypothesis-driven medical education research: Task force report from the Millennium Conference 2007 on educational research. *Academic Medicine*, *85*(5), 821–828. doi:10.1097/ACM.0b013e3181d73f9e PMID:20520035

Gross, I. T., Whitfill, T., Redmond, B., Couturier, K., Bhatnagar, A., Joseph, M., Joseph, D., Ray, J., Wagner, M., & Auerbach, M. (2020). Comparison of Two Telemedicine Delivery Modes for Neonatal Resuscitation Support: A Simulation-Based Randomized Trial. *Neonatology*, *117*(2), 159–166. doi:10.1159/000504853 PMID:31905354

Hayden, E. M., Khatri, A., Kelly, H. R., Yager, P. H., & Salazar, G. M. (2018). Mannequin-based Telesimulation: Increasing Access to Simulation-based Education. *Academic Emergency Medicine: Official Journal of the Society for Academic Emergency Medicine, 25*(2), 144-147. doi:10.1111/acem.13299

Honda, R., & McCoy, C. E. (2020). Teledebriefing in Medical Simulation. In *StatPearls*. StatPearls Publishing. https://pubmed.ncbi.nlm.nih.gov/31536193 https://www.ncbi.nlm.nih.gov/books/NBK546584/

Intelligence, A. A. (2020). *U.S. Telehealth Market - Industry Outlook and Forecast 2020-2025*. Retrieved February 28 from https://www.arizton.com/market-reports/telehealth-market-in-united-states-2025

Jain, A., Agarwal, R., Chawla, D., Paul, V., & Deorari, A. (2010). Tele-education vs classroom training of neonatal resuscitation: A randomized trial. *Journal of Perinatology*, *30*(12), 773–779. doi:10.1038/jp.2010.42 PMID:20357810

Jones-Bamman, C., Niermeyer, S., McConnell, K., Thomas, J. F., & Olson, C. (2019). Teaching Helping Babies Breathe via Telehealth: A New Application in Rural Guatemala. *Biomedicine Hub*, *4*(3), 1–6. doi:10.1159/000502934 PMID:31993430

Katzman, J. G., Galloway, K., Olivas, C., McCoy-Stafford, K., Duhigg, D., Comerci, G., Kalishman, S., Buckenmaier, C. C. III, McGhee, L., Joltes, K., Bradford, A., Shelley, B., Hernandez, J., & Arora, S. (2016). Expanding health care access through education: Dissemination and implementation of the ECHO model. *Military Medicine*, *181*(3), 227–235. doi:10.7205/MILMED-D-15-00044 PMID:26926747

Keilman, A. E., Umoren, R., Lo, M., Roberts, J., Yoshida, H., Hartford, E., Patrao, F., Burns, B., Fenstermacher, S., & Masse, E. (2020). Virtual protective equipment: paediatric resuscitation in the COVID-19 era. *BMJ Simulation and Technology Enhanced Learning*.

Kolbe, M., Grande, B., & Spahn, D. R. (2015). Briefing and debriefing during simulation-based training and beyond: Content, structure, attitude and setting. *Best Practice & Research. Clinical Anaesthesiology*, *29*(1), 87–96. doi:10.1016/j.bpa.2015.01.002 PMID:25902470

Kononowicz, A. A., Woodham, L. A., Edelbring, S., Stathakarou, N., Davies, D., Saxena, N., Tudor Car, L., Carlstedt-Duke, J., Car, J., & Zary, N. (2019). Virtual Patient Simulations in Health Professions Education: Systematic Review and Meta-Analysis by the Digital Health Education Collaboration. *Journal of Medical Internet Research*, *21*(7), e14676. doi:10.2196/14676 PMID:31267981

McCoy, C. E., Alrabah, R., Weichmann, W., Langdorf, M. I., Ricks, C., Chakravarthy, B., Anderson, C., & Lotfipour, S. (2019). Feasibility of Telesimulation and Google Glass for Mass Casualty Triage Education and Training. *The Western Journal of Emergency Medicine*, *20*(3), 512–519. doi:10.5811/westjem.2019.3.40805 PMID:31123554

McCoy, C. E., Sayegh, J., Alrabah, R., & Yarris, L. M. (2017). Telesimulation: An innovative tool for health professions education. *AEM Education and Training*, *1*(2), 132–136. doi:10.1002/aet2.10015 PMID:30051023

McCoy, C. E., Sayegh, J., Rahman, A., Landgorf, M., Anderson, C., & Lotfipour, S. (2017). Prospective randomized crossover study of telesimulation versus standard simulation for teaching medical students the management of critically ill patients. *AEM Education and Training*, *1*(4), 287–292. doi:10.1002/aet2.10047 PMID:30051046

McGaghie, W. C., Issenberg, S. B., Petrusa, E. R., & Scalese, R. J. (2016). Revisiting 'A critical review of simulation-based medical education research: 2003-2009'. *Medical Education*, *50*(10), 986–991. doi:10.1111/medu.12795 PMID:27628715

Mikrogianakis, A., Kam, A., Silver, S., Bakanisi, B., Henao, O., Okrainec, A., & Azzie, G. (2011). Telesimulation: An innovative and effective tool for teaching novel intraosseous insertion techniques in developing countries. *Academic Emergency Medicine*, *18*(4), 420–427. doi:10.1111/j.1553-2712.2011.01038.x PMID:21496146

Pearl, A. (1992). *System support for integrated desktop video conferencing*. Citeseer.

Ponsky, T. A., Bobanga, I. D., Schwachter, M., Stathos, T. H., Rosen, M., Parry, R., Nalugo, M., & Rothenberg, S. S. (2014). Transcontinental telementoring with pediatric surgeons: Proof of concept and technical considerations. *Journal of Laparoendoscopic & Advanced Surgical Techniques. Part A.*, *24*(12), 892–896. doi:10.1089/lap.2014.0363 PMID:25423091

Poore, J. A., Dawson, J. C., Dunbar, D.-M., & Parrish, K. (2019). Debriefing Interprofessionally: A Tool for Recognition and Reflection. *Nurse Educator*, *44*(1), 25–28. doi:10.1097/NNE.0000000000000518 PMID:29538051

Rosser, J. C., Fleming, J. P., Legare, T. B., Choi, K. M., Nakagiri, J., & Griffith, E. (2017). Design and Development of a Novel Distance Learning Telementoring System Using Off-the-Shelf Materials and Software. *Surgical Technology International, 31*, 41–49. https://pubmed.ncbi.nlm.nih.gov/29301168 PMID:29301168

Rudolph, A., Vaughn, J., Crego, N., Hueckel, R., Kuszajewski, M., Molloy, M., Brisson, R. III, & Shaw, R. J. (2017). Integrating Telepresence Robots Into Nursing Simulation. *Nurse Educator, 42*(2), E1–E4. doi:10.1097/NNE.0000000000000329 PMID:27892900

Salik, I., & Paige, J. T. (2020). Debriefing the Interprofessional Team in Medical Simulation. In *StatPearls*. StatPearls Publishing. https://pubmed.ncbi.nlm.nih.gov/32119413 https://www.ncbi.nlm.nih.gov/books/NBK554526/

Sampsel, D., Vermeersch, P., & Doarn, C. R. (2014). Utility and effectiveness of a remote telepresence robotic system in nursing education in a simulated care environment. *Telemedicine Journal And E-Health: The Official Journal of the American Telemedicine Association, 20*(11), 1015-1020. doi:10.1089/tmj.2014.0038

Sartori, D. J., Olsen, S., Weinshel, E., & Zabar, S. R. (2019). Preparing trainees for telemedicine: A virtual OSCE pilot. *Medical Education, 53*(5), 517–518. doi:10.1111/medu.13851 PMID:30859605

Sawyer, T., Eppich, W., Brett-Fleegler, M., Grant, V., & Cheng, A. (2016). More Than One Way to Debrief: A Critical Review of Healthcare Simulation Debriefing Methods. *Simulation in Healthcare: Journal of the Society for Simulation in Healthcare, 11*(3), 209-217. doi:10.1097/SIH.0000000000000148

Sawyer, T., Loren, D., & Halamek, L. P. (2016). Post-event debriefings during neonatal care: why are we not doing them, and how can we start? *Journal of Perinatology: Official Journal of the California Perinatal Association, 36*(6), 415-419. doi:10.1038/jp.2016.42

Schlachta, C. M., Nguyen, N. T., Ponsky, T., & Dunkin, B. (2016). Project 6 Summit: SAGES telementoring initiative. *Surgical Endoscopy, 30*(9), 3665–3672. doi:10.100700464-016-4988-5 PMID:27270593

Shur, N., Atabaki, S. M., Kisling, M. S., Tabarani, A., Williams, C., Fraser, J. L., Regier, D., & Summar, M. (2021). Rapid deployment of a telemedicine care model for genetics and metabolism during COVID-19. *American Journal of Medical Genetics. Part A*, *185*(1), 68–72. doi:10.1002/ajmg.a.61911 PMID:33051968

Solutions, T. (n.d.). *Video Conferencing Standards and Terminology*. http:// www. teamsolutions. co. uk/tsstds. html

Thomas, A., Burns, R., Sanseau, E., & Auerbach, M. (2021). Tips for Conducting Telesimulation-Based Medical Education. *Cureus*, *13*(1). PMID:33552792

Umoren, R. A., Gray, M. M., Schooley, N., Billimoria, Z., Smith, K. M., & Sawyer, T. L. (2018). Effect of Video-based Telemedicine on Transport Management of Simulated Newborns. *Air Medical Journal*, *37*(5), 317–320. doi:10.1016/j.amj.2018.05.007 PMID:30322635

Umoren, R. A., Poore, J. A., Sweigart, L., Rybas, N., Gossett, E., Johnson, M., Allen, M., Scott, P. J., Truman, B., & Das, R. (2017). TeamSTEPPS Virtual Teams: Interactive Virtual Team Training and Practice for Health Professional Learners. *Creative Nursing*, *23*(3), 184–191. doi:10.1891/1078-4535.23.3.184 PMID:28789739

Wang, J. J., Lavigueur, O., Sheridan, M., & Stern, E. (2017). Implementation of a simulation-based telemedicine curriculum. *Medical Education*, *51*(11), 1178–1179. doi:10.1111/medu.13433 PMID:28913892

Winter, B., Wendt, M., Waldschmidt, C., Rozanski, M., Kunz, A., Geisler, F., Grittner, U., Kaczmarek, S., Ebinger, M., Audebert, H. J., & Stroke Emergency Mobile, C. (2019). 4G versus 3G-enabled telemedicine in prehospital acute stroke care. *International Journal of Stroke: Official Journal of the International Stroke Society*, *14*(6), 620-629. doi:10.1177/1747493019830303

Zhou, C., Crawford, A., Serhal, E., Kurdyak, P., & Sockalingam, S. (2016). The impact of project ECHO on participant and patient outcomes: A systematic review. *Academic Medicine*, *91*(10), 1439–1461. doi:10.1097/ ACM.0000000000001328 PMID:27489018

Zigmont, J. J., Kappus, L. J., & Sudikoff, S. N. (2011). Theoretical foundations of learning through simulation. *Seminars in Perinatology*, *35*(2), 47–51. doi:10.1053/j.semperi.2011.01.002 PMID:21440810

KEY TERMS AND DEFINITIONS

Augmented Reality: Computer generated holographic images can be viewed by the learner in the physical environment using a mobile device or specially designed headset.

High-Fidelity Manikin: This term refers to a technology-enabled manikin with features such as mechanical respiration and heart rate.

Low-Fidelity Manikin: This is typically a low cost, low technology manikin with minimal features.

Objective Structured Clinical Examination (OSCE): An approach to assessment that involves defined objectives and anticipated actions, often with an accompanying checklist for assessment.

Simulation Debriefer: A simulation instructor who leads the learners through a reflective analysis of simulation events.

Simulation Facilitator: A simulation instructor who guides the learners through the scenario with the goal of meeting learning objectives.

Simulation Technician/Specialist: An individual who supports the practice of simulation through setting up and managing simulation manikins and supplies.

Teledebriefing: Teledebriefing describes a process in which learners who are participating in a simulation scenario undergo debriefing with a facilitator located at an off-site location.

Telefacilitation: The conduct of a telesimulation by a remote facilitator.

Telesimulation: Telesimulation is a process by which telecommunication and simulation resources are utilized to provide education, training, and/or assessment to learners at an off-site location.

Video-Assisted Debriefing: The practice of using video captured during simulation sessions for reflective discussions on learner and team performance.

Virtual Environment: 3D computer generated objects that can be viewed on a screen or in a head-mounted display.

Virtual Reality: Computer generated 3D images viewed by a learner in a virtual environment using a low-cost or high-end head mounted display.

Section 3

Sustainability and Global Dissemination of Simulation Education

Chapter 8
Translation of Skills From Simulation to Clinical Practice:
The Role of Academic-Industry-Community Collaboration

ABSTRACT

Simulation education is a technique for skills acquisition, skills practice, evaluation, and research. The goal of any educational strategy is to support learning and, with healthcare simulation, transfer to clinical practice. There is increasing emphasis on research that demonstrates how simulation supports the transfer of skills from the educational setting to the clinical setting with the goal of improving patient outcomes. The approach and setting in which the simulation is conducted may facilitate skills transfer. The enabling environment created by academic-industry-community collaborations supports the establishment and equipping of simulation facilities and the conduct of in situ simulation in clinical environments. This chapter discusses the role of school-industry-community collaboration and its impact on translation of skills from simulation to clinical practice with an emphasis on patient safety outcomes and health system improvements.

DOI: 10.4018/978-1-7998-4378-8.ch008

INTRODUCTION

Academic-industry partnerships for simulation education have become increasingly common and with this, their impact on patients and communities. In the 1970s, specific policies such as the Office of Science and Technology Policy of the United States Department of Energy enabled partnerships between scientific researchers from academia and industry in order to drive innovation. Since that time, collaboration between industry and institutions of higher learning has been a common practice in the United States (Norberg-Bohm, 2000). Universities continue to serve as hubs for education and research across a diverse range of fields, despite the fact that over time they have received less funding for research. Educational opportunities for students, as well as ground-breaking research and innovation that can help solve complex problems, improve the delivery of healthcare, support public health initiatives, and propel economic growth can be produced as a result of partnerships between universities, industry, and communities that are beneficial to all parties involved. Collaboration between academic institutions and private businesses can be beneficial in a number of ways, including the generation of new ideas, savings in operational expenses, and advancement in a given field. Academic institutions are becoming increasingly capable of forging partnerships with various industries, particularly in the information technology sector. This is because healthcare programs are collaborating with technology and simulation companies to build facilities, obtain simulation equipment, and share technical expertise for the purpose of research and development. These partnerships make it possible for educators to broaden their professional networks and share their knowledge and expertise with one another, which is of mutual benefit. If optimized, collaboration between universities and industry accelerates the translation of research into practice with new technologies and therapies that improve the lives of patients in communities around the world.

Academic-Industry-Community Collaboration for Simulation Education

When it comes to education through simulation, a partnership that is of particular interest is the one between medical schools and the healthcare industry. This partnership between an academic institution that has a health professional school and a hospital or clinic that serves as a site for patients and the patient care setting that is required for comprehensive health professional training provides the essential access to patients and the patient care setting. The scope and structure of academic institutions' partnerships with healthcare organizations can look very different from one another. When academic institutions want to launch new health professional schools, they frequently seek support from regional healthcare organizations. Likewise, when hospitals want to form long-term research partnerships, they frequently approach academic institutions. The process by which an academic institution collaborates with a hospital to establish a simulation center can be as straightforward as the academic institution presenting a solution to a problem that the hospital is attempting to solve, such as improving patient outcomes, enhancing employee training, reducing the risk of infection, or patient safety concerns. A great number of healthcare simulation centers have been constructed and staffed with the support of the affiliated hospital institutions. The purpose of these partnerships is to assist academic institutions in the process of educating pre-service and in-service healthcare professionals through simulation-based teaching methods for the purpose of providing better and safer patient care in the healthcare organization with which the partnership is affiliated. Collaboration between academic institutions and other industry partners, such as manufacturers of simulation manikins and medical equipment, is both possible and commonplace.

Interprofessional teams consist of healthcare professionals from various professions including medicine, nursing, pharmacy, respiratory therapy, occupational and physical therapy. Physicians work with advanced practice providers including physician assistants and nurse practitioners. Ad hoc teams assemble in response to routine day-to-day clinical care and code events. These dynamic teams must function based on their roles to provide safe and effective patient care. Interprofessional team simulations are facilitated by academic-healthcare organization partnerships to support interprofessional training for health professionals working together in the healthcare setting. Simulation-enhanced interprofessional education occurs when participants and facilitators from two or more professions are engaged in a simulated health care experience to achieve shared or linked objectives and outcomes (Decker et al., 2015).

This approach has been advocated at the undergraduate and postgraduate level for health professional students to prepare learners for clinical practice. It is thought that interprofessional simulation-based education may promote more open communication, mutual respect and trust which could reduce stereotypes and improve cooperation between healthcare professionals (Liaw et al., 2014; Wong et al., 2016). The timing of introduction of interprofessional simulation into health professional curricula may vary and typically coincides with clinical exposure. However, early opportunities to work with learners of other professions may provide additional benefit (van Gessel et al., 2018).

Simulation and Patient Safety in Academic-Industry-Community Partnerships

The impact of educational interventions can be measured through initial classroom or simulation laboratory outcomes (T1), improved patient care practices and processes (T2), improved patient outcomes in a clinical setting (T3) and outcomes that impact the healthcare system including system improvements, cost savings, and skill retention (T4).(McGaghie, 2010) See Figure 1. For many years, investigators focused on the role of simulation in improving knowledge and skills in the classroom and simulation laboratory setting (DiMiceli et al., 2020; Heskin et al., 2019; Huang et al., 2019; Keddington & Moore, 2019; Kyaw et al., 2019). This resulted in simulation being identified as one of the best ways to learn. Simulation also has a significant role in improving patient care practices and processes, leading to improved patient outcomes in the clinical setting. The educational benefits of simulation have been described in Chapter 1 on "Introduction to simulation in the healthcare professions" and Chapter 2 on "Theory of simulation and gaming for health professional education".

Figure 1. Measuring the impact of simulation education

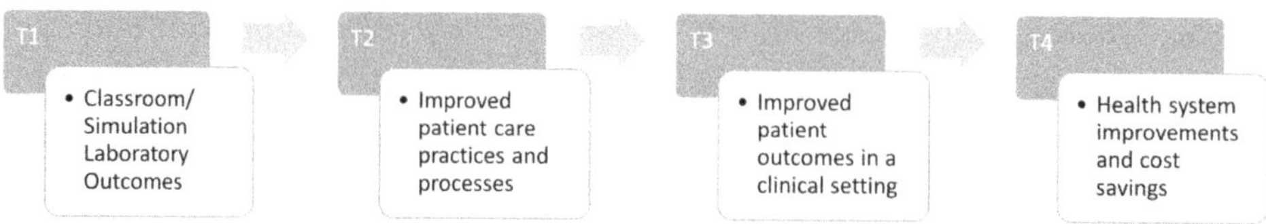

Meeting educational requirements for in-service health professionals, such as those pertaining to resuscitation education and updating their skills through continuing education, is one of the short-term benefits of academic-healthcare organization partnerships for the purpose of simulation education. In addition, the simulation centers have the potential to both cut costs and bring in additional revenue. Simulation centers have the potential to increase their revenue by providing educational courses to healthcare professionals working at other facilities. These courses might include simulation facilitation and curriculum development. This enables healthcare organizations to provide the necessary training to their staff at a cost that is more manageable. However, the long-term effects of simulation-oriented partnerships may be of greater consequence as healthcare organizations seek to improve outcomes for patients under their care by improving patient safety. This, in turn, will ultimately enhance their reputation and increase the number of patients who refer their friends and family to their practice. In the remaining sections of this chapter, we will concentrate on how simulation helps to bring about these outcomes, as well as the partnerships that help to create an environment that is conducive to putting the knowledge gained from simulation into practice in the form of safe patient care, and on the role that simulation plays in the improvement of health systems and the reduction of associated costs. In addition, we will discuss the partnerships that help to create an environment that is conducive to putting the knowledge gained from simulation into practice in the form of safe patient care.

Patient safety has been defined as the prevention of harm to patients (Erickson et al., 2003). Healthcare organizations are tasked with providing a system of care delivery that is built on a culture of safety that involves healthcare professionals. This requires that the healthcare system commit to preventing errors and learning from the errors that do occur (Erickson et al., 2003). The root causes of patient harm have been classified into latent failures (staff shortages, room set-up), active failures (poor hand hygiene, medication errors), system failures (no policies, poor safety culture), and technology failure (monitors, equipment) (Hughes, 2008). Simulation has been used to address the latent failures by defining the appropriate room set-up, increased awareness and training on policies, identifying potential for technology failures and building non-technical skills needed to strengthen the safety culture. In a simulated crisis, non-technical skills such as teamwork, task management and decision-making can be practiced in a safe and supportive environment. Simulation has been associated with increases in the number of specialized procedures performed, improvements in procedure performance, task success, patient discomfort, procedure time, complication rates, and costs (Griswold-Theodorson et al., 2015; Tejos et al., 2019).

Simulation and Procedural Success

The use of simulation has been described in improving procedural success, including overall success, first pass success, improved nursing procedural competence and reduction in central line infection rates (Scholtz et al., 2013). Simulation training has been used in the context of use of advanced surgical techniques such as laparoscopic and robotic procedures (Zendejas et al., 2012). While some studies showed no significant difference in performance with the use of different exercises, the majority of reports have demonstrated that the use of ergonomically appropriate simulation platforms improves performance in the manipulation of laparoscopic devices (Phipps et al., 2012; Placek et al., 2017; Walliczek-Dworschak et al., 2017). A simulation-based mastery learning program improved performance, decreased complications and overnight stays after laparoscopic inguinal hernia repair (Zendejas et al., 2011). Cardiovascular fellows performed better at diagnostic coronary angiography after simulation-based education with a significant reduction in procedure time and radiation exposure from fluoroscopy (Schimmel et al., 2016). Nephrology fellows were found to similar success rates in temporary hemodialysis catheter placement with simulation-based training and fewer complications when compared to the traditional apprenticeship model of training (Tan et al., 2018).

Even in very low resource settings where high-risk deliveries are common, increased performance of neonatal resuscitation and improved newborn survival have been attributed to the teaching of neonatal resuscitation procedures using simulation-based methods. This has resulted in improved patient level outcomes including increased performance of neonatal resuscitation (Budhathoki et al., 2019; Mduma et al., 2019; Riley et al., 2019). The risk of a mother passing away after giving birth as a result of postpartum hemorrhage is high, and this risk is exacerbated in settings with limited resources and a risk that deliveries will not be attended by trained medical professionals. The provision of clinical care was successfully improved through the use of simulation-based training in low-resource settings. This was accomplished by successfully reducing postpartum hemorrhage through active management of labor, as well as improving the performance of other birth practices, such as early skin-to-skin contact for the mother and the baby (Fritz et al., 2017; Nelissen et al., 2017).

Simulation and Latent Safety Threats

Latent safety threats such as poor availability of equipment, inadequate emergency call buttons, inappropriate room arrangement or unsafe obstacles interfere with safe patient care. It is believed that simulation that is conducted in situ (that is, in the actual patient care setting), as opposed to simulation that is conducted in a dedicated center, results in an experience that is more realistic and authentic. This training is especially suited for work environments that are confined in space and/or have a lot of background noise, such as an ambulance (Guise et al., 2010; Ullman et al., 2016). However, it is possible that there is not much of a difference in knowledge, patient safety attitude, motivation, or stress when using in situ simulations when compared to simulations in non-clinical spaces (Srensen et al., 2015). The advantage of conducting process-oriented simulations in situ may rather be in determining and addressing latent safety threats (or risks) as a result of the availability and location of specific resources, room set up, and team organization. These simulations focus on determining and addressing latent safety threats (or risks) (Patterson et al., 2013; Wetzel et al., 2013).

Simulation and Active Failures

Active failure of healthcare professionals to act resulting in medical errors can be addressed using cognitive aids such as checklists. By encouraging the use of checklists by medical professionals, simulation has the potential to cut down on the number of times patients are hurt as a result of medical mistakes. These tools cut down on misunderstandings, mistakes, and oversights, which in turn leads to better outcomes for patients (Geeraerts & Le Guen, 2018). In the past, it was reported that using checklists that included information such as the patient's name, the surgical site, and the procedure could reduce the mortality rate among surgical patients (Haynes et al., 2009). One example of a straightforward safety checklist is that which is provided by the World Health Organization (WHO). Surgical Safety Checklist (Lacassie et al., 2016). An additional illustration of this would be the WHO Safe Childbirth Checklist (SCC), which is a facility-based reminder tool designed to improve the quality of intrapartum care. It was also found that birth attendants who used the SCC checklist had a higher rate of adhering to essential birth practices (Semrau et al., 2017). According to the findings of a study that was conducted in India, there was a significant reduction in the number of stillbirths and deaths that occurred in very young neonates when the SCC was utilized (Varghese et al., 2019). When performing neonatal resuscitation, the use of checklists streamlines the preparation of the team and boosts the level of communication between members of the team (Katheria et al., 2013). It has been demonstrated that the pre-anesthetic induction patient safety (PIPS) checklist can improve performance in a simulated setting (Wetmore et al., 2016). In addition, it has been demonstrated that the use of a preprocedural checklist can improve the safety of intubation procedures carried out in emergency departments on patients suffering from trauma (Smith et al., 2015).

Simulation and Systems Improvements

Simulation has been described to be more effective for root cause analysis than conventional approaches (Slakey et al., 2014). In the research carried out by Slakey and colleagues, simulation scenarios were utilized in order to investigate the factors that led to undesirable surgical outcomes. The cases were run multiple times in order to identify potential sources of error; the findings were then compared with the events that were documented, and the decision-making abilities of the test subjects were evaluated (Slakey et al., 2014). The use of this method was linked to the identification of a greater number of errors that were system-based in comparison to traditional root cause analysis, which has a tendency to place more of an emphasis on individual errors (Slakey et al., 2014). In addition to this, the investigators were able to investigate, in greater depth, the process by which difficult decisions were made (Slakey et al., 2014). The use of electronic checklists to reduce the amount of work that needs to be done and the number of errors made while simultaneously improving patient safety is yet another method that has been informed by simulation. In this respect, electronic checklists performed better than paper checklists, especially in surgical and intensive care unit settings (Thongprayoon et al., 2016; Wetmore et al., 2016).

In the realm of patient care, simulation has been utilized to enable and support the introduction and application of technologies such as ultrasound and telemedicine. A quick evaluation of the heart's function can be performed with the help of focus cardiac ultrasound, even by individuals with only a basic understanding of echocardiography. Learners were able to obtain high-quality ultrasound views in a short amount of time on actual patients by participating in a self-training simulation program that is based on focus cardiac ultrasound (Bernard et al., 2019). One study that was carried out in a medical intensive care unit found that residents who had received simulation-based training on ultrasound guided procedures as well as supervised training on the placement of central venous catheters were able to achieve better clinical outcomes while simultaneously shortening the amount of time needed for the procedure (Corvetto et al., 2017; Koh et al., 2014). In a similar vein, simulation training significantly improved both the knowledge and skills required for ultrasound-guided regional anesthesia (Chen et al., 2017).

Telemedicine stroke care training simulations led to a significant increase in the number of patients diagnosed with stroke and a reduction in the amount of time it took for these patients to receive treatment at community hospital sites that were part of a Brazilian telestroke network (Carvalho et al., 2019). Following simulation-based training, another study demonstrated improved recognition of out-of-hospital cardiac arrest and time to initiation of telephone-assisted chest compressions in an emergency medical communication center (Hardeland et al., 2017). In addition, simulation has been utilized in research concerning the influence of video telemedicine on decision-making, as well as in the presentation of innovative methods, such as coaching strategies, intended to enhance the performance of positive pressure ventilation (Sawyer et al., 2019; Umoren, Gray, et al., 2018).

Simulation and Non-Technical Skills

Interprofessional simulations are also used to facilitate communication through emphasizing values such as teamwork and crisis management skills among practicing healthcare professionals (George & Quatrara, 2018; Merchant, 2012). Simulations including nursing, pharmacy and medicine have been used to improve teamwork attitudes and highlight the role of each profession in reducing medical errors (Motycka et al., 2018). Through interprofessional training on team interactions and the use of cognitive aids and checklists, team members are empowered to improve patient care through enhanced individual and team performance (West et al., 2016).

In the perinatal setting a cluster randomized trial showed an improvement of 37% in perinatal morbidity in using simulation-based training on nontechnical skills as compared to didactic training alone (Riley et al., 2011). Simulation programs have been demonstrated to improve teamwork and team communication overall among members of a multidisciplinary trauma team in emergency room settings (Miller et al., 2012). Similar findings of improved teamwork and communication skills were seen in staff caring for perioperative patients (Paull et al., 2013). While the improvements in team communication may be as a result of increased knowledge of communication skills, attitude changes that impact the patient safety culture of a unit or team may be equally impactful (Sweigart et al., 2016; Umoren, Scott, et al., 2018; Wong et al., 2016). While the transfer of communication skills learned in simulation to actual clinical practice may not always occur, learners with lower baseline scores may show larger improvements and could be the focus of greater training resources (Bylund et al., 2018).

Sustainable Academic-Industry-Community Collaboration for Simulation Education

Considering the sustainability of simulation programs is critical for success in translating simulation education to patient level outcomes. While the initial focus of simulation education may be on specific aspects of patient care or the patient experience, these goals shift over time and new goals may need to be identified. Studies show that the gains achieved by simulation education are not sustained after the training ceases and refresher training is needed to support improvements in care (Mduma et al., 2019; Miller et al., 2012). As simulation programs grow, they may require more space, upgrades to equipment, or the incorporation of new technologies to achieve their mission. There is a growing need to create ways to maximize the use of limited resources while maintaining high performance, which is why programs have explored alternatives such as standardized virtual patients and virtual simulations to reduce the need for personnel, alleviate the need for instructor and learner travel, and deal with space constraints. Cost constraints and tight budgets in academic institutions mean that there is a growing need to create ways to maximize the use of limited resources while maintaining high performance. However, as a result of competition for resources from other programs, technologies, and initiatives, the majority of academic institutions have limited opportunities to invest in technology for simulation programs. This has resulted in simulation programs becoming more reliant than ever before on funding from outside sources.

Good communication between academic and industry partners is important for identifying opportunities to translate identified needs from both partners into successful ventures. These conversations between academic and industry experts are important to promote translation of ideas and prototypes into usable products and devices. While pursuing formal agreements may be a lengthy process, it is important for key individuals from each sector to establish relationships and build trust. Confidentiality agreements are an important part of this process. While most universities have technology transfer offices that help researchers file patents and copyrights and collaborate with industry, researchers in academia and industry face differences in institutional culture with respect to approach to translating knowledge to solutions for communities. One of the key differences can be in timeline. While academic researchers may receive grants to pursue a particular project for years, industrial laboratories expect faster results and abandon projects that aren't immediately promising. While academic research is altruistic and seeks knowledge for the benefit of society, industry has a vested interest in securing outcomes that are profitable and can be used to the company's benefit. However, with collaboration, the new knowledge gained by working with academia can contribute significantly to an organization's performance.

While cost has been referred to the missing outcome in simulation-based medical education research, there is increasing evidence that the use of simulation for health professional training can and does save cost to healthcare organizations (Hippe et al., 2020; Zendejas et al., 2013). Simulation education necessitates an initial investment of funds for the purchase of manikins, equipment, and space. However, the payments made for ongoing simulation activities and training programs are how the majority of simulation centers make their living. It is possible to create a pathway to sustainability by mandating the training of preservice healthcare workers as well as the recertification of inservice healthcare workers, both of which must frequently include education that is based on in-person simulations. In most cases, hospital systems or the individuals receiving training will be responsible for making payment. Another potential source of funding is the completion of simulation-based coursework in order to earn continuing medical or nursing education credits. When evaluating the performance of the center, directors of the center are required to develop metrics for assessing the costs and benefits related to sustainability. Because of this, the management team is able to adapt and improve strategies, communicate results with stakeholders, track costs, and evaluate activities that create value. In the end, best practices will emerge, which can then be used to inform decisions regarding the future. Examples of these cost-savings can be found in multiple specialties. Simulation in pediatric hospital wards was associated with savings from improved patient outcomes and reduced length of intensive care stay (Theilen et al., 2017). Simulation was used in obstetric care to improve perinatal outcomes and reduce litigation claims (Smith et al., 2013). In surgery, a study demonstrated that proficiency-based robotic training for general surgeons was associated with shorter operating room times and a 20% reduction in costs per robotic hernia case (Tam et al., 2019). For additional discussion on the costs of simulation education, see Chapter 10 on "Strategies for Sustainability and Global Dissemination of Simulation Education".

Even in cases where there is clear evidence that simulation education is beneficial, such as when there is a reduction in costs and an improvement in patient outcomes, the success of academic-industry-community collaborations is not a given. In point of fact, just like any other kind of relationship, these collaborations may go through periods of both success and failure. It is essential to the continuation of the partnership to acknowledge the values and cultures that differ from one another as well as any that may conflict with those values. When it comes to the use of limited resources like personnel and time for education, the values of academic faculty may conflict with those of hospital leaders. This is especially likely to be the case when it comes to education. It is essential for the partners to recognize the unique ways in which they approach problems, the ways in which they work, the demands placed on their time, and the information they use.

The Role of the Community in Academic-Industry-Community Collaborations for Simulation Education

One of the primary goals of simulation education, improved patient safety outcomes, tangibly benefits communities in which the healthcare and academic organizations are based. As outlined above, simulation methods can be leveraged beyond skills development to process evaluation and root cause analysis in which the outcome is new learning or insights to enable organizations better adapt and more effectively respond to community needs (Kelly et al., 2002). Simulation faculty may also work with community partners to create and share educational resources with a broader group of community stakeholders, enabling healthcare and academic institutions to understand the impact of simulation education on the broader community. Mechanisms that engage members of the community including community-based participatory research, patient-centered outcomes research, and other engaged research collaborations for collaborative research can be tools to determine the ways in which simulation education can be used at the community level to impact public health outcomes beyond hospital walls (Skizim et al., 2017).

Other types of community engagement supported by industry may involve supplying equipment and initiating and advancing simulation education in smaller community-based facilities with the support of grants programs. The increased learning and collegial relationships promoted between academic institutions and community hospital organizations through these efforts support referral networks and produce tangible and intangible benefits for the communities in which these facilities are based.

SOLUTIONS AND RECOMMENDATIONS

Exploring common interests, and goals, and overcoming organizational cultural differences and geographic constraints to build trusting relationships, establish a common language, and understand the problem or problems from multiple perspectives is essential to achieving partnership goals. There must be significant time invested in developing trusting mutual relationships between the healthcare organization, academic institution, and the community. The success of academic-industry-community collaborations is not a given, even in circumstances where there is clear evidence that simulation education is beneficial, such as when there is a reduction in costs and an improvement in patient outcomes. In point of fact, these collaborations can go through periods of both success and failure, just like any other kind of relationship. It is essential to the continuation of the partnership to acknowledge the values and cultures that differ from one another, as well as any that may be in conflict with those values. There may be tension between the priorities of academic faculty and those of hospital administrators regarding the allocation of scarce resources, such as personnel and time, for educational purposes. This is especially likely to be the case with regard to educational opportunities. It is essential for the partners to recognize the unique ways in which they approach problems, the ways in which they work, the demands that are placed on their time, and the information that they use.

FUTURE RESEARCH DIRECTIONS

The role of academic-industry-community collaborations in supporting and fostering simulation programs is an area for future study. While the opportunities appear significant for organizations that partner in support of simulation education and research, little is known about the challenges and barriers to achieving these goals. The input of the host communities in guiding targets of simulation education that are tailored to patients and caregivers would be invaluable as academic-industry partnerships expand from educating hospital and clinic staff to patients and caregivers as the target of simulation education. In the field of patient care, simulation has been used to facilitate and provide support for the implementation of technologies such as ultrasound and telemedicine. Future research on academic-industry-community collaborations should explore the ways that simulation can enhance the uptake of new technologies and approaches.

CONCLUSION

In conclusion, academic-industry-community partnerships are indispensable for the success and sustainability of simulation education. These relationships can be leveraged for securing simulation space within healthcare organizations, obtaining simulation and medical equipment for realistic simulation experiences, and supporting simulation events. The improvement of patient outcomes is the primary focus of simulation education. This can be accomplished in a number of different ways, including increasing technical skills through procedural competency, supporting team communication and non-technical skills, and increasing system performance by identifying and addressing the root causes of failure, thereby reducing active failures and latent safety threats. These are just a few of the ways that this goal can be accomplished. To ensure equity and sustainability, partnerships between academic institutions, healthcare organizations, and community partners need to be cultivated through open communication, exploration, and periodic reevaluation of partner goals and objectives.

REFERENCES

Bernard, A., Chemaly, P., Dion, F., Laribi, S., Remerand, F., Angoulvant, D., & Ivanes, F. (2019). Evaluation of the efficacy of a self-training programme in focus cardiac ultrasound with simulator. *Archives of Cardiovascular Diseases*, *112*(10), 576–584. doi:10.1016/j.acvd.2019.06.001 PMID:31350012

Budhathoki, S. S., Gurung, R., Ewald, U., Thapa, J., & Kc, A. (2019). Does the Helping Babies Breathe Programme impact on neonatal resuscitation care practices? Results from systematic review and meta-analysis. *Acta Paediatrica, 108*(5), 806-813. doi:10.1111/apa.14706

Bylund, C. L., Banerjee, S. C., Bialer, P. A., Manna, R., Levin, T. T., Parker, P. A., Schofield, E., Li, Y., Bartell, A., Chou, A., Hichenberg, S. A., Dickler, M., & Kissane, D. W. (2018). A rigorous evaluation of an institutionally-based communication skills program for post-graduate oncology trainees. *Patient Education and Counseling, 101*(11), 1924–1933. doi:10.1016/j.pec.2018.05.026 PMID:29880404

Carvalho, V. S., Jr., Picanço, M. R., Volschan, A., & Bezerra, D. C. (2019). Impact of simulation training on a telestroke network. *International Journal of Stroke: Official Journal of the International Stroke Society, 14*(5), 500-507. doi:10.1177/1747493018791030

Chen, X. X., Trivedi, V., AlSaflan, A. A., Todd, S. C., Tricco, A. C., McCartney, C. J. L., & Boet, S. (2017). Ultrasound-Guided Regional Anesthesia Simulation Training: A Systematic Review. *Regional Anesthesia and Pain Medicine, 42*(6), 741–750. doi:10.1097/AAP.0000000000000639 PMID:28759501

Corvetto, M., Pedemonte, J., Varas, D., Fuentes, C., & Altermatt, F. (2017). Simulation-based training program with deliberate practice for ultrasound-guided jugular central venous catheter placement. *Acta Anaesthesiologica Scandinavica, 61*(9), 1184–1191. doi:10.1111/aas.12937 PMID:28685812

Decker, S. I., Anderson, M., Boese, T., Epps, C., McCarthy, J., Motola, I., Palaganas, J., Perry, C., Puga, F., & Scolaro, K. (2015). Standards of best practice: Simulation standard VIII: Simulation-enhanced interprofessional education (Sim-IPE). *Clinical Simulation in Nursing, 11*(6), 293–297. doi:10.1016/j.ecns.2015.03.010

DiMiceli, M., Banerjee, A., Newton, M. W., & McEvoy, M. D. (2020). Simulation in Low-Resource Settings: A Review of the Current State and Practical Implementation Strategies. *Comprehensive Healthcare Simulation: Anesthesiology*, 313-321.

Erickson, S. M., Wolcott, J., Corrigan, J. M., & Aspden, P. (2003). *Patient safety: Achieving a new standard for care*. Academic Press.

Fritz, J., Walker, D. M., Cohen, S., Angeles, G., & Lamadrid-Figueroa, H. (2017). Can a simulation-based training program impact the use of evidence based routine practices at birth? Results of a hospital-based cluster randomized trial in Mexico. *PLoS One*, *12*(3), e0172623–e0172623. doi:10.1371/journal.pone.0172623 PMID:28319122

Geeraerts, T., & Le Guen, M. (2018). Checklists and cognitive aids in simulation training and daily critical care practice: Simple tools to improve medical performance and patient outcome. *Anaesthesia Critical Care & Pain Medicine*, *37*(1), 3–4. doi:10.1016/j.accpm.2017.12.004 PMID:29362161

George, K. L., & Quatrara, B. (2018). Interprofessional Simulations Promote Knowledge Retention and Enhance Perceptions of Teamwork Skills in a Surgical-Trauma-Burn Intensive Care Unit Setting. *Dimensions of critical care nursing. Dimensions of Critical Care Nursing*, *37*(3), 144–155. doi:10.1097/DCC.0000000000000301 PMID:29596291

Griswold-Theodorson, S., Ponnuru, S., Dong, C., Szyld, D., Reed, T., & McGaghie, W. C. (2015). Beyond the simulation laboratory: A realist synthesis review of clinical outcomes of simulation-based mastery learning. *Academic Medicine*, *90*(11), 1553–1560. doi:10.1097/ACM.0000000000000938 PMID:26375271

Guise, J.-M., Lowe, N. K., Deering, S., Lewis, P. O., O'Haire, C., Irwin, L. K., Blaser, M., Wood, L. S., & Kanki, B. G. (2010). Mobile in situ obstetric emergency simulation and teamwork training to improve maternal-fetal safety in hospitals. *Joint Commission Journal on Quality and Patient Safety*, *36*(10), 443–453. doi:10.1016/S1553-7250(10)36066-1 PMID:21548505

Hardeland, C., Skåre, C., Kramer-Johansen, J., Birkenes, T. S., Myklebust, H., Hansen, A. E., Sunde, K., & Olasveengen, T. M. (2017). Targeted simulation and education to improve cardiac arrest recognition and telephone assisted CPR in an emergency medical communication centre. *Resuscitation*, *114*, 21–26. doi:10.1016/j.resuscitation.2017.02.013 PMID:28236428

Haynes, A. B., Weiser, T. G., Berry, W. R., Lipsitz, S. R., Breizat, A.-H. S., Dellinger, E. P., Herbosa, T., Joseph, S., Kibatala, P. L., Lapitan, M. C. M., Merry, A. F., Moorthy, K., Reznick, R. K., Taylor, B., & Gawande, A. A. (2009). A surgical safety checklist to reduce morbidity and mortality in a global population. *The New England Journal of Medicine*, *360*(5), 491–499. doi:10.1056/NEJMsa0810119 PMID:19144931

Heskin, L., Simms, C., Holland, J., Traynor, O., & Galvin, R. (2019). A Systematic Review of the Educational Effectiveness of Simulation Used in Open Surgery. *Simulation in Healthcare: Journal of the Society for Simulation in Healthcare, 14*(1), 51-58. doi:10.1097/SIH.0000000000000349

Hippe, D. S., Umoren, R. A., McGee, A., Bucher, S. L., & Bresnahan, B. W. (2020). A targeted systematic review of cost analyses for implementation of simulation-based education in healthcare. *SAGE Open Medicine, 8*, 2050312120913451. doi:10.1177/2050312120913451 PMID:32231781

Huang, J., Tang, Y., Tang, J., Shi, J., Wang, H., Xiong, T., Xia, B., Zhang, L., Qu, Y., & Mu, D. (2019). Educational efficacy of high-fidelity simulation in neonatal resuscitation training: A systematic review and meta-analysis. *BMC Medical Education, 19*(1), 323–323. doi:10.118612909-019-1763-z PMID:31464614

Hughes, R. (2008). *Patient safety and quality: An evidence-based handbook for nurses*. Academic Press.

Katheria, A., Rich, W., & Finer, N. (2013). Development of a strategic process using checklists to facilitate team preparation and improve communication during neonatal resuscitation. *Resuscitation, 84*(11), 1552–1557. doi:10.1016/j.resuscitation.2013.06.012 PMID:23810750

Keddington, A. S., & Moore, J. (2019). Simulation as a Method of Competency Assessment Among Health Care Providers: A Systematic Review. *Nursing Education Perspectives, 40*(2), 91–94. doi:10.1097/01.NEP.0000000000000433 PMID:30601272

Kelly, M. J., Schaan, J. L., & Joncas, H. (2002). Managing alliance relationships: Key challenges in the early stages of collaboration. *R & D Management, 32*(1), 11–22. doi:10.1111/1467-9310.00235

Koh, J., Xu, Y., Yeo, L., Tee, A., Chuin, S., Law, J., Noor, I. B. M., Poulose, V., Raghuram, J., Verma, A., & Ng, A. (2014). Achieving optimal clinical outcomes in ultrasound-guided central venous catheterizations of the internal jugular vein after a simulation-based training program for novice learners. *Simulation in Healthcare: Journal of the Society for Simulation in Healthcare, 9*(3), 161-166. doi:10.1097/SIH.0000000000000010

Kyaw, B. M., Saxena, N., Posadzki, P., Vseteckova, J., Nikolaou, C. K., George, P. P., Divakar, U., Masiello, I., Kononowicz, A. A., Zary, N., & Tudor Car, L. (2019). Virtual Reality for Health Professions Education: Systematic Review and Meta-Analysis by the Digital Health Education Collaboration. *Journal of Medical Internet Research, 21*(1), e12959. doi:10.2196/12959 PMID:30668519

Lacassie, H. J., Ferdinand, C., Guzmán, S., Camus, L., & Echevarria, G. C. (2016). World Health Organization (WHO) surgical safety checklist implementation and its impact on perioperative morbidity and mortality in an academic medical center in Chile. *Medicine, 95*(23), e3844. doi:10.1097/MD.0000000000003844 PMID:27281092

Liaw, S. Y., Siau, C., Zhou, W. T., & Lau, T. C. (2014). Interprofessional simulation-based education program: A promising approach for changing stereotypes and improving attitudes toward nurse-physician collaboration. *Applied nursing research. ANR, 27*(4), 258–260. doi:10.1016/j.apnr.2014.03.005 PMID:24849067

McGaghie, W. C. (2010). Medical education research as translational science. *Science Translational Medicine, 2*(19).

Mduma, E., Kvaloy, J. T., Soreide, E., Svensen, E., Mdoe, P., Perlman, J., Johnson, C., Kidanto, H. L., & Ersdal, H. L. (2019). Frequent refresher training on newborn resuscitation and potential impact on perinatal outcome over time in a rural Tanzanian hospital: An observational study. *BMJ Open, 9*(9), e030572. doi:10.1136/bmjopen-2019-030572 PMID:31562152

Merchant, D. C. (2012). Does high-fidelity simulation improve clinical outcomes? *Journal for Nurses in Staff Development, 28*(1), E1-E10. doi:10.1097/NND.0b013e318240a728

Miller, D., Crandall, C., Washington, C., 3rd, & McLaughlin, S. (2012). Improving teamwork and communication in trauma care through in situ simulations. *Academic Emergency Medicine: Official Journal of the Society for Academic Emergency Medicine, 19*(5), 608-612. doi:10.1111/j.1553-2712.2012.01354.x

Motycka, C., Egelund, E. F., Gannon, J., Genuardi, F., Gautam, S., Stittsworth, S., Young, A., & Simon, L. (2018). Using interprofessional medication management simulations to impact student attitudes toward teamwork to prevent medication errors. *Currents in Pharmacy Teaching & Learning*, *10*(7), 982–989. doi:10.1016/j.cptl.2018.04.010 PMID:30236437

Nelissen, E., Ersdal, H., Mduma, E., Evjen-Olsen, B., Twisk, J., Broerse, J., van Roosmalen, J., & Stekelenburg, J. (2017). Clinical performance and patient outcome after simulation-based training in prevention and management of postpartum haemorrhage: An educational intervention study in a low-resource setting. *BMC Pregnancy and Childbirth*, *17*(1), 301–301. doi:10.118612884-017-1481-7 PMID:28893211

Norberg-Bohm, V. (2000). Creating incentives for environmentally enhancing technological change: Lessons from 30 years of US energy technology policy. *Technological Forecasting and Social Change*, *65*(2), 125–148. doi:10.1016/S0040-1625(00)00076-7

Patterson, M. D., Geis, G. L., Falcone, R. A., LeMaster, T., & Wears, R. L. (2013). In situ simulation: Detection of safety threats and teamwork training in a high risk emergency department. *BMJ Quality & Safety*, *22*(6), 468–477. doi:10.1136/bmjqs-2012-000942 PMID:23258390

Paull, D. E., Deleeuw, L. D., Wolk, S., Paige, J. T., Neily, J., & Mills, P. D. (2013). The effect of simulation-based crew resource management training on measurable teamwork and communication among interprofessional teams caring for postoperative patients. *Journal of Continuing Education in Nursing*, *44*(11), 516–524. doi:10.3928/00220124-20130903-38 PMID:24024501

Phipps, M. G., Lindquist, D. G., McConaughey, E., O'Brien, J. A., Raker, C. A., & Paglia, M. J. (2012). Outcomes from a labor and delivery team training program with simulation component. *American Journal of Obstetrics and Gynecology*, *206*(1), 3–9. doi:10.1016/j.ajog.2011.06.046 PMID:21840493

Placek, S. B., Franklin, B. R., Haviland, S. M., Wagner, M. D., O'Donnell, M. T., Cryer, C. T., Trinca, K. D., Silverman, E., & Matthew Ritter, E. (2017). Outcomes of Fundamentals of Laparoscopic Surgery (FLS) mastery training standards applied to an ergonomically different, lower cost platform. *Surgical Endoscopy*, *31*(6), 2616–2622. doi:10.100700464-016-5271-5 PMID:27734202

Riley, C., Spies, L. A., Prater, L., & Garner, S. L. (2019). Improving Neonatal Outcomes Through Global Professional Development. *Advances in Neonatal Care: Official Journal of the National Association of Neonatal Nurses, 19*(1), 56-64. doi:10.1097/ANC.0000000000000550

Riley, W., Davis, S., Miller, K., Hansen, H., Sainfort, F., & Sweet, R. (2011). Didactic and simulation nontechnical skills team training to improve perinatal patient outcomes in a community hospital. *Joint Commission Journal on Quality and Patient Safety, 37*(8), 357–364. doi:10.1016/S1553-7250(11)37046-8 PMID:21874971

Sawyer, T., Motz, P., Schooley, N., & Umoren, R. (2019). Positive pressure ventilation coaching during neonatal bag-mask ventilation: A simulation-based pilot study. *Journal of Neonatal-Perinatal Medicine, 12*(3), 243–248. doi:10.3233/NPM-18119 PMID:30909252

Schimmel, D. R., Sweis, R., Cohen, E. R., Davidson, C., & Wayne, D. B. (2016). Targeting clinical outcomes: Endovascular simulation improves diagnostic coronary angiography skills. *Catheterization and Cardiovascular Interventions: Official Journal of the Society for Cardiac Angiography & Interventions, 87*(3), 383-388. doi:10.1002/ccd.26089

Scholtz, A. K., Monachino, A. M., Nishisaki, A., Nadkarni, V. M., & Lengetti, E. (2013). Central venous catheter dress rehearsals: translating simulation training to patient care and outcomes. *Simulation in Healthcare: Journal of the Society for Simulation in Healthcare, 8*(5), 341-349. doi:10.1097/SIH.0b013e3182974462

Semrau, K. E. A., Hirschhorn, L. R., Marx Delaney, M., Singh, V. P., Saurastri, R., Sharma, N., Tuller, D. E., Firestone, R., Lipsitz, S., Dhingra-Kumar, N., Kodkany, B. S., Kumar, V., & Gawande, A. A. (2017). Outcomes of a Coaching-Based WHO Safe Childbirth Checklist Program in India. *The New England Journal of Medicine, 377*(24), 2313–2324. doi:10.1056/NEJMoa1701075 PMID:29236628

Skizim, M., Harris, N., Leonardi, C., & Scribner, R. (2017). Academic-community partnership development to enhance program outcomes in underserved communities: A case study. *Ethnicity & Disease, 27*(Suppl 1), 321. doi:10.18865/ed.27.S1.321 PMID:29158657

Slakey, D. P., Simms, E. R., Rennie, K. V., Garstka, M. E., & Korndorffer, J. R., Jr. (2014). Using simulation to improve root cause analysis of adverse surgical outcomes. *International Journal for Quality in Health Care: Journal of the International Society for Quality in Health Care, 26*(2), 144-150. doi:10.1093/intqhc/mzu011

Smith, A., Siassakos, D., Crofts, J., & Draycott, T. (2013). Simulation: Improving patient outcomes. *Seminars in Perinatology, 37*(3), 151–156. doi:10.1053/j.semperi.2013.02.005 PMID:23721770

Smith, K. A., High, K., Collins, S. P., & Self, W. H. (2015). A preprocedural checklist improves the safety of emergency department intubation of trauma patients. *Academic Emergency Medicine, 22*(8), 989–992. doi:10.1111/acem.12717 PMID:26194607

Sørensen, J. L., van der Vleuten, C., Rosthøj, S., Østergaard, D., LeBlanc, V., Johansen, M., Ekelund, K., Starkopf, L., Lindschou, J., Gluud, C., Weikop, P., & Ottesen, B. (2015). Simulation-based multiprofessional obstetric anaesthesia training conducted in situ versus off-site leads to similar individual and team outcomes: A randomised educational trial. *BMJ Open, 5*(10), e008344–e008344. doi:10.1136/bmjopen-2015-008344 PMID:26443654

Sweigart, L. I., Umoren, R. A., Scott, P. J., Carlton, K. H., Jones, J. A., Truman, B., & Gossett, E. J. (2016). Virtual TeamSTEPPS(®) Simulations Produce Teamwork Attitude Changes Among Health Professions Students. *The Journal of Nursing Education, 55*(1), 31–35. doi:10.3928/01484834-20151214-08 PMID:26812380

Tam, V., Borrebach, J., Dunn, S. A., Bellon, J., Zeh, H. J., & Hogg, M. E. (2019). Proficiency-based training and credentialing can improve patient outcomes and decrease cost to a hospital system. *American Journal of Surgery, 217*(4), 591–596. doi:10.1016/j.amjsurg.2018.07.053 PMID:30098709

Tan, R. Y., Lee, K. G., Gan, S. W. S., Li, H., Yeon, W., Pang, S. C., Teh, S. P., Htay, H., Teo, S. H., Kwek, J. L., Tok, P. L., Poh, C. B., Ng, C. Y., Liu, P., Tay, H. B., Koniman, R., Foo, M. W. Y., Choong, L. H. L., & Tan, C. S. (2018). Impact of simulation-based learning on immediate outcomes of temporary haemodialysis catheter placements by nephrology fellows. *Nephrology (Carlton, Vic.), 23*(10), 933–939. doi:10.1111/nep.13156 PMID:28833793

Tejos, R., Avila, R., Inzunza, M., Achurra, P., Castillo, R., Rosberg, A., Cordero, O., Kusanovich, R., Bellolio, F., Varas, J., & Martínez, J. (2019). Impact of a simulated laparoscopic training program in a three-year general surgery residency. *Arquivos Brasileiros de Cirurgia Digestiva*, *32*(2), e1436–e1436. doi:10.1590/0102-672020190001e1436 PMID:31038561

Theilen, U., Fraser, L., Jones, P., Leonard, P., & Simpson, D. (2017). Regular in-situ simulation training of paediatric Medical Emergency Team leads to sustained improvements in hospital response to deteriorating patients, improved outcomes in intensive care and financial savings. *Resuscitation*, *115*, 61–67. doi:10.1016/j.resuscitation.2017.03.031 PMID:28359769

Thongprayoon, C., Harrison, A. M., O'Horo, J. C., Berrios, R. A. S., Pickering, B. W., & Herasevich, V. (2016). The Effect of an Electronic Checklist on Critical Care Provider Workload, Errors, and Performance. *Journal of Intensive Care Medicine*, *31*(3), 205–212. doi:10.1177/0885066614558015 PMID:25392010

Ullman, E., Kennedy, M., Di Delupis, F. D., Pisanelli, P., Burbui, A. G., Cussen, M., Galli, L., Pini, R., & Gensini, G. F. (2016). The Tuscan Mobile Simulation Program: A description of a program for the delivery of in situ simulation training. *Internal and Emergency Medicine*, *11*(6), 837–841. doi:10.100711739-016-1401-2 PMID:26861702

Umoren, R. A., Gray, M. M., Schooley, N., Billimoria, Z., Smith, K. M., & Sawyer, T. L. (2018). Effect of Video-based Telemedicine on Transport Management of Simulated Newborns. *Air Medical Journal*, *37*(5), 317–320. doi:10.1016/j.amj.2018.05.007 PMID:30322635

Umoren, R. A., Scott, P. J., Sweigart, L., Gossett, E., Hodson-Carlton, K., Johnson, M., Jones, J. A., Poore, J. A., Rybas, N., Truman, B., & Das, R. (2018). A comparison of teamwork attitude changes with virtual TeamSTEPPS® simulations in health professional students. *Journal of Interprofessional Education & Practice*, *10*, 51–55. doi:10.1016/j.xjep.2017.12.001

van Gessel, E., Picchiottino, P., Doureradjam, R., Nendaz, M., & Mèche, P. (2018). Interprofessional training: Start with the youngest! A program for undergraduate healthcare students in Geneva, Switzerland. *Medical Teacher*, *40*(6), 595–599. doi:10.1080/0142159X.2018.1445207 PMID:29519173

Varghese, B., Copas, A., Kumari, S., Bandyopadhyay, S., Sharma, J., Saha, S., Yadav, V., & Kumar, S. (2019). Does the safe childbirth checklist (SCC) program save newborn lives? Evidence from a realistic quasi-experimental study, Rajasthan, India. *Maternal Health, Neonatology and Perinatology, 5*(1), 3. doi:10.118640748-019-0098-4 PMID:30867935

Walliczek-Dworschak, U., Schmitt, M., Dworschak, P., Diogo, I., Ecke, A., Mandapathil, M., Teymoortash, A., & Güldner, C. (2017). The effect of different training exercises on the performance outcome on the da Vinci Skills Simulator. *Surgical Endoscopy, 31*(6), 2397–2405. doi:10.100700464-016-5240-z PMID:27651354

West, C., Graham, L., Palmer, R. T., Miller, M. F., Thayer, E. K., Stuber, M. L., Awdishu, L., Umoren, R. A., Wamsley, M. A., Nelson, E. A., Joo, P. A., Tysinger, J. W., George, P., & Carney, P. A. (2016). Implementation of interprofessional education (IPE) in 16 U.S. medical schools: Common practices, barriers and facilitators. *Journal of Interprofessional Education & Practice, 4*, 41–49. doi:10.1016/j.xjep.2016.05.002 PMID:28184380

Wetmore, D., Goldberg, A., Gandhi, N., Spivack, J., McCormick, P., & DeMaria, S. Jr. (2016). An embedded checklist in the Anesthesia Information Management System improves pre-anaesthetic induction setup: A randomised controlled trial in a simulation setting. *BMJ Quality & Safety, 25*(10), 739–746. doi:10.1136/bmjqs-2015-004707 PMID:26590199

Wetzel, E. A., Lang, T. R., Pendergrass, T. L., Taylor, R. G., & Geis, G. L. (2013). Identification of latent safety threats using high-fidelity simulation-based training with multidisciplinary neonatology teams. *Joint Commission Journal on Quality and Patient Safety, 39*(6), 268–273. doi:10.1016/S1553-7250(13)39037-0 PMID:23789165

Wong, A. H.-W., Gang, M., Szyld, D., & Mahoney, H. (2016). Making an "Attitude Adjustment": Using a Simulation-Enhanced Interprofessional Education Strategy to Improve Attitudes Toward Teamwork and Communication. *Simulation in Healthcare: Journal of the Society for Simulation in Healthcare, 11*(2), 117-125. doi:10.1097/SIH.0000000000000133

Zendejas, B., Cook, D. A., Bingener, J., Huebner, M., Dunn, W. F., Sarr, M. G., & Farley, D. R. (2011). Simulation-based mastery learning improves patient outcomes in laparoscopic inguinal hernia repair: A randomized controlled trial. *Annals of Surgery, 254*(3), 502–511. doi:10.1097/SLA.0b013e31822c6994 PMID:21865947

Zendejas, B., Hernandez-Irizarry, R., & Farley, D. R. (2012). Does simulation training improve outcomes in laparoscopic procedures? *Advances in Surgery*, *46*(1), 61–71. doi:10.1016/j.yasu.2012.03.004 PMID:22873032

Zendejas, B., Wang, A. T., Brydges, R., Hamstra, S. J., & Cook, D. A. (2013). Cost: the missing outcome in simulation-based medical education research: a systematic review. *Surgery*, *153*(2), 160–176. doi:10.1016/j.surg.2012.06.025 PMID:22884087

KEY TERMS AND DEFINITIONS

Augmented Reality: Computer generated holographic images can be viewed by the learner in the physical environment using a mobile device or specially designed headset.

High-Fidelity Manikin: This term refers to a technology-enabled manikin with features such as mechanical respiration and heart rate.

Low-Fidelity Manikin: This is typically a low cost, low technology manikin with minimal features.

Objective Structured Clinical Examination (OSCE): An approach to assessment that involves defined objectives and anticipated actions, often with an accompanying checklist for assessment.

Simulation Debriefer: A simulation instructor who leads the learners through a reflective analysis of simulation events.

Simulation Facilitator: A simulation instructor who guides the learners through the scenario with the goal of meeting learning objectives.

Simulation Technician/Specialist: An individual who supports the practice of simulation through setting up and managing simulation manikins and supplies.

Teledebriefing: Teledebriefing describes a process in which learners who are participating in a simulation scenario undergo debriefing with a facilitator located at an off-site location.

Telefacilitation: The conduct of a telesimulation by a remote facilitator.

Telesimulation: Telesimulation is a process by which telecommunication and simulation resources are utilized to provide education, training, and/or assessment to learners at an off-site location.

Video-Assisted Debriefing: The practice of using video captured during simulation sessions for reflective discussions on learner and team performance.

Virtual Environment: 3D computer generated objects that can be viewed on a screen or in a head-mounted display.

Virtual Reality: Computer generated 3D images viewed by a learner in a virtual environment using a low-cost or high-end head mounted display.

Chapter 9
Research and Data Collection Strategies for Simulation Educators

ABSTRACT

This chapter introduces basic research concepts and strategies for simulation faculty conducting research or other scholarly work. These include an overview of how to initiate a scholarly project, ask well-refined research questions, and clearly define study objectives. The chapter also presents an introduction to quantitative and qualitative data collection during simulation sessions and strategies for understanding and reporting simulation data. Other considerations include the process for obtaining institutional review board approval for research in human subjects and participating in simulation research network collaborations.

INTRODUCTION

Research is the conduct of a systematic investigation to establish new facts and research new conclusions. The use of simulation methodologies in research is intended to generate new information about simulation education and its outcomes that can be generalized to other populations in various educational settings. The purpose of simulation research is to improve an area or field by generating knowledge through the introduction or evaluation of scientific theories, concepts and ideas. Indeed, high-quality simulation research produces

DOI: 10.4018/978-1-7998-4378-8.ch009

evidence that informs the practice of simulation instructors around the world. This may lead to major advances in learning and retention of patient care knowledge that influences healthcare practice and important patient level outcomes (McGuire & Halliday, 2018).

Patient safety is one of the most important downstream impacts of simulation education, particularly in high-risk but infrequently occurring events. This is especially true in emergency situations. These kinds of occurrences are frequently depicted in simulation cases and investigated as a part of research pertaining to simulation. Participants in simulation research can include students, teachers, and even patients whose care is provided by medical professionals who have been trained to perform their jobs using simulation methods (J.-M. Koivisto et al., 2018). When designing a study, it is essential to take into account a variety of perspectives, and there is a lot of value in collaborating with people from a variety of fields, especially when planning and carrying out research that crosses professional boundaries (Hall et al., 2018; J. M. Koivisto et al., 2018).

BACKGROUND

The scope of research in simulation involves the collection, organization, and analysis of quantitative and/or qualitative data to increase understanding of a topic or issue (Grayson-Sneed & Smith, 2018). However, there are some clear areas of distinction in the approach to data collection and reporting that are different from other kinds of research. The approach to research and data collection during simulation has many similarities with other types of educational or clinical research. It is of the utmost importance to carry out simulation research of a high quality in order to both validate the practice of simulation and assess the influence that it has on educational and clinical outcomes. This chapter reviews the fundamentals of simulation research and data collection strategies in order to provide an overview for simulation educators who are just getting started in the field of simulation research. By conducting an in-depth literature review at the beginning of a simulation research project, the simulation educator should familiarize themselves with the prior research that has been carried out in this field. This will reveal gaps in the literature and enable the researcher to ask more thoughtful and concise questions as they proceed to conduct a problem analysis and develop specific study objectives.

Simulation research, much like other types of research, builds on the foundation laid by earlier work done in the field. In order to accomplish this, it is essential to conduct an in-depth literature review that identifies any gaps in the existing literature on the topic of your research. These gaps may take the form of questions that have not been answered regarding the impact of simulation research on education or clinical outcomes, best practices for utilizing simulation as an educational approach, types of simulation platforms which may include manikin or virtual simulation, location of facilitators or learners as described in telesimulation and teledebriefing, and the availability of validated surveys, observation checklists, and other evaluation tools. Additionally, these gaps may concern the availability of validated surveys, observation checklists, and other evaluation tools. Beginning any kind of literature review, whether it's targeted or systematic, can feel overwhelming, especially considering how rapidly the simulation literature base has been expanding across all disciplines over the course of the past two decades. When researching a topic, you might find that you can only access the relevant literature by using specialized databases, such as PubMed or CINAHL to research topics related to medicine or nursing, respectively. An approach to the literature review that is methodical, with the assistance of your local librarian if one is available, and in which all databases are searched for the topic that is being considered is one way to avoid taking a limited, specialty-specific point of view.

LITERATURE REVIEW

Literature review is valuable to understanding how simulation studies are conducted including typical research questions, approaches and methodologies, previous results and potential areas for follow-up studies. Find some systematic reviews that cover the subject you're interested in reading about to get a head start on your literature review. Almeida et al. (Almeida 2018) conducted a review of nursing simulation research and found that out of 160 articles, 68 percent used simulated teaching to develop clinical reasoning in learners, and 32 percent used simulation to train learners in specific nursing skills. The summary tables that the authors of the review have provided offer illuminating information regarding the study's population, population size, methodology for data collection, and findings. When it comes to relevant studies, a review of the study's limitations (which is typically done at the end of the discussion section) and conclusion may shed light on the gaps in the literature that the study did not answer or that the authors see as potential directions for future research. For instance, Almeida and colleagues (Almeida 2018) came to the conclusion that "appropriate tools are needed to measure the true impact of simulation on the teaching of nursing care and the training needed to use simulation as a teaching strategy." Validation of the learner evaluation tools in the learner population that will be studied is necessary for the success of the research study on the educational outcomes of simulation. These tools are essential to the success of the study. Further discussion on the approach to evaluation in simulation education is undertaken in Chapter 6 on "Evaluation of Simulation Performance".

Organizing the Literature Review

Many researchers will organize their literature review using databases or citation managers like Zotero, EndNote, RefWorks and others. These citation managers will allow you to easily organize the references and include them in the background of your study protocol and eventually in your study report.

Table 1. Simple literature review table

S/N	Author(s)	Year	Title	Design	Study Population	Results

If you do not have access to a citation manager, a simple table or spreadsheet can be used to keep track of your findings on literature review. See Table 1.

PROBLEM ANALYSIS

Clinical simulation has been used to study how to improve quality and safety in healthcare (Lamé & Dixon-Woods, 2020). Along with your literature review, you may also explore your own environment or hospital setting for potential areas of interest. Is there an opportunity to improve patient care through simulation education or research in your facility? Has a medical error occurred due to communication failure or human factors issue? This might be a subject of a simulation study to find ways to show why the mistake occurred and test whether an intervention may be able to prevent it from happening again. Further literature review should identify the theoretical frameworks and concepts underpinning the research question and approach. For example, the learning curve theory is a scientific theory that has been applied to simulation research and may have implications for longitudinal study designs (Pusic et al., 2018). See Chapter 2 on the "Theory of simulation and gaming for health professional education". A review of adult learning theory as it applies to simulation can help the researcher make key decisions about refining the study question and the design of the study. This is also a good stage to obtain viewpoints from patients (if appropriate) and the public. Involvement of patients and the public is considered to be essential for good conduct of research. While this is a growing area of focus, research priority setting that seeks the input of patients and communities potentially affected by the research can lead to greater alignment of researcher's goals with the priorities of the communities in which they work (Franck et al., 2018).

FRAMING THE RESEARCH QUESTION

When your literature review and problem analysis is complete, you may have come up with a number of potential areas for study. Next, you must frame your research question in a clear, concise way that defines the problem, the study population and the research design. The PICO format has been described as a way to ask a good clinical research question.
This acronym stands for:

P (Problem or Population or Patient)
I (Intervention/Indicator)
C (Comparison)
O (Outcome of interest)

Table 2. Asking a simulation research question

	Problem or Patient or Population (Learner/ Instructor/ Patient)	Intervention (or indicator)	Comparison (optional)	Outcome
Element of the simulation research question	Describe as accurately as possible the study participant or group of study participants of interest	What is the main educational intervention you wish to consider? This may include an exposure to a simulation or debriefing technique, use of specific simulation cases or equipment, learner perceptions, a checklist or tool, a learning facilitator or barrier, etc.	Is there an alternative educational approach to compare? This includes no training, placebo, a different learning strategy, absence of a learning facilitator or barrier, etc.	What is the educational outcome, including a time horizon if relevant?
Example 1	In simulation instructors	does training on debriefing techniques plus the use of debriefing checklists	training on debriefing techniques alone	increase learner satisfaction with debriefing?
Example 2	In health professional students	does the use of virtual teamwork simulations	lecture on teamwork principles	increase learner positive attitudes towards teamwork?
Example 3	In respiratory therapists	does positive pressure ventilation coaching during simulated positive pressure ventilation	none	decrease the percentage of mask leak during positive pressure ventilation?
Example 4	According to simulation center directors	how frequently is virtual simulation used		for training distance learners?
Example 5	In pediatric patients	does virtual reality simulation training of hospital staff	manikin-based simulation training	more timely evacuation in the event of a fire on the patient care unit?

For example: In pediatric residents (Population), does using a standardized pre-briefing checklist (Intervention), compared to no intervention (Comparison), decrease the number of endotracheal intubation attempts (Outcome of interest). This approach can also be applied to many aspects of simulation research. See Table 2 for additional examples.

Once the question has been drafted, it should be further refined to ensure that it targets the appropriate study population and if the optional comparison is selected, it is an appropriate comparison intervention for a rigorous study.

In Example 1, both the intervention and the comparison group of simulation instructors received training on debriefing techniques, so the main intervention being studied is the use of the debriefing checklist. In some cases, there is no comparator. In others, such as in Example 4, there is no intervention, but rather the question is about the use of an educational indicator.

DEFINING STUDY OBJECTIVES

The next step is to determine what you want to get out of your study. Even

Figure 1. SMART objectives for simulation research

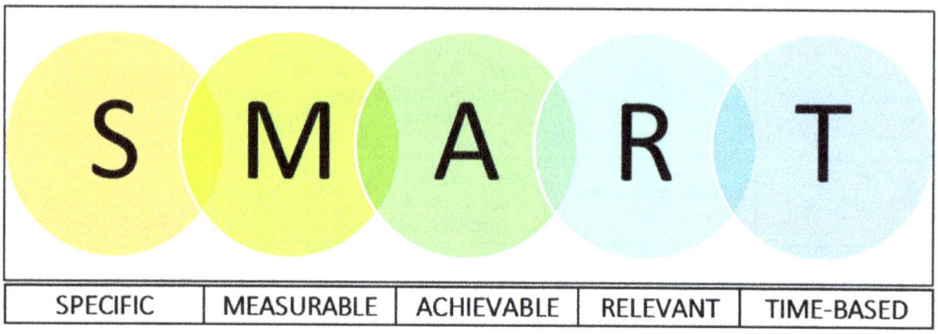

though it might seem simple on the surface, one of the most challenging aspects of conducting research is formulating a research question that is both specific and comprehensive. Simulation researchers need to put a lot of thought into their study objectives, as well as how those objectives will be stated and measured, before they can even start a study. Utilizing the SMART approach to the creation of objectives and goals is one method that can be utilized to clearly define the study's intended outcomes. Figure 1.

If learning objectives are clearly stated and measurable, the study outcomes will often mirror the learning objectives. See Chapters 3 and 4 on "Scenario Development for Manikin-based Simulation" and "Scenario Development for Virtual Simulation" respectively. This is an area in which the connection between the scholarly work of a simulation educator can be harnessed and translated to fulfill the demands of education research.

DATA COLLECTION

Types of Research Studies

Educational research can be performed using observational or interventional study designs or through qualitative methods. It is beyond the scope of this chapter to provide a detailed description of all of the various study designs that are possible; however, such information is typically included in textbooks on research methods. Nevertheless, it is essential to ensure that the methodology chosen for a simulation research study is congruent with the objective (or objectives) of the study as well as the learning objective (s). Historically, a significant number of simulation researchers have relied on observational methods, such as cohort studies and case-control studies. It is important to conduct observational research, but this method is not as reliable as conducting a study in which an intervention is implemented and the effects of the intervention are compared in a group that experiences it and a group that does not experience it. A randomized controlled trial, also known as an RCT, is a type of research design that can produce high-quality evidence regarding the efficacy of an educational intervention. The use of simulation as an intervention is possible in certain circumstances. For instance, a study could be conducted to investigate the efficacy of using a virtual reality simulation as an intervention in manikin-based pediatric resuscitation training in order to achieve better results. In other situations, simulation can be utilized to determine how effective an intervention actually was. For instance, a study may use manikin-based simulation as an evaluation tool in order to assess the impact that virtual simulation has on the level of preparedness of practicing nurses working in emergency departments and neonatal intensive care units in comparison to training that is didactic (Gray et al., 2020). In another study, the performance of nursing students who were given a self-learning module on the prevention of healthcare associated infections was compared to the performance of nursing students who were taught the same material in traditional in-person classes using post-training knowledge tests and simulations (Kappes Ramirez, 2018).

However, if other students in the same group do not participate in the educational intervention, it may be difficult to randomly assign one learner to receive the educational intervention. Because of this, some researchers may choose to conduct historical cohort studies. In these studies, a new intervention is implemented, and the results are compared with those of students who attended school in years prior, when the intervention was not available. In a "crossover" study design, each participant acts as their own control and may be exposed to more than one intervention following a "washout" period. This is another approach that can be taken to engage the entire group of students in the learning process. Learners who were not initially selected at random to receive the intervention but who participated in the study may be given access to the intervention once it has been determined whether or not the study has a time limit. This could happen after one day, after one month, or even later in the year, depending on the length of time that was spent on the study.

On the other hand, qualitative studies seek to answer a research question through the use of qualitative methods such as observation, interviews, and focus groups. It is beyond the scope of this chapter to go into detail on how to carry out a qualitative research study; however, such a discussion can be found in textbooks on qualitative research methods. It is possible for qualitative studies to investigate the benefits of simulation for certain aspects of training, such as the acquisition of new skills, or they may be used to understand how simulation experiences can be improved through better preparation of instructors or instructional methods (Craft-Blacksheare & Frencher, 2018).

Human Subjects Protections in Simulation Research

The International Compilation of Human Research Standards is a listing of over 1,000 laws, regulations, and guidelines on human subjects' protections in 133 countries. These laws, regulations and guidelines are classified into nine categories. The categories applicable to simulation research are: 1) General i.e. applicable to all types of human subjects research; 2) Research injury; 3) Social-Behavioral research; 4) Privacy/Data protection; and 5) Clinical Trial Registries. Human subjects' protections in simulation research are the same as those for other fields of study. Researchers working with simulations ought to have some sort of training in ethics and human subjects research. This training can be obtained through educational establishments of a higher level in addition to being offered online at www.citiprogram.org. Before beginning a research study, the primary investigator on the project should have first completed any necessary training. In the event that you intend to have other people, such as research assistants or collaborators, take part in the gathering of data for your study, those other people should also receive training. The purpose of fundamental training is to raise awareness of the rights of human research subjects and to familiarize participants with fundamental research processes. These processes include informed consent, privacy and confidentiality, and data security. Courses at the advanced level might focus on a particular aspect of research, such as recruiting participants through social media or conducting research with wearable technologies.

All research protocols should be reviewed and approved by your institution's Institutional Review Board (IRB) or Institutional Review Ethics Committee before any subjects are recruited or enrolled in a research study. The research protocol typically consists of a brief study background and detailed description of study methods including the number of subjects you intend to recruit, how and where recruitment will take place, how informed consent will be documented, what the subjects will do in the study, how long the study intervention will take and whether there will be repeated visits, what compensation is available (if applicable) and what will be done to ensure the comfort and safety of subjects as well as the privacy and confidentiality of study data. If there are recruitment flyers, surveys or educational material e.g., videos, educational modules that the subjects will see, these will need to be submitted along with the study protocol for IRB review. In cases where the material is unable to be submitted in full e.g., a virtual simulation, it may be acceptable to submit pictures or a short video showing the key elements of the activity. Some IRBs have specially designed paper or electronic forms to capture the information needed for the IRB submission, while others do not. It is important to contact your local Institutional Research Office for more details to guide your IRB application submission.

Once your research protocol and application to the IRB has been submitted, it will undergo review by the members of the IRB. The study will be classified into "Exempt" from further review, "Expedited" review or "Full Board" review. This classification is made based on whether the study is considered by the IRB to be less than "minimal risk", not greater than "minimal risk" or more than "minimal risk" to the participating subjects. See Figure 2. The Institutional Review Board (IRB) will determine that the proposed research is "Exempt" from further review in the majority of simulation studies; however, if sensitive and/or identifiable data is collected, the review of the study may need to be "Expedited" or even "Full Board." After the preliminary evaluation, the Institutional Review Board (IRB) may have questions for the researchers to ask in order to further clarify the study intervention and assign risk. Because getting approval from the IRB can take anywhere from a few weeks to several months, it is essential to plan ahead. It is possible in the United States for a single IRB to give the study its blessing at the primary institution, while the IRBs at the other institutions "rely" on the decision made by the IRB at the primary institution. This occurs when there are multiple institutions involved in the research project. After the initial approval of a study that is

Figure 2. Institutional review board classification of simulation research studies

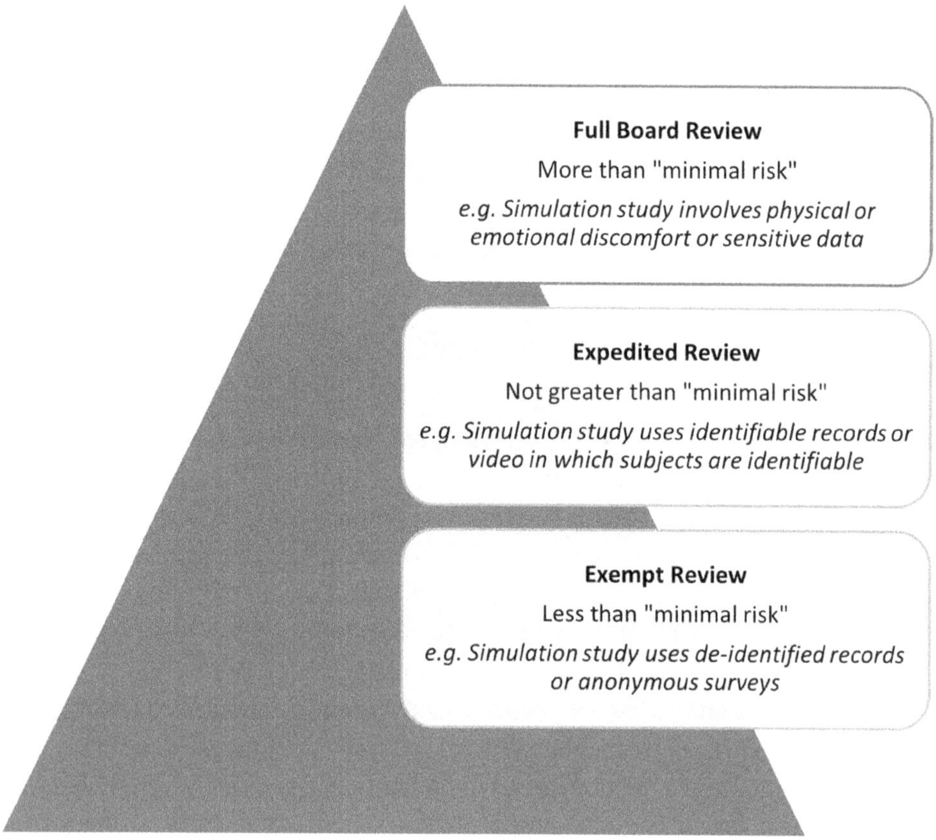

categorized as more than "minimal risk," the Institutional Review Board (IRB) may require annual reports and timely updates if any unexpected events take place. A number of IRBs will also provide an approval period, which, if necessary, can be extended upon inquiry. Before any modifications are made to the previously approved study methods and personnel, they must first be submitted to the Institutional Review Board (IRB) as a modification for approval.

In order to give the general public participating in research studies approved by the IRB the confidence that the studies are being carried out in a safe and ethical manner, it is necessary to take these necessary steps. When conducting a research study, if institutional review board (IRB) approval is not obtained, the researcher will have difficulty conducting the study and reporting the findings because the majority of journals require the IRB approval number for studies prior to publication. You are required to register your study in the Clinical Trials Registry if it includes a clinical trial, such as one that evaluates the effects of an educational intervention on patients. In 2004, the International Committee of Medical Journal Editors came to the conclusion that in order for clinical trials to be published, they must first be registered in a public registry before they can be considered for publication.

Data Collection Approaches and Tools

Determine, for each research question, the data sources to which you already have access or to which you can gain access in order to answer the question. Consider all of the possible sources of data, and categorize them as primary, secondary, tertiary, and so on, depending on how dependable and valid the source of the data is, as well as how easily the data can be accessed. Choose the data source that will provide you with the most reliable and valid information while still being easily accessible. Existing datasets, surveys, automatically generated data from high-fidelity manikins and virtual simulations, validated observer checklists, and physiologic data such as gaze tracking, galvanic skin responses, and heart rate variability from wearable devices and smart clothing are some examples of the different types of data sources that may be utilized. In the event that there are a number of research questions, you may make use of a data collection matrix that contains a row for each research question. Table 3.

Table 3. Example of a data source matrix

Data source/ Characteristic	Data source A	Data source B	Data source C
Reliable (yes/no)			
Valid (yes/no)			
Accessible (yes/no)			

Data collection approaches for simulation include:

Surveys

Surveys are question sets which may include multiple choice questions, short answer and essay open-ended questions. Surveys and questionnaires can be used for collection of demographic data, subject attitudes and perceptions, cognitive load and self-efficacy. Some examples of validated surveys used for evaluation during simulations are provided in Chapter 6 on "Evaluation of Simulation Performance".

Observer Checklists

Standardized checklists which may be validated or unvalidated can be used for in-person or video review of subject performance. When checklists are utilized, it is common practice for two raters to conduct an independent review of the session and submit their findings. Before the actual data collection takes place, it is essential for the investigator to conduct rater training in order to make an assessment of intra-rater and interrater differences. Significant differences, also known as a low kappa score, indicate that two raters would assign different ratings to the subject. This causes errors to be produced in the results. Before the study can move forward, there must first be additional rater training or discussion to settle any discrepancies that have arisen between the results of the two groups. Observer checklists include things like the NRP Performance Checklist and the TEAM checklist, among other things. Although there is a correlation between team stress and team performance, it is not clear which way the correlation should be read. It's possible that successful teamwork during a simulation will result in a more cohesive group, which will result in less stress for the team. On the other hand, ineffective teamwork during the simulation may result in elevated levels of stress for the team. On the other hand, it is possible that, high team stress levels may decrease teamwork behaviors and team perspective(Driskell et al., 1999; Harvey et al., 2010; Hunziker et al., 2011; Leonard et al., 2004; Weaver et al., 2001).

Physiologic Data

Smart shirts or standalone heart rate, gaze and activity trackers can be used for data collection during simulation studies. For a number of years, these instruments have been utilized in the context of a laboratory setting to investigate the relationship between attention, cognitive load, stress, and performance. It is possible that certain tasks require a certain amount of stress in order to be completed successfully; however, studies have shown that excessive stress brought on by time pressure, performance pressure, role conflict, and fatigue can impair the performance of healthcare teams. The Yerke-Dodson Law is responsible for describing the U-shaped curve that results from performance while under pressure. The level of performance is inversely proportional to the level of stress. This rises to a certain optimal level, above which performance begins to decline, and then continues to rise until it reaches a point where it no longer does. These factors have the effect of lessening the focus of the team and increasing negative behaviors that may be detrimental to the team's ability to function effectively (Dietz et al., 2017; Weaver et al., 2001).

It has been demonstrated through research that it is possible to foster resilience by means of stress inoculation. In a similar vein, the treatment of phobias has made use of exposure studies that have been conducted in simulated virtual environments (Maples-Keller et al., 2017; Parsons & Rizzo, 2008; Raghav et al., 2016). It is possible that learners can be adequately prepared to carry out clinical tasks such as resuscitation, which are performed under stressful conditions, by participating in realistic simulations of clinical events. These simulations could achieve the same purpose as traditional clinical training.

It is also possible that reducing team stress by defining team member roles and standardizing information-sharing can be accomplished by encouraging improved teamwork and team communication using tools such as briefs, huddles, and pre-procedural checklists (Hatch et al., 2016; Sawyer et al., 2013; Sawyer et al., 2014; Smith et al., 2015). It's possible that reducing stress and ultimately improving team performance can be achieved through the use of checklists. According to the findings of Hatch and colleagues, the utilization of a standardized pre-intubation checklist for neonatal tracheal intubations was associated with a decrease in the number of adverse safety events. The use of video is yet another strategy for information sharing that can be implemented during tracheal intubation as well as other procedures such as laparoscopy. Because all members of the team are able to view the airway anatomy during the procedure, shared video during procedures, such as with the use of video laryngoscopy, may decrease team stress by information sharing. This is because experienced team members are able to provide additional support and coaching to those on the team who have less experience. The utilization of these tools might make it easier for teams to communicate and engage in behaviors that are beneficial to both their stress levels and their overall performance.

Manikin-Based and Virtual Simulations

Simulation based research scenarios need to be as standardized as possible to maintain internal validity. Alterations in performance can be traced back to the component of the simulation that is the focus of this analysis this way. Research involving virtual simulations is frequently carried out as a comparison intervention to research involving manikin-based simulations or education delivered in a conventional classroom setting. Because simulation as a mode of education and research is still relatively new, many studies have concentrated on its characteristics, such as immersion, learner engagement, and comparative effectiveness to more traditional methods of instruction. A comparative analysis of virtual reality telepresence and more conventional simulation techniques was conducted by Dang and colleagues (Dang, 2020). Studies have been conducted to evaluate the effects of virtual reality immersion on the attitudes and behaviors of learners as they experience different environments or personas. This concept is based on the idea of virtual reality immersion. For example, the subjects who participated in a Virtual Dementia Tour program which provided an opportunity to "imagine what it is like to live with dementia" reported more empathetic responses(Slater et al., 2019).

Data on selections made during manikin or virtual simulations can reveal individual and group trends with a high level of detail. This data can be captured through direct user interaction with the manikin, virtual characters or objects within the simulation environment (Kononowicz et al., 2019). While some virtual simulations may generate performance reports, many are not designed for research data collection and reporting. The approach for designing virtual simulations to capture data related to learning objectives is described in Chapter 4 on "Scenario Development for Virtual Simulations".

Systems Simulation Models

In the field of simulation research, discrete event simulations and other applications of system dynamics modeling, such as agent-based simulation, can be used to represent and explain the behavior of healthcare systems, track the journeys of individual patients as they move through the care system, capture the complex interactions of patients at every stage from diagnosis to the various forms of treatment, and model the limited availability of system resources. Research in the field of simulation is expanding, and one of its subfields, systems simulations, focuses on how to make the best and most economical use of the scarce resources available in the health care system. For several decades, these methods have been put to extensive use in the field of engineering, as well as in the field of business; however, until relatively recently, their application in the field of health services has been relatively limited. (Chahal et al., 2013; Pitt et al., 2016)

PREPARING REPORTS

After collecting your data, you must analyze it and put your findings in context. Then it is time to share it with other simulation colleagues and interested parties in the form of research abstracts, publications and presentations.

Understanding Your Data

The first step to understanding your data is to organize it. Your data may have been collected on paper or in an electronic database. If you used paper data collection methods, then the data should be entered into a spreadsheet (paper or electronic) that will allow you to analyze the outcomes of interest. Electronic databases such as REDCap (Harris et al., 2009) or survey tools such as Survey Monkey® will often have options to visualize or export data to spreadsheets for analysis. Discrete data such as counts may be described using total, percentage, median and range. Continuous data is often described using mean and standard deviation. Tables, figures or charts represent your data and this will allow others to understand it better. If you used simulation as an intervention or are studying the impact of an intervention using simulation in different groups, use statistical methods to compare the outcomes of interest between groups. A full description of analytical methods is beyond the scope of this chapter.

Putting Your Findings in Context

After organizing and analyzing your data, review the literature for similarities and differences with your results. It is highly likely that you will find some results that are comparable to those discovered by other researchers who have studied the same population; however, it is also possible that you will find similarities between populations. Take note of whether or not the inclusion and exclusion criteria, setting, and research methods of the study were identical to those of your own. In addition to this, give the analysis and any data that were left out careful consideration. You might be able to account for varying findings by pointing to differences in the study population or the procedures used. You should provide a summary of your findings because these will come in handy when responding to questions regarding your findings or when forming the discussion section of a manuscript.

Publishing Your Results

There are many educational outlets for simulation research. Some journals like MedED portal will publish simulation scenarios. Journals like Simulation in Healthcare, Medical Teacher, Medical Education and others, will publish studies that use simulation methods. A first step to identifying a suitable journal is to explore the literature you reviewed for journals that may accept similar work. Think about the people who read each journal to determine whether or not they are the kind of people who would be interested in the results of your research. Your audience may be determined by the people in your study population. For instance, the results of a study conducted on residents will be of interest to the directors of residency programs, but it is possible that practicing clinicians working in facilities that do not have residency programs will not find the findings of interest. Entering the journal's title and abstract into a search field is yet another method that can be utilized to find an appropriate journal among those that are presently being provided by particular publishers. The publisher will then give you a list of possible journals to which you could submit your manuscript, along with a rating that indicates how closely it matches your manuscript.

The submission of an abstract to a local, regional, national, or international conference whose primary focus is on medical education or simulation is another option to take into account when thinking about how to disseminate your work. International Meeting on Simulation in Healthcare (IMSH), International Pediatric Simulation Symposia and Workshops (IPSSW), Association of Pediatric Program Directors (APPD), and American Association of Medical Colleges (AAMC) conferences are some examples of national and international conferences that accept educational abstracts. An education or simulation track will likely be offered at the majority of specialty-specific conferences.

Simulation Research Collaborations

Significant growth has been seen in the field of simulation research, and the ability to conduct multicenter, collaborative research has been made easier by the establishment of simulation research networks such as the International Network for Simulation-Based Pediatric Innovation Research and Education (INSPIRE) (INSPIRE). These efforts to collaborate on research provide support for the meticulous planning and execution of simulation research. The INSPIRE Network was established in 2011, and since then, it has finished and published a significant number of research projects in collaboration with institutions and academics located all over the world. (Cheng et al., 2018)

FUTURE RESEARCH DIRECTIONS

Areas for future research in the area of simulation include the exploration of the role of simulation educators in improving the learner experience, increasing the rigor of simulation research studies through integrating physiologic data collection during the simulation to facilitate learner assessment. Simulation research, like other types, builds on earlier work. To do this, you must conduct a thorough literature review to identify any gaps in the existing research. These gaps may include questions about the impact of simulation research on education or clinical outcomes, best practices for using simulation as an educational approach, types of simulation platforms such as manikin or virtual simulation, location of facilitators or learners in telesimulation and teledebriefing, and availability of validated surveys, observation checklists, and other evaluation tools. However, researchers who study simulations will have access to a wide variety of tools with which to investigate the effects of simulations on both small and large groups of students as the availability of simulation modeling, systems simulation, virtual simulations, and virtual simulated patients continues to grow. When it comes to real-time and video observation during simulation research, there have been an increasing number of validated tools developed in recent years. Simulation researchers have more options than ever before to choose tools that are relevant to the context of their research and the subjects they are examining. Both research in simulation and evaluation will benefit from novel and cutting-edge methods of data analysis.

CONCLUSION

In conclusion, the process of designing an education study, collecting data and disseminating results is similar to that of a clinical research project. Research systematically investigates new facts and new conclusions. Simulation research aims to generate new information about simulation education and its outcomes that can be applied to other populations and educational settings. Simulation research improves a field by introducing or evaluating scientific theories, concepts, and ideas. Indeed, high-quality simulation research informs simulation instructors worldwide. This could improve learning and retention of patient care knowledge, influencing healthcare practice and patient outcomes (McGuire & Halliday, 2018).

Simulation education can improve patient safety, especially in high-risk but infrequent events. Especially in emergencies. These events are often depicted in simulation cases and studied in simulation research. Students, teachers, and even patients cared for by medical professionals trained using simulation methods can participate in simulation research. Appropriate attention needs to be paid to ethical principles of research including human subjects' protections and to organizing and analyzing the data collected. Finally, the choice of an outlet to disseminate your results to other educators and educational audiences will continue to grow the field of simulation expands. One of the greatest areas of progress is the emergence of networks of simulation educators and researchers. Collaborative simulation research which will continue to propel the field in discovering best practices for learner teaching and evaluation.

REFERENCES

Almeida, R. G. D. S., Jorge, B. M., Souza-Junior, V. D., Mazzo, A., Martins, J. C. A., Negri, E. C., & Mendes, I. A. C. (2018). Trends in Research on Simulation in the Teaching of Nursing: An Integrative Review. *Nursing Education Perspectives*, *39*(3), E7–E10. doi:10.1097/01.NEP.0000000000000292 PMID:29505502

Chahal, K., Eldabi, T., & Young, T. (2013). A conceptual framework for hybrid system dynamics and discrete event simulation for healthcare. *Journal of Enterprise Information Management*, *26*(1/2), 50–74. doi:10.1108/17410391311289541

Cheng, A., Auerbach, M., Calhoun, A., Mackinnon, R., Chang, T. P., Nadkarni, V., Hunt, E. A., Duval-Arnould, J., Peiris, N., & Kessler, D. (2018). Building a Community of Practice for Researchers: The International Network for Simulation-Based Pediatric Innovation, Research and Education. *Simulation in Healthcare: Journal of the Society for Simulation in Healthcare, 13*(3S Suppl 1), S28-S34. doi:10.1097/SIH.0000000000000269

Craft-Blacksheare, M., & Frencher, Y. (2018). Using high fidelity simulation to increase nursing students' clinical postpartum and newborn assessment proficiency: A mixed-methods research study. *Nurse Education Today*, *71*, 198–204. doi:10.1016/j.nedt.2018.09.031 PMID:30296730

Dang, B. K., O'Leary-Kelley, C., Palicte, J. S., Badheka, S., & Vuppalapati, C. (2020). Comparing Virtual Reality Telepresence and Traditional Simulation Methods: A Pilot Study. *Nursing Education Perspectives*, *41*(2), 119–121. doi:10.1097/01.NEP.0000000000000496 PMID:31107394

Dietz, A. S., Driskell, J. E., Sierra, M. J., Weaver, S. J., Driskell, T., & Salas, E. (2017). Teamwork under Stress. The Wiley Blackwell Handbook of the Psychology of Team Working and Collaborative Processes, 297-315.

Driskell, J. E., Salas, E., & Johnston, J. (1999). Does stress lead to a loss of team perspective? *Group Dynamics*, *3*(4), 291–302. doi:10.1037/1089-2699.3.4.291

Franck, L. S., McLemore, M. R., Cooper, N., De Castro, B., Gordon, A. Y., Williams, S., Williams, S., & Rand, L. (2018). A Novel Method for Involving Women of Color at High Risk for Preterm Birth in Research Priority Setting. *Journal of Visualized Experiments*, (131). Advance online publication. doi:10.3791/56220 PMID:29364217

Gray, M. M., Thomas, A. A., Burns, B., & Umoren, R. A. (2020). Evacuation of vulnerable and critical patients: Multimodal simulation for nurse-led patient evacuation. *Simulation in Healthcare*, *15*(6), 382–387. doi:10.1097/SIH.0000000000000451 PMID:32371747

Grayson-Sneed, K. A., & Smith, R. C. (2018). A research coding method to evaluate medical clinicians conduct of behavioral health care in patients with unexplained symptoms. *Patient Education and Counseling*, *101*(4), 743–749. doi:10.1016/j.pec.2017.10.006 PMID:29050952

Hall, K. L., Vogel, A. L., Huang, G. C., Serrano, K. J., Rice, E. L., Tsakraklides, S. P., & Fiore, S. M. (2018). The science of team science: A review of the empirical evidence and research gaps on collaboration in science. *The American Psychologist*, *73*(4), 532–548. doi:10.1037/amp0000319 PMID:29792466

Harris, P. A., Taylor, R., Thielke, R., Payne, J., Gonzalez, N., & Conde, J. G. (2009). Research electronic data capture (REDCap)—A metadata-driven methodology and workflow process for providing translational research informatics support. *Journal of Biomedical Informatics*, *42*(2), 377–381. doi:10.1016/j.jbi.2008.08.010 PMID:18929686

Harvey, A., Nathens, A. B., Bandiera, G., & Leblanc, V. R. (2010). Threat and challenge: Cognitive appraisal and stress responses in simulated trauma resuscitations. *Medical Education*, *44*(6), 587–594. doi:10.1111/j.1365-2923.2010.03634.x PMID:20604855

Hatch, L. D., Grubb, P. H., Lea, A. S., Walsh, W. F., Markham, M. H., Maynord, P. O., Whitney, G. M., Stark, A. R., & Ely, E. W. (2016). Interventions to improve patient safety during intubation in the neonatal intensive care unit. *Pediatrics*, *138*(4), e20160069. doi:10.1542/peds.2016-0069 PMID:27694281

Hunziker, S., Laschinger, L., Portmann-Schwarz, S., Semmer, N. K., Tschan, F., & Marsch, S. (2011). Perceived stress and team performance during a simulated resuscitation. *Intensive Care Medicine*, *37*(9), 1473–1479. doi:10.100700134-011-2277-2 PMID:21695475

Kappes Ramirez, M. S. (2018). Influence of undergraduate nursing student teaching methods on learning standard precautions and transmission-based precautions: Experimental research. *Nurse Education Today*, *61*, 101–105. doi:10.1016/j.nedt.2017.11.007 PMID:29195210

Koivisto, J. M., Haavisto, E., Niemi, H., Haho, P., Nylund, S., & Multisilta, J. (2018). Design principles for simulation games for learning clinical reasoning: A design-based research approach. *Nurse Education Today*, *60*, 114–120. doi:10.1016/j.nedt.2017.10.002 PMID:29096383

Koivisto, J.-M., Hannula, L., Bøje, R. B., Prescott, S., Bland, A., Rekola, L., & Haho, P. (2018). Design-based research in designing the model for educating simulation facilitators. *Nurse Education in Practice*, *29*, 206–211. doi:10.1016/j.nepr.2018.02.002 PMID:29433039

Kononowicz, A. A., Woodham, L. A., Edelbring, S., Stathakarou, N., Davies, D., Saxena, N., Tudor Car, L., Carlstedt-Duke, J., Car, J., & Zary, N. (2019). Virtual Patient Simulations in Health Professions Education: Systematic Review and Meta-Analysis by the Digital Health Education Collaboration. *Journal of Medical Internet Research*, *21*(7), e14676. doi:10.2196/14676 PMID:31267981

Lamé, G., & Dixon-Woods, M. (2020). Using clinical simulation to study how to improve quality and safety in healthcare. *BMJ Simulation & Technology Enhanced Learning*, *6*(2), 87–94. doi:10.1136/bmjstel-2018-000370 PMID:32133154

Leonard, M., Graham, S., & Bonacum, D. (2004). The human factor: The critical importance of effective teamwork and communication in providing safe care. *Quality & Safety in Health Care*, *13*(suppl 1), i85–i90. doi:10.1136/qshc.2004.010033 PMID:15465961

Maples-Keller, J. L., Yasinski, C., Manjin, N., & Rothbaum, B. O. (2017). Virtual Reality-Enhanced Extinction of Phobias and Post-Traumatic Stress. *Neurotherapeutics; the Journal of the American Society for Experimental NeuroTherapeutics*, *14*(3), 554–563. doi:10.100713311-017-0534-y PMID:28512692

McGuire, W., & Halliday, H. L. (2018). The Research Cycle: Improving Care and Outcomes for Newborn Infants. *Neonatology*, *114*(1), 2–6. doi:10.1159/000487990 PMID:29566381

Parsons, T. D., & Rizzo, A. A. (2008). Affective outcomes of virtual reality exposure therapy for anxiety and specific phobias: A meta-analysis. *Journal of Behavior Therapy and Experimental Psychiatry*, *39*(3), 250–261. doi:10.1016/j.jbtep.2007.07.007 PMID:17720136

Pitt, M., Monks, T., Crowe, S., & Vasilakis, C. (2016). Systems modelling and simulation in health service design, delivery and decision making. *BMJ Quality & Safety*, *25*(1), 38–45. doi:10.1136/bmjqs-2015-004430 PMID:26115667

Pusic, M. V., Boutis, K., & McGaghie, W. C. (2018). Role of Scientific Theory in Simulation Education Research. *Simulation in Healthcare: Journal of the Society for Simulation in Healthcare, 13*(3S Suppl 1), S7-S14. doi:10.1097/SIH.0000000000000282

Raghav, K., Van Wijk, A. J., Abdullah, F., Islam, M. N., Bernatchez, M., & De Jongh, A. (2016). Efficacy of virtual reality exposure therapy for treatment of dental phobia: A randomized control trial. *BMC Oral Health, 16*(1), 25–25. doi:10.118612903-016-0186-z PMID:26920573

Sawyer, T., Laubach, V. A., Hudak, J., Yamamura, K., & Pocrnich, A. (2013). Improvements in teamwork during neonatal resuscitation after interprofessional TeamSTEPPS training. *Neonatal Network, 32*(1), 26–33. doi:10.1891/0730-0832.32.1.26 PMID:23318204

Sawyer, T., Leonard, D., Sierocka-Castaneda, A., Chan, D., & Thompson, M. (2014). Correlations between technical skills and behavioral skills in simulated neonatal resuscitations. *Journal of Perinatology, 34*(10), 781–786. doi:10.1038/jp.2014.93 PMID:24831522

Slater, P., Hasson, F., Gillen, P., Gallen, A., & Parlour, R. (2019). Virtual simulation training: Imaged experience of dementia. *International Journal of Older People Nursing, 14*(3), e12243–e12243. doi:10.1111/opn.12243 PMID:31070851

Smith, K. A., High, K., Collins, S. P., & Self, W. H. (2015). A preprocedural checklist improves the safety of emergency department intubation of trauma patients. *Academic Emergency Medicine, 22*(8), 989–992. doi:10.1111/acem.12717 PMID:26194607

Weaver, J. L., Bowers, C. A., & Salas, E. (2001). Stress and teams: Performance effects and interventions. *Stress, Workload, and Fatigue.*

ADDITIONAL READING

Cypress, B. (2018, November 1). Qualitative research methods: A phenomenological focus. *Dimensions of Critical Care Nursing, 37*(6), 302–309. doi:10.1097/DCC.0000000000000322 PMID:30273215

Lamé, G., & Dixon-Woods, M. (2020, March 1). Using clinical simulation to study how to improve quality and safety in healthcare. *BMJ Simulation & Technology Enhanced Learning*, *6*(2), 87–94. doi:10.1136/bmjstel-2018-000370 PMID:32133154

KEY TERMS AND DEFINITIONS

Augmented Reality: Computer generated holographic images can be viewed by the learner in the physical environment using a mobile device or specially designed headset.

High-Fidelity Manikin: This term refers to a technology-enabled manikin with features such as mechanical respiration and heart rate.

Low-Fidelity Manikin: This is typically a low cost, low technology manikin with minimal features.

Objective Structured Clinical Examination (OSCE): An approach to assessment that involves defined objectives and anticipated actions, often with an accompanying checklist for assessment.

Simulation Debriefer: A simulation instructor who leads the learners through a reflective analysis of simulation events.

Simulation Facilitator: A simulation instructor who guides the learners through the scenario with the goal of meeting learning objectives.

Simulation Technician/Specialist: An individual who supports the practice of simulation through setting up and managing simulation manikins and supplies.

Teledebriefing: Teledebriefing describes a process in which learners who are participating in a simulation scenario undergo debriefing with a facilitator located at an off-site location.

Telefacilitation: The conduct of a telesimulation by a remote facilitator.

Telesimulation: Telesimulation is a process by which telecommunication and simulation resources are utilized to provide education, training, and/or assessment to learners at an off-site location.

Video-Assisted Debriefing: The practice of using video captured during simulation sessions for reflective discussions on learner and team performance.

Virtual Environment: 3D computer generated objects that can be viewed on a screen or in a head-mounted display.

Virtual Reality: Computer generated 3D images viewed by a learner in a virtual environment using a low-cost or high-end head mounted display.

Chapter 10
Strategies for Sustainability and Global Dissemination of Simulation Education

ABSTRACT

For simulation to be effective and achieve long-term sustainability as an educational strategy, institutions must have adequate and ongoing availability of training resources, trained educators, and curricula. This chapter explores stakeholder considerations in adoption and implementation of simulation programs. The chapter then discusses the cost considerations of manikin-based and virtual simulations, revenue generation, and return on investment. Ultimately, the widespread use of simulation education at the pre-service and in-service training levels is driven by health professional schools, hospitals, accreditation bodies, and health professional associations. This chapter discusses the role of faculty development and outcomes-based research in the global dissemination of simulation education.

INTRODUCTION

Simulation education has global application in healthcare education. Consideration of the dimensions of simulation education influence how adoption and expansion of simulation education occur in a healthcare system. This chapter explores how the policies of healthcare agencies, healthcare organizations and other stakeholders influence the use of simulation in the

DOI: 10.4018/978-1-7998-4378-8.ch010

U.S. and globally. In the two decades since the landmark Institute of Medicine report "To err is human", there has been increased adoption of simulation by healthcare organizations with a focus on improving healthcare delivery and patient outcomes (Donaldson et al., 2000). The cost of medical malpractice, estimated at U.S. $55.6 billion per year (2008), represents about 2.4% of annual healthcare spending (Mello et al., 2010). The global healthcare simulation market is anticipated to reach between $3.19 billion and $7.7 billion by 2027, with a compound annual growth rate (CAGR) between 14.6% and 17.8% between 2020 and 2027. The acknowledgment and funding of simulation education by the leadership of an organization is essential to the development of simulation as a method. However, acknowledging the savings made possible by simulation as well as the return on investment (ROI) made possible by simulation is a significant contributor to the long-term viability of the method. After all, the ratio of instructors to students in simulations is quite high, and the demands placed on the logistics of the situation in terms of equipment, space, and time are considerable. The value proposition of simulation in comparison to various other educational approaches needs to be presented to decision-makers.

BACKGROUND

To better understand the aspects that healthcare stakeholders and decision-makers must consider, the following section reviews the key implementation elements or dimensions of simulation education.

Dimensions of Simulation Education

The key considerations for implementing simulation can be classified into 11 dimensions described by Gaba and in part by Miller (Gaba, 2007; Miller, 1990):

- The *aims* of the simulation activity. These may range from education to performance assessment and research.
- The *participation unit*. The participation unit in the simulation can be described as individual, team, or organization (for systems simulations).

- The *experience level.* Experience of participants ranges from undergraduate level learners to continuing education and training for in-service health professionals.
- The *healthcare domain.* This refers to the setting in which the simulation scenario occurs and can be described as in-hospital, clinic-based, intensive care, public health, etc.
- The *profession* of the learner. Learners may be of various disciplines including nurse, physician, manager, technician, etc. or multiple professions may participate in an interprofessional simulation.
- The *knowledge, skill, attitudes, or behaviors addressed.* The focus of the simulation may range from technical skills or decision-making skills (meta-cognition) to attitudes and behaviors (teamwork).
- The *simulated patient.* Patient characteristics drive the content and tempo of the scenario and may range from newborns to geriatric patients.
- The *applicable technology.* Scenarios may require minimal to no technology (verbal role playing or low-fidelity task trainer) or high technology (high-fidelity manikin, screen-based virtual simulation, virtual or augmented reality simulator).
- The *simulation site.* The location where the learner experiences the simulation can be described as home, classroom, simulation laboratory, or clinical environment (in situ).
- The *participation level.* The level of learner participation refers to the extent of direct participation which may range from minimal direct participation through remote viewing of the simulation event with no interaction, to significant direct participation through in person, hands-on participation.
- The *feedback method.* The approach to learner feedback may be of various types from automatic, individualized feedback from the

Figure 1. Dimensions of healthcare simulation

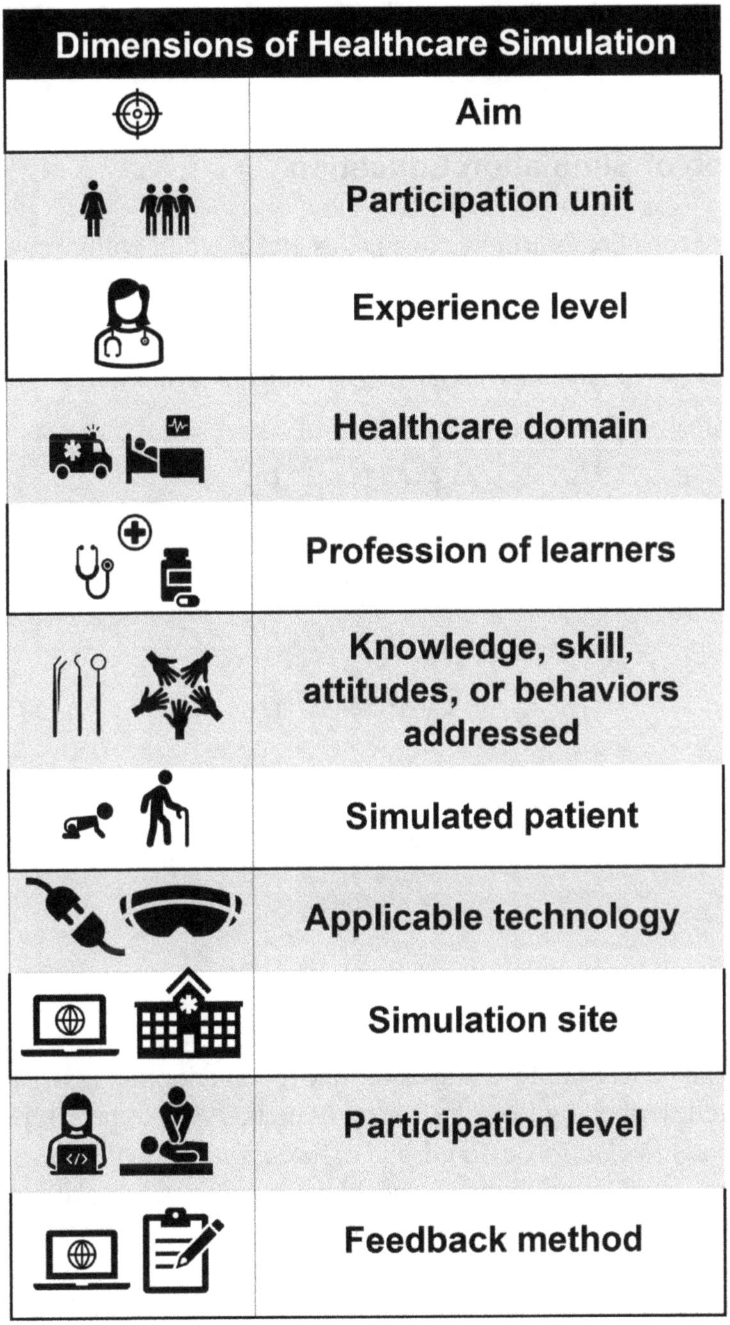

simulator to real-time or delayed instructor feedback or video-based debriefing and feedback of individuals or groups (Gaba, 2007; Miller, 1990). See Figure 1.

Adoption of Simulation Education

Taking into consideration these dimensions, stakeholders within organizations begin the process of adopting innovations such as simulation for health

Figure 2. Stages of simulation adoption by healthcare organizations

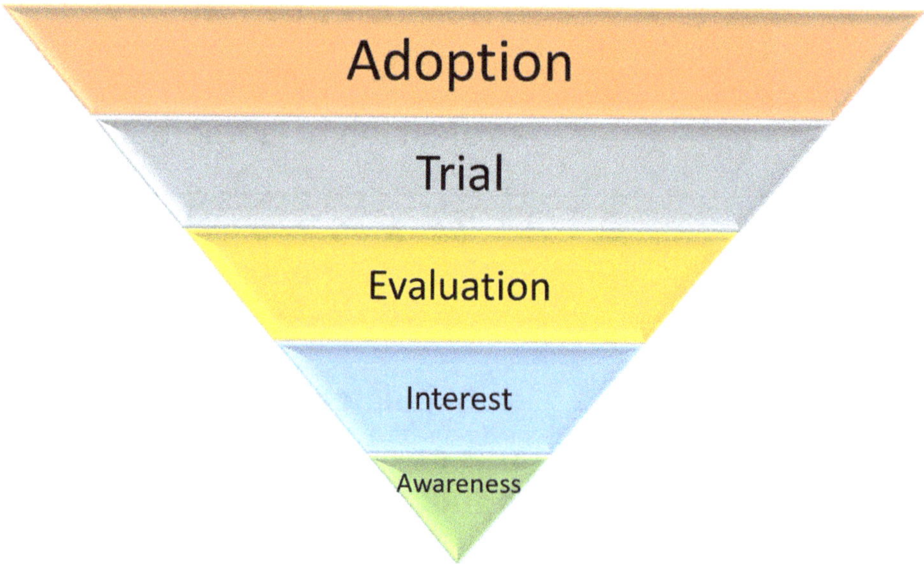

professional education. Five stages of innovation adoption in organizations have been described by Rogers (Rogers Everett, 1995) to be: a) *Awareness*, b) *Interest*, c) *Evaluation*, d) *Trial*, and e) *Adoption*. Applying these stages of innovation to simulation education, healthcare organizations take similar steps in their progression to simulation adoption (Issenberg, 2006). See Figure 2.

At the beginning of the Awareness and Interest stages, instructors and students become familiar with the idea and methodology of simulation, perhaps through exposure to its use in other institutions or at professional meetings, and develop an interest in teaching or learning through simulation in their own institution or setting. This may occur as a result of exposure to simulation's use in other institutions or at professional meetings (Umoren et al., 2020). In the subsequent stages of Evaluation and Trial, early adopters are typically tasked with investigating various options for acquiring additional training in simulation methods and putting those methods into practice within their own organizations with specific groups of students. The results of these early tests of simulation use in a new setting may lead to adoption or to further stages of evaluation. [Case in point:] [Case in point:] Eventually, once a critical mass of trained simulation educators has been attained and the leadership of the organization is either in favor of (or not opposed to) the adoption of simulation, curricular integration will be proposed.

Role of Curricular Institutionalization

The process known as "curricular institutionalization" refers to the incorporation of simulation-based education into every aspect of an organization's mission and culture. This is typically done in conjunction with the objectives of enhancing the quality of care provided to patients by graduating students who have a higher level of proficiency in the skills and teamwork necessary for entry-level positions in the healthcare industry (Issenberg, 2006). The pursuit of curricular institutionalization needs to be accompanied by the creation of evidence-based simulation curricula and the development of faculty. As a result of the implementation of simulation education within an institutional setting by institutional champions, additional faculty and learners are exposed to simulation concepts and applications, which ultimately leads to widespread integration across a variety of fields. At this point, the implementation of simulation education within the organization is extremely likely to take place. However, ongoing work is required to implement a structure of administrative support and faculty and staff development in order to guarantee the ongoing availability of simulation equipment, space, and time. This work must be carried out in a continuous manner. The recognition of the work done by faculty members in simulation education and recognition through the development of divisions of healthcare simulation science, opportunities for grant funding, and opportunities for faculty advancement make up the final pillar of adoption.

Role of Institutional Accreditation

In a similar manner, academic institutions have the potential to earn recognition for their efforts toward the establishment of simulation centers of excellence. At the beginning of the twenty first century, professional societies started developing procedures for health care providers to earn accreditation through the use of training programs that incorporated simulation and cutting-edge technology. The Workgroup on Simulation Education of the American Society of Anesthesiologists (ASA) developed formal recognition and accreditation processes for simulation training programs in 2006. (Issenberg, 2006). Through the American College of Surgeons' (ACS) Program for Accreditation of Education Institutes, similar accreditation criteria were developed in order to recognize surgical simulation programs (AEI). In 2014, the National Council of State Boards of Nursing (NCSBN) made public the research findings from a seminal study conducted by Hayden et al. (Hayden et al., 2014). The findings indicated that traditional clinical practice for nursing students could be partially or completely replaced by simulation for up to fifty percent of the prelicensure nursing curriculum. While there is variability in the degree to which U.S. state boards of nursing apply these recommendations, these findings kicked off the process of establishing guidelines for the use of simulation in the curriculum for nursing students in their first year of schooling. In general, these accreditation criteria demand the availability of training and administrative resources, technical support, curricula, and trained faculty in order to establish an environment that is conducive to the successful implementation of simulation-based education.

Costs of Simulation Education

Costs of Manikin-Based Simulation

Simulation costs are incurred by dedicated personnel, space, manikins, new, repurposed, or expired healthcare devices, equipment, supplies. Purchases of manikins and the creation of scenarios are examples of fixed costs. There is a correlation between the number of students and the variable costs, which include things like staffing costs, space charges, and consumable supplies. A review of cost analyses of simulation education found that procedurally based specialties such as surgery and urology had more reports (60%) than other medical fields such as obstetrics, gynecology, or pediatrics (11%) (Hippe et al., 2020). Many pediatric simulation cost studies have focused on a standard curriculum for neonatal resuscitation training in low resource settings called Helping Babies Breathe. Despite the fact that the majority of reports were published by investigators based in either North America or Europe, this curriculum has been the subject of many of the studies (Chaudhury et al., 2016; Wilson et al., 2020).

Small cost-utility studies that have been conducted have compared lower fidelity manikins to higher fidelity manikins. The results of these studies suggest that using manikins with medium fidelity required only $1.14 per learner in comparison to $6.17 per learner for high-fidelity manikins (Lapkin & Levett-Jones, 2011). This difference in cost can be attributed to the fact that higher fidelity manikins are more realistic. According to the findings of other research, the cost of setting up a simulation can range anywhere from $165 to $17,000, and this disparity is directly related to the type of manikin that is employed (Bulamba et al., 2019). The cost of self-debriefing vs. instructor debriefing have been compared in mathematical models with self-debriefing found to be cost-effective in crew resource management simulation training when compared to instructor debriefing, particularly with lower willingness-to-pay.

The cost of constructing or establishing a simulation center is one of the most significant costs that must be incurred initially. The initial investment is substantial, so educational institutions typically carry out economic analyses to determine the minimum number of students who must utilize the simulation center in order to "break even" with the costs associated with its establishment (Maloney & Haines, 2016). When choosing a space for simulation, it is important to consider whether or not it is accessible to both students and teachers. Instead of designing a new building from the ground up, it might be more beneficial to retrofit an existing structure or make use of clinical spaces for in situ simulation. However, if a new building is being designed, it is essential to take into account the "building adaptability," which refers to the structure's capacity for being put to a variety of uses and accessed in a number of different ways. In addition to this, it is essential to incorporate into the planning stages the capacity for establishments to integrate access to audio-video recording and virtual simulation technology platforms. To ensure the success of their projects, architects must collaborate with other professionals, including constructors, educators, and end-users such as students, whether they are designing a brand-new building or modifying an existing one. When it comes to the ability to achieve reductions in energy consumption, water consumption, and waste generation, new structures may have an advantage over existing structures.

Costs of Virtual Simulation

Newer additions to simulation costs include the cost of purchasing or developing in-house virtual simulation platforms. This is because many educational institutions are transitioning to hybrid offerings for both in-person and online learners. The requirement for trained faculty is a significant factor that drives up the cost of simulation-based education. Additionally, the cost of compensating in-service personnel for the time they have to spend away from their clinical practice in order to attend the session needs to be taken into consideration. Because of increased access, automated feedback, and the elimination of travel time, faculty and personnel time spent away from patient care may be significantly reduced in virtual simulations. Virtual simulations also eliminate the need for travel time. When compared to other forms of education, such as lectures, in which one instructor may teach hundreds of students at a time, the relative ratio of instructors to students participating in simulation-based education tends to be high, with one instructor teaching an average of five or six students at a time. The requirement for hands-on instruction and direct interaction with learners in order to facilitate and debrief in-person simulation sessions is the reason for this high instructor to learner ratio. Learners must be able to interact directly with their instructors. The initial development costs of well-designed virtual simulation courses are the same as those of in-person simulation courses, but the ongoing costs of faculty instruction may be significantly lower than those of in-person simulation courses due to the significantly lower instructor to learner ratios. An examination of the cost-utility ratio of manikin-based simulation versus virtual simulation found that manikin-based simulation had a cost-utility ratio of $3.62, while virtual simulation had a cost-utility ratio of $1.08, suggesting that virtual simulation may be a more cost-effective option (Haerling, 2018).

Return on Investment

Obtaining Value through Improved Patient Outcomes

The costs of simulation need to be analyzed in an objective manner and through the lens of return on investment, which should include both tangible and intangible benefits. Along with the direct and indirect costs, the potential savings from events or complications that did not occur as a result of the simulation, such as central line infections or pericardial effusions, must be considered. When compared with didactic lectures, simulation education has the potential to help students retain more information and transfer that information more effectively into their professional lives. This is the primary argument in favor of simulation education. Previous chapters have provided a description of the typical applications as well as the short-term and long-term effects that simulation has on clinical practice and the outcomes at the patient level. The value of academic-industry collaboration can be in the form of knowledge, cost-savings or innovation to advance the field and stay ahead of competitors. Academic institutions are increasingly establishing partnerships with industries, particularly in the information technology sector as healthcare programs collaborate with technology and simulation companies to build facilities, obtain simulation equipment, and share technical expertise for research and development. See Chapter 1 on "Introduction to Simulation in the Healthcare Professions" and Chapter 8 on "Translation of Skills from Simulation to Clinical Practice: the Role of Academic-Industry-Community Collaboration".

When compared to other types of education, the return on investment for simulation education is higher because it has a longer-term impact on the safety of patients and the outcomes of their care. However, investors in simulation training may need to adjust their expectations for returns because a commitment to the sustainable development of human resources may have more modest earnings results in the near term. This adjustment may be necessary because of the potential for the commitment to have an impact on future earnings. In order for simulation to be a desirable investment, the directors of simulation centers need to take a long-term view of performance with regard to the outcomes for patients, while at the same time meeting the short-term training expectations of organizations with which they partner. For instance, economic evaluations of clinical outcomes as a result of simulation education may review either the direct costs or the costs avoided of healthcare services or goods that were not used as a result of a successful treatment or a reduction in the number of days spent in the intensive care unit.

Revenue Generation by Simulation Centers

In order for educational institutions to get the most out of their investments in simulation facilities and equipment and to guarantee the continuity of their material and human resources, the construction and operation of simulation centers should be guided by an awareness of and commitment to sustainability. The creation of sustainability value, also known as "what we must do," is made possible for simulation directors by taking into account execution capacity, also known as "how we must do it." This enables the creation of a sustainability performance system. Establishing and integrating capabilities in these five essential areas is a requirement for organizations: leadership, assessment, strategy development, management integration, and reporting and communication. To provide the service that is required now and to capitalize on the opportunities for regional, national, and international expansion of service opportunities, simulation centers require an approach that is holistic and that integrates strategy, design, and execution. The leadership team is tasked with formulating a vision and mission, assessing opportunities, and determining the relative magnitudes of benefits and risks. When evaluating the performance of the center, directors of the center are required to develop metrics for assessing the costs and benefits related to sustainability. Because of this, the management team is able to adapt and improve strategies, communicate results with stakeholders, track costs, and evaluate activities that create value. In the end, best practices will emerge, which can then be used to inform decisions regarding the future.

As was mentioned earlier, simulation education necessitates an initial investment of funds for the purchase of manikins, equipment, and space. However, the payments made for ongoing simulation activities and training programs are how the majority of simulation centers make their living. It is possible to create a pathway to sustainability by mandating the training of preservice healthcare workers as well as the recertification of inservice healthcare workers, both of which must frequently include education that is based on in-person simulations. In most cases, hospital systems or the individuals receiving training will be responsible for making payment. Another potential source of funding is the completion of simulation-based coursework in order to earn continuing medical or nursing education credits. The continuing education credits, which must be completed in order to maintain a valid license to practice, can be paid for using either institutional or individual resources (Breaud et al., 2019; Bulamba et al., 2019).

Global Dissemination of Simulation Education

Faculty Development in Simulation Education

The training of knowledgeable simulation facilitators in each nation is the first step toward the global dissemination of simulation education. These simulation facilitators are equipped with the knowledge, skills, and attitudes necessary to advocate for and ensure the spread of simulation education by training other simulation educators and providing simulation facilitation for their institution. The development of faculty is essential in settings with both high and low resources (Bulamba et al., 2019). Areas that are critical to faculty development in simulation include a solid grasp of the theoretical foundations of simulation education. Adult learners have a need to know why they must learn something. Learning must have a value for them and help them improve their lives (Knowles et al., 2005). Further, it is important for instructors to emphasize the advantages that adult learners will have once they have learned the material (Knowles et al., 2005). Simulation is a place where learners and instructors can interact and dialogue. For an overview of adult learning theory applications to simulation education, see Chapter 2 on "Theory of Simulation and Gaming for Health Professional Education". There are a lot of different approaches to making a solid scenario. In point of fact, simulation scenarios for common scenarios involving basic life support, adult and pediatric advanced life support, and neonatal resuscitation have already been developed and are available for facilitators to use. These scenarios cover a range of medical specialties, including basic life support, advanced life support, and neonatal resuscitation. However, as a simulation facilitator, you may need to modify these scenarios to fit the environment of your own hospital or clinic, or if your learners are emergency medical technicians, you may need to adapt them to the pre-hospital setting. Scenario development is an important skill for simulation educators and is covered in Chapter 3 "Approach to Scenario Development for Manikin-based Simulation" and Chapter 4, "Approach to Scenario Development for Virtual Simulation". See also the overview on organization of simulation sessions in Chapter 5, "Organizing Simulations for Interprofessional Learners". Also, of relevance in tracking the impact of simulation education is the ability to evaluate learners' performance described in Chapter 6 on "Evaluation of Simulation Performance" and how to translate this evaluation into scholarly activity that can be disseminated discussed in Chapter 9 on "Research and Data

Collection Strategies for Simulation Educators". It is possible for individual or institutional funds to be used for the training of simulation facilitators. Workshops for Simulation Facilitators can be held at national conferences as well as educational institutions of higher learning. Training in the facilitation of remote simulations may take place in environments in which the trainee is situated in a geographically remote location.

Integration of Simulation Education into Pre-Service Education

The progressive integration of simulation education into undergraduate and postgraduate training has led to the wide dissemination of simulation methods in many countries. To accomplish this health professional educators must first identify opportunities for simulation-based education within existing curricula, then develop or adapt in-person or virtual simulation scenarios to be used in support of the curriculum. Interprofessional simulation-based training at all levels of training supports collaborative health professional practice. Shared training spaces that accommodate learners with differing schedules or in different geographical locations (virtual simulation spaces) are essential to provide learners with the interprofessional simulation experiences to prepare them for both common and rare events.

Optimally Utilizing Simulation Facilities for Large Groups

The adoption of simulation globally may hinge on the efficient delivery of simulation education to large groups. Simulations with large numbers of learners currently require maintenance of a strict facilitator to learner ratio that may not be feasible in settings where there are fewer trained instructors (Ersdal et al., 2013; Mduma et al., 2015). Some healthcare scenarios may require even more resources than typical. For example, in a simulated mass casualty event, deploying observers to different locations in the event such as the accident scene, the ambulance, the emergency room and the operating room would be needed to be able to adequately track learner performance throughout during the simulation.

Large scale simulation experiences can be conducted in-person in simulation centers by dividing learners into groups and using multiple simulation rooms and manikins or virtually using simulation environments that allow for learner groups to form within simulation spaces. For example, the web-based e-simulation program FIRST2ACT effectively enhanced knowledge, virtual clinical performance, and self-assessed knowledge, skills, confidence, and competence in final-year nursing students (Bogossian et al., 2015). From 2016-2021, the Neonatal Resuscitation Program eSim was used for neonatal resuscitation simulation training nationally in the U.S. (Ghoman et al., 2020). The eHBB virtual reality simulation program was used in a study of neonatal resuscitation retention in nurses and midwives in Nigeria and Kenya (Umoren et al., 2021).

Debriefing large scale simulation experiences can be challenging. When instructors are unavailable for real time debriefing, it is possible to conduct debriefing asynchronously using video captured during the simulation and through online discussion groups with pre-specified questions for discussion (Sawyer et al., 2016; Sawyer et al., 2012). However, some virtual environments include an artificial intelligence generated general or specific instructions and feedback to help support a synchronous learning experience (Motz et al., 2018; Umoren et al., 2021).

Accreditation Requirements Support Simulation Education

In addition to the internal processes driven by learners and faculty who may be early adopters or champions of simulation within institutions, external driving forces "push" or "pull" an institution or group toward the use of simulation. These pressures are not unique to any educational or healthcare setting and apply to institutions around the world. They may come from other institutions, professional societies, professional licensing bodies, healthcare organizations, healthcare insurers, liability insurers, accrediting organizations, government agencies and the public (Issenberg, 2006). National and international professional organizations including the Society for Simulation in Healthcare, International Nursing Association for Clinical Simulation and Learning (INACSL), National League for Nursing, the American Association of Medical Colleges (AAMC) and American Association for Colleges of Nursing (AACN) have taken the lead in their support for simulation education (Hayden et al., 2014). Over the years, efforts from these groups have driven the evolution of clinical training from an unsystematic apprenticeship to structured, systematic training, performance assessment and continuing education with opportunities for mastery learning and practice. These organizations play a significant role in developing guidelines and best practices on the optimal use of simulation education (Dieckmann et al., 2011). They also establish and evaluate the effectiveness of coordinating mechanisms for collecting, sharing, and communicating statistics among national, regional and international settings. Other opportunities for professional associations include the development of harmonization tools and databases for tracking outcomes needed for quality improvement and research.

Industry Support for Simulation

The role industry plays in support of healthcare simulation has been explored in detail in Chapter 8, "Translation of Skills from Simulation to Clinical Practice: the Role of Academic-Industry-Community Collaboration." These collaborations arise from technological innovation or research opportunities that support mutual goals and provide a business advantage. Input from educators and learners can enable companies that develop manikin-based and virtual simulators to redesign selected products or services to optimize their performance, decreasing product failures and inefficiencies. These collaborations may also provide benefits for academic partners in access to new simulators and technologies. Ultimately, the expansion in the use of virtual simulations has been driven by increased access to devices such as headsets and software that have been made accessible to educators in academic institutions through academic grants from various industries.

Scholarly Work and Dissemination

The expansion of simulation education can be attributed to the vast efforts of researchers to explore the applications, process, and outcomes of simulation education. Case studies and simulation scenarios along with evaluation checklists and worksheets for session organization are available through various mechanisms including online repositories and platforms such as MedED Portal (mededportal.org) to faculty who are new to simulation. The dissemination of research in simulation provides insight into the methods and best practices for success in simulation education. Support offered by internal and external grant mechanisms for simulation researchers enables them to conduct multi-center research projects and answer increasingly sophisticated research questions with a focus on increasing knowledge in this area and creating a research portfolio.

SOLUTIONS AND RECOMMENDATIONS

While much is known about the short-term and long-term impact of simulation education in high resource settings, there are gaps in awareness and adoption of simulation education in lower resource environments (Bulamba et al., 2019). While there is little doubt that simulation is effective, the cost of providing it may be prohibitive, particularly in these settings. Some of the considerations outlined by Bulamba et al., were equipment costs, difficulty in procurement, lack of context-appropriate curricula, unreliable power, limited local teaching capacity, and lack of coordination among user groups (Bulamba et al., 2019). Even in high resource settings with adequate support for the fixed and variable costs of simulation, economic evaluations that support greater efficiency are recommended and will add value to the current practice of simulation education (Maloney & Haines, 2016). It can be difficult to carry out economic studies, particularly those focused on educational outcomes at the undergraduate education level, due to the fact that health professional students are exposed to a wide variety of educational programs and may not be fully responsible for the care of patients or the decisions they make, amongst other potential confounders (Asche et al., 2018). In addition, educators working with simulations might not have a background in economics, and administrators might not be familiar with education or clinical practice. It is necessary to bridge the gap that this lack of expertise creates between the stakeholders who hold the responsibility for the delivery of simulation education and the allocation of resources needed in order for these two groups to realize their shared objective of improving the outcomes for patients. To successfully carry out comprehensive economic evaluations of educational simulations, interdisciplinary teams consisting of administrators, educators, clinicians, and economists are required to collaborate.

FUTURE RESEARCH DIRECTIONS

The expansion of simulation to different disciplines and it's use in high and low resource settings has provided significant opportunity for scholarly evaluation of the short and long-term impact of simulation education as a strategy for healthcare worker skill's acquisition and maintenance. Increased attention is needed to explore the dimensions of simulation education as they apply to low resource settings and to understand the facilitators and barriers to adoption of simulation in low resource settings (Wackernagel et al., 2017). In addition, exploration of the stages of adoption of simulation in various settings and ways in which they may be expedited will increase the global dissemination of simulation. Additional areas of investigation include the mechanisms for enhancing the sustainability of simulation education in different environments and populations, the use of evaluation modeling to explore the impact and outcome of simulation education and greater attention to rigorous economic evaluations of the use of simulation in various capacities for education, process evaluation and research.

CONCLUSION

In conclusion, simulation-based education is a highly effective strategy for health professional training. However, cost considerations play a significant role in organizational adoption of simulation education. Healthcare organizations that prioritize patient safety must factor both short and long-term outcomes of simulation education as they determine the return on investment. The global expansion of simulation is supported by faculty development opportunities, accreditation requirements, the expansion of evidence-based curricula, industry support and the increase in the evidence base supporting the use of simulation methods.

REFERENCES

Asche, C. V., Kim, M., Brown, A., Golden, A., Laack, T. A., Rosario, J., Strother, C., Totten, V. Y., & Okuda, Y. (2018). Communicating value in simulation: Cost–benefit analysis and return on investment. *Academic Emergency Medicine*, *25*(2), 230–237. doi:10.1111/acem.13327 PMID:28965366

Bogossian, F. E., Cooper, S. J., Cant, R., Porter, J., Forbes, H., & Team, F. A. R. (2015). A trial of e-simulation of sudden patient deterioration (FIRST2ACT WEB) on student learning. *Nurse Education Today*, *35*(10), e36–e42. doi:10.1016/j.nedt.2015.08.003 PMID:26296543

Bulamba, F., Sendagire, C., Kintu, A., Hewitt-Smith, A., Musana, F., Lilaonitkul, M., Ayebale, E. T., Law, T., Dubowitz, G., Kituuka, O., & Lipnick, M. S. (2019). Feasibility of Simulation-Based Medical Education in a Low-Income Country: Challenges and Solutions From a 3-year Pilot Program in Uganda. *Simulation in Healthcare: Journal of the Society for Simulation in Healthcare, 14*(2), 113-120. doi:10.1097/SIH.0000000000000345

Dieckmann, P., Phero, J. C., Issenberg, S. B., Kardong-Edgren, S., Ostergaard, D., & Ringsted, C. (2011). The first Research Consensus Summit of the Society for Simulation in Healthcare: conduction and a synthesis of the results. *Simulation in Healthcare: Journal of the Society for Simulation in Healthcare, 6*, S1-S9. doi:10.1097/SIH.0b013e31822238fc

Donaldson, M. S., Corrigan, J. M., & Kohn, L. T. (2000). *To err is human: building a safer health system*. Academic Press.

Ersdal, H. L., Vossius, C., Bayo, E., Mduma, E., Perlman, J., Lippert, A., & Soreide, E. (2013). A one-day "Helping Babies Breathe" course improves simulated performance but not clinical management of neonates. *Resuscitation, 84*(10), 1422–1427. doi:10.1016/j.resuscitation.2013.04.005 PMID:23612024

Gaba, D. M. (2007). The future vision of simulation in healthcare. *Simulation in Healthcare, 2*(2), 126–135. doi:10.1097/01.SIH.0000258411.38212.32 PMID:19088617

Ghoman, S. K., Patel, S. D., Cutumisu, M., von Hauff, P., Jeffery, T., Brown, M. R., & Schmölzer, G. M. (2020). Serious games, a game changer in teaching neonatal resuscitation? A review. *Archives of Disease in Childhood. Fetal and Neonatal Edition, 105*(1), 98–107. doi:10.1136/archdischild-2019-317011 PMID:31256010

Hayden, J. K., Smiley, R. A., Alexander, M., Kardong-Edgren, S., & Jeffries, P. R. (2014). The NCSBN national simulation study: A longitudinal, randomized, controlled study replacing clinical hours with simulation in prelicensure nursing education. *Journal of Nursing Regulation, 5*(2), S3–S40. doi:10.1016/S2155-8256(15)30062-4

Isaranuwatchai, W., Alam, F., Hoch, J., & Boet, S. (2017). A cost-effectiveness analysis of self-debriefing versus instructor debriefing for simulated crises in perioperative medicine in Canada. *Journal of Educational Evaluation for Health Professions*, 13. PMID:28028288

Issenberg, S. B. (2006). The scope of simulation-based healthcare education. *Simulation in Healthcare, 1*(4), 203–208. doi:10.1097/01.SIH.0000246607.36504.5a PMID:19088590

Knowles, M. S., Holton, E., & Swanson, R. (2005). *The adult learner: the definitive classic in adult education and human resource development (6th ed.)*. Elsevier. doi:10.4324/9780080481913

Maloney, S., & Haines, T. (2016). Issues of cost-benefit and cost-effectiveness for simulation in health professions education. *Advances in Simulation (London, England), 1*(1), 1–6. doi:10.118641077-016-0020-3 PMID:29449982

Mduma, E., Ersdal, H., Svensen, E., Kidanto, H., Auestad, B., & Perlman, J. (2015). Frequent brief on-site simulation training and reduction in 24-h neonatal mortality—An educational intervention study. *Resuscitation, 93*, 1–7. doi:10.1016/j.resuscitation.2015.04.019 PMID:25957942

Mello, M. M., Chandra, A., Gawande, A. A., & Studdert, D. M. (2010). National costs of the medical liability system. *Health Affairs, 29*(9), 1569–1577. doi:10.1377/hlthaff.2009.0807 PMID:20820010

Miller, G. E. (1990). The assessment of clinical skills/competence/performance. *Academic Medicine, 65*(9), S63–S67. doi:10.1097/00001888-199009000-00045 PMID:2400509

Motz, P., Gray, M., Sawyer, T., Kett, J., Danforth, D., Maicher, K., & Umoren, R. (2018). Virtual Antenatal Encounter and Standardized Simulation Assessment (VANESSA): Pilot Study. *JMIR Serious Games, 6*(2), e8. doi:10.2196/games.9611 PMID:29752249

Rogers Everett, M. (1995). Diffusion of innovations (Vol. 12). Academic Press.

Sawyer, T., Eppich, W., Brett-Fleegler, M., Grant, V., & Cheng, A. (2016). More Than One Way to Debrief: A Critical Review of Healthcare Simulation Debriefing Methods. *Simulation in Healthcare: Journal of the Society for Simulation in Healthcare, 11*(3), 209-217. doi:10.1097/SIH.0000000000000148

Sawyer, T., Gray, M. M., & Umoren, R. (2022). The Global Healthcare Simulation Economy: A Scoping Review. *Cureus, 14*(2). Advance online publication. doi:10.7759/cureus.22629 PMID:35371834

Sawyer, T., Sierocka-Castaneda, A., Chan, D., Berg, B., Lustik, M., & Thompson, M. (2012). The effectiveness of video-assisted debriefing versus oral debriefing alone at improving neonatal resuscitation performance: a randomized trial. *Simulation in Healthcare: Journal of the Society for Simulation in Healthcare, 7*(4), 213-221. doi:10.1097/SIH.0b013e3182578eae

Umoren, R., Bucher, S., Hippe, D. S., Ezenwa, B. N., Fajolu, I. B., Okwako, F. M., Feltner, J., Nafula, M., Musale, A., Olawuyi, O. A., Adeboboye, C. O., Asangansi, I., Paton, C., Purkayastha, S., Ezeaka, C. V., & Esamai, F. (2021). eHBB: A randomised controlled trial of virtual reality or video for neonatal resuscitation refresher training in healthcare workers in resource-scarce settings. *BMJ Open, 11*(8), e048506. doi:10.1136/bmjopen-2020-048506 PMID:34433598

Wackernagel, M., Hanscom, L., & Lin, D. (2017). Making the sustainable development goals consistent with sustainability. *Frontiers in Energy Research, 5*, 18. doi:10.3389/fenrg.2017.00018

KEY TERMS AND DEFINITIONS

Augmented Reality: Computer generated holographic images can be viewed by the learner in the physical environment using a mobile device or specially designed headset.

High-Fidelity Manikin: This term refers to a technology-enabled manikin with features such as mechanical respiration and heart rate.

Low-Fidelity Manikin: This is typically a low cost, low technology manikin with minimal features.

Objective Structured Clinical Examination (OSCE): An approach to assessment that involves defined objectives and anticipated actions, often with an accompanying checklist for assessment.

Simulation Debriefer: A simulation instructor who leads the learners through a reflective analysis of simulation events.

Simulation Facilitator: A simulation instructor who guides the learners through the scenario with the goal of meeting learning objectives.

Simulation Technician/Specialist: An individual who supports the practice of simulation through setting up and managing simulation manikins and supplies.

Teledebriefing: Teledebriefing describes a process in which learners who are participating in a simulation scenario undergo debriefing with a facilitator located at an off-site location.

Telefacilitation: The conduct of a telesimulation by a remote facilitator.

Telesimulation: Telesimulation is a process by which telecommunication and simulation resources are utilized to provide education, training, and/or assessment to learners at an off-site location.

Video-Assisted Debriefing: The practice of using video captured during simulation sessions for reflective discussions on learner and team performance.

Virtual Environment: 3D computer generated objects that can be viewed on a screen or in a head-mounted display.

Virtual Reality: Computer generated 3D images viewed by a learner in a virtual environment using a low-cost or high-end head mounted display.

About the Author

Rachel Umoren is an Associate Professor of Pediatrics in the Division of Neonatology at the University of Washington, Seattle, U.S.A. where she is Associate Division Head for Research, Director of Research for the Neonatal Education and Simulation-based Training (NEST) program and Inpatient Medical Director for Telehealth at Seattle Children's Hospital. She serves as Program Director for the International Community Access to Child Health (ICATCH) Program of the American Academy of Pediatrics and Chair of the Virtual Simulation Section of the Society for Simulation in Healthcare. Dr. Umoren received her medical degree from the University of Calabar, Nigeria, and completed her pediatric residency and neonatal fellowship training at Indiana University Health Riley Children's Hospital where she also earned a Masters' degree in Clinical Research. Her NIH and AHRQ-funded research focus is on improving neonatal resuscitation and care practices through simulation education and telemedicine in high and low resource settings.

Index

A

C

D

E

F

G

H

I

L

M

O

P

R

S

T

www.ingramcontent.com/pod-product-compliance
Lightning Source LLC
LaVergne TN
LVHW060002031026
849161LV00025B/1271